VEGETABLES
and
FRUITS

Nutritional and Therapeutic Values

Thomas S.C. Li

CRC Press
Taylor & Francis Group
Boca Raton London New York

CRC Press is an imprint of the
Taylor & Francis Group, an **informa** business

CRC Press
Taylor & Francis Group
6000 Broken Sound Parkway NW, Suite 300
Boca Raton, FL 33487-2742

© 2008 by Taylor & Francis Group, LLC
CRC Press is an imprint of Taylor & Francis Group, an Informa business

No claim to original U.S. Government works
Printed in the United States of America on acid-free paper
10 9 8 7 6 5 4 3 2 1

International Standard Book Number-13: 978-1-4200-6871-9 (Hardcover)

Library of Congress Cataloging-in-Publication Data

Li, Thomas S. C.
    Vegetables and fruits : nutritional and therapeutic values / Thomas S.C. Li.
        p. cm.
    Includes bibliographical references and index.
    ISBN 978-1-4200-6871-9 (hardback : alk. paper)
        1. Vegetables--Composition. 2. Vegetables--Therapeutic use. 3.
Fruit--Composition. 4. Fruit--Therapeutic use. I. Title.

    QP144.V44L5 2006
    613.2'8--dc22   2007035791

Visit the Taylor & Francis Web site at
http://www.taylorandfrancis.com

and the CRC Press Web site at
http://www.crcpress.com

Contents

Foreword

Until the achievements of agriculture, sanitation, and medicine, most humans died of starvation or disease. In recent centuries, advancing scientific knowledge and technology have progressively reduced mortality, improved health, and increased longevity. However, an embarrassing crisis has now developed in human affairs: despite the unprecedented availability of medicines and medical treatments, as well as an astonishing variety of food offerings, in most countries people are becoming less healthy, due in considerable part to rising epidemics of obesity and diabetes. The next generation is not expected to live as long as their parents.

What has gone wrong? First, for most people, life has become more sedentary and stressful. Second, the marketplace has become saturated with fast food, and relentless advertising has resulted in a predominance of "synthetic foods" that combine dozens if not hundreds of ingredients, diabolically concocted to appeal to mankind's inherent attraction to sugar, salt, fat, and calories, all the while minimizing or ignoring the basic needs for nutrition and health. Much of the current health crisis is due to ignorance of the nutritional and therapeutic values of vegetables and fruits, the traditional foundation of a healthy diet. The importance of this unique book in addressing the dietary problems of modern society cannot be exaggerated.

Just what natural foods should be the basis of a healthy diet? Modern dieticians are now in agreement that plant foods should comprise the major part of the human diet. Moreover, while cereals and legumes are clearly indispensable, vegetables and fruits are the key to obtaining essential phytochemicals. Humans are dependent on obtaining tiny amounts of essential compounds from plants — not just vitamins and minerals, but a wide variety of other constituents.

A considerable proportion of human disease appears to be related simply to a diet that is inadequate in these constituents. Before the age of pharmaceutical medicine, herbal doctors learned from trial and error how certain foods rich in particular chemicals possessed curative properties. Almost certainly, humans have been ingesting and benefiting from these chemicals for hundreds of thousands of years. This highlights the problem with the modern synthetic diet: it is deficient in these essential natural compounds (in ways that we still do not appreciate), and so contributes to, rather than alleviates, disease.

The "Father of Medicine," the Greek physician Hippocrates (460–377 BC), reflected on the essential medical wisdom of a diet rich in nutritional plants by saying, "Let food be thy medicine." The same thought was captured by the equally long-lived Benjamin Franklin (1706–1790): "An apple a day keeps the doctor away." While the foods of all cultures undoubtedly offer healthful benefits, those of Asia are of particular significance. Asian cultures (notably Chinese and Indian) are ancient, having accumulated vast wisdom. Moreover, Asian cultures in recent centuries have added to their food repertoires by adopting numerous fruit and vegetable species indigenous to other countries, particularly from the New World. Most importantly, Asians have a tradition of using food plants for improving or maintaining health. The

Chinese in particular have historically combined their concepts of food and therapeutic plants, emphasizing the intimate link between medicine and diet.

This book represents a milestone in that it introduces North Americans to the
healthful properties of more than 100 each of vegetables and fruits that are available
to the general public. This is an authoritative and comprehensive reference guide,
providing critical information on nutritional as well as other health-related constituents and their therapeutic applications. Much of the information and interpretations
are presented in user-friendly chapters. This comprehensive treatment is important
because undoubtedly the book will be extremely useful to a diverse range of healthcare and food professionals with different backgrounds.

Dr. Li's book will provide those in the applied food and health industries with
key information that will assist in the provision of nutritious food, particularly in
relation to countering disease. It will also assist in the creation of health-related con-
sumer goods. Finally, those who produce, process, and market vegetables and fruits,
as well as their nutraceutical and pharmacological extracts, would be well advised
to carefully study Dr. Li's information. Many of the species documented have the
potential to become extremely profitable in areas where they are not presently grown
or utilized.

Dr. Li, one of the world's most knowledgeable and well-known researchers on
medicinal and food plants, is the author of numerous authoritative reference books.
This latest scholarly, authoritative, and comprehensive effort achieves the extremely
high standards for which his publications are renowned. *Vegetables and Fruits: Nutritional and Therapeutic Values* is a superb and invaluable synthesis that will undoubtedly be a standard reference on food plants and human nutrition for many years.

Ernest Small
Agriculture and Agri-Food Canada

Preface

This book provides comprehensive information on vegetables and fruits. It includes nutritional and therapeutic values on more than 100 species each of vegetables and fruits. The objective of this book was to assemble in one volume the large amount of information that is not familiar to the general public about the healthful properties of vegetables and fruits that are available in the North America market. Vegetables and fruits have more than just nutritional value. Some may contain therapeutic compounds that are beneficial to consumers.

This book is designed to provide researchers, manufacturers, and producers easy access to information on vegetables and fruits in user-friendly tables. It begins with a general introduction regarding their essential human nutritional values such as protein, vitamins, minerals, and fiber contents as well as the presence of non-nutrient phytochemicals such as sulfur-containing compounds. Chapters 1 and 4 present currently available information on the major constituents and therapeutic values in more than 100 each of vegetables and fruits, respectively. Chapters 2 and 5 present the vitamins and minerals that are contained in, respectively, vegetables and fruits. Chapter 3 presents flavonoid, isoflavone, and carotenoid contents in raw vegetables. Chapter 6 indicates how the use of vegetables and fruits can protect or improve human health.

The information in this book is primarily for reference and education. It is not intended to be a substitute for the advice of a physician. The uses of vegetables and fruits described in this book are not recommendations, and the author is not responsible for liability arising directly or indirectly from the use of information in this book.

Acknowledgments

The author thanks Paul Ferguson for his word-processing assistance, Barry Butler for his technical computer assistance, and Lynne Boyd for her efforts in the literature search. I also thank my colleagues, Drs. Tom Beveridge, Dave Oomah, Peter Sholberg, Ernest Small, and numerous scientists and researchers overseas, for their valuable assistance and contributions. Finally, I would like to thank my wife Rose for her encouragement.

Introduction

Vegetables and fruits have been used in many parts of the world for hundreds of years as herbal medicines with broad ranges of nutritional and therapeutic values (Chapters 1 and 4). Recent studies indicate that consumption of adequate amounts of vegetables and fruits may have disease-preventive properties (Chapter 6).

The demand for varieties of vegetables and fruits has expanded in the North American marketplace recently. The situation is due not only to increases in the population, but also to significant interest from the general public, with their higher standard of living and their desire to have a variety of healthy foods in their diet. On the other hand, consumers are well-aware that consumption of a variety of vegetables and fruits is as important as the quantity consumed, as no single vegetable or fruit provides all of the nutrients needed.

Vegetables can be considered as chemical reagents (Cordell et al. 2007) that are essential to improve human nutrition and health with various phytochemicals and different bioactivities. Vegetables and fruits provide excellent sources of nutrients, such as protein, vitamins, minerals, and fiber, as well as nonnutrient phytochemicals such as sulfur-containing compounds (Chapter 3). The nonnutrient phytochemicals may contribute to the normal functioning of the human body (Wettasinghe et al. 2002). Epidemiological studies have demonstrated the beneficial effects on human health from consumption of vegetables and fruits. The antioxidant composition and capacity of vegetables and fruits relative to intake data are important to understand the health implications of various dietary patterns. It has been reported that vegetables ranked in the top ten in an antioxidant assay included sweet potato leaf, ginger, amaranth, spinach, eggplant, pak choi (bok choy), leafy Chinese cabbage, tomato, onion and Welsh onion (Easdown and Kalb 2004).

It would appear that major public health benefits could be achieved by substantially increasing consumption of vegetables and fruits. Numerous studies (128 out of 135 dietary studies) indicated that increased vegetable and fruit consumption by humans significantly reduced the risk of cancer (Block et al. 1992).

Vegetables are rich in valuable nutritional components (Chapter 2) that vary with the plant species, but no single species contains all the required nutrients. Therefore, consumption of a variety of vegetables and fruits is important, since nutrients act together, with optimal levels of several nutrients being required to be functional (Frei et al. 1988).

Proteins: In a balanced diet, protein should be supplied from different sources. In addition to the common sources from milk, cheese, eggs, and meats, vegetable and fruit such as broad bean can also provide adequate amounts of protein. It has reported that broad bean contains up to 31.8 g/100 g of protein (Chapter 2). Other abundant sources of proteins are glycinin in soybean and glutenin in wheat, pulses, beans, and peas.

Fat: Almost all vegetables and fruits contain some fat or oil. However, the amount is not significant except in certain groundnuts, such as peanuts, soybeans, and the seeds of the sunflower, pumpkin, watermelon, and sesame. The fat in peanut and soybean is rich in both unsaturated fatty acids and in sterol precursors of vitamin D; therefore, even in a small amount, vegetable fat is a valuable component of a balanced diet.

Sugar: Vegetable sugar is mainly glucose and sucrose. The contents vary from 1.6 (water dropwort) to 56.6 g/100 g (lotus) (Chapter 2). This natural source of sugar is an important component in the human diet.

Minerals: All vegetables and fruits contain important minerals, such as potassium, calcium, magnesium, phosphorus, iron, and zinc (Chapter 2). Minerals are basic components in secondary metabolic pathways that produce valuable phytochemicals for normal human health. The contents of minerals in vegetables is variable. Green vegetables have higher amounts of calcium and iron than root vegetables. Calcium is not only associated with preventing osteoporosis, but it also appears to have protective effects in some types of cancer, most recently colon cancer (Boik 1996).

Vitamin A: Vegetables and fruits are the main source of vitamin A for human health. Provitamin A carotenes account for the yellow, orange, red, and green color in many vegetables and fruits, including carrot, spinach, sweet potato, pumpkin, broccoli, squash, lettuce, green pepper, tomato, green bean, garden pea, cabbage, and sweet corn (B. H. Chen et al. 1995). Dietary approaches to the prevention of vitamin A deficiency can include consumption of ivy gourd, kale, Chinese swamp cabbage, and pumpkin. (Charoenkiatkul et al. 1985). The highest concentrations of β-carotene are found in sweet potato (*Ipomoea batatas*, *Batatas edulis*) and green leafy vegetables such as kale (*Brassica oleracea*) and spinach (*Spinacia oleracea*). The highest concentrations of lutein and zeaxanthin are found in cooked kale and raw spinach. Carrots and pumpkin were the main contributors of alpha-carotene and beta-carotene equivalent intakes, whereas broccoli and green beans contributed substantially to lutein and zeaxanthin intake. The main contributors to lycopene intake were tomatoes (Manzi et al. 2002).

Vitamin B_1: It is most abundantly present in seeds and grains, particularly in the outer layers and in the germ. Sunflower seeds contain 0.92 mg/100 g of vitamin B_1 (Chapter 2). Vitamin B_1 is unstable at high temperatures, and a considerable amount may be lost during cooking or processing, especially in the presence of an alkali such as sodium bicarbonate.

Vitamin B_2: It was first found in milk, eggs, and livers, and later in plant tissues. It is most abundant in actively growing green leaves and stems. It accumulates to a significant extent in seeds and grains. Cooking may affect the folate content in vegetables. Boiled spinach and pak choy on average only retained 30% of vitamin B_2; nonleafy vegetables retained 50–90%; stir-fried leafy vegetables retained 43–70%; and 9–15% was retained in soup. Stir-fried nonleafy vegetables retained nearly 100% of the folate (B. Lin and Lin 1999). Folic acid was found in vegetables, such as spinach (115 µg/100 g), parsley (116 µg/100 g), broccoli (110 µg/100 g), pea (78 µg/100 g), and watercress (200 µg/100 g).

Vitamin C: It is an essential phytonutrient for the metabolism of living cells. There is compelling evidence that a diet rich in fruits and vegetables can lower the risk of heart disease, a leading cause of death in the United States. Vegetables, especially green leafy vegetables, are rich in vitamin C. There are 94–141 mg/100 g of vitamin C in *Capsicum* spp. and 34–73 mg/100 g in *Brassica* spp. (Chapter 2). Cole crops have long been recognized as important sources of vitamin C and other water-soluble vitamins in the diet, including riboflavin, niacin, and thiamine. Cole crops are also a good source of the fat-soluble vitamins generally grouped together as vitamin A (β-carotene). As shown in Chapter 2, dietary contributions of individual vitamins differ among species of cole crops (C. Xue 2001a; 2001b).

Vitamin D: It does not occur in plants, but its precursors, such as phytosterols, are widely distributed in plants. It was reported that vitamin D protects against colon cancer by helping to detoxify cancer-triggering chemicals that are released during the digestion of high-fat foods (Boik 1996).

Vitamin E: It is an effective lipid-soluble antioxidant. Vitamin E is obtained mainly from nuts, from vegetable seed oils of canola, soybean, corn, safflower, and cotton; and from cereals. It will be beneficial to use a variety of oils in the diet to ensure that different forms of vitamin E are consumed.

Diets with an adequate amount of vegetable consumption increase antioxidant activity, which behaves as a free-radical scavenger in the human body, thereby reducing or retarding oxidation (Boik 1996). Little is known about the activity of antioxidant components isolated from vegetables. Research has focused mostly on the activity of antioxidant compounds, such as flavonoids, phenolic acids, tocopherol, carotenoid, ascorbic acid, and sulfur-containing compounds. It may not be well-known, however, that phytocompounds are present in vegetables. Examples are quercetin in bell peppers and onion (Pratt and Watts 1964), phenolic compounds in cole vegetables (Vinson et al. 1998), allicin in onions (Pratt and Watts 1964), caffeic acid derivatives, chlorogenic acid, and patatin in potato (Al-Saikhan et al. 1995), and peonidin glycoside in purple sweet potatoes (Sang et al. 1997).

Vegetables such as root and tuberous crops (carrot, potato, sweet potato, red beet, onion, etc.), cole vegetables (cabbage, Brussels sprouts, broccoli, etc.), green leafy vegetables (lettuce, spinach, etc.), solanaceous fruits (tomato, pepper), and other vegetables have been screened for antioxidant activity (Gazzani et al. 1998). It was reported that antioxidant activities of broccoli and potato are higher than onion, carrot, and green pepper (Al-Saikhan et al. 1995), and green onion tops were twice as potent as antioxidants than potato peel, green pepper, and green onion and four times more potent than potatoes in inhibiting the coupled oxidation of β-carotene and linoleic acid (Pratt and Watts 1964). Vegetable extracts from green onion, green pepper, celery, potato peels, and tomato peel also exhibited antioxidant activity (Pratt and Watts 1964). Total phenolic (mg of GAE/g dry wt.) may play a major role as a source of antioxidant. It can be extracted from vegetables including onion (2.5), cucumber leaf (3.8), carrot (0.6), tomato (2.0), pea (0.4), potato peel (4.3), and sugar beet peel (4.2) (Kahkonen et al. 1999). Some vegetables, such as onion, celery, pepper, alfalfa, watercress, and parsley, have a tonic effect and may maintain or improve health (T. Li 2003). Cole, alliums, and other vegetable crops contain a variety of biologically active phytochemicals. Scientific evidence for their role in the prevention of disease, such as cancer, is growing rapidly.

In the case of carrot, celery, garlic, mushroom, zucchini, tomato, and particularly eggplant juice, it was reported that the antioxidant activity of the vegetables was increased by boiling. This suggests that the prooxidant activity was due to peroxides that were inactivated at high temperature (Maslarova and Heinonen 2003). Cao et al. (1996) reported that the antioxidant score decreased in the following order: kale > garlic > spinach > Brussels sprout > alfalfa sprout > broccoli flower > beet > red bell pepper > onion > corn > eggplant > cauliflower > sweet potato > cabbage > leaf lettuce > string bean > carrot > yellow squash > iceberg lettuce > celery > cucumber. Carotenoids are antioxidants and could prevent free-radical damage to cellular DNA and other molecules. The immunomodulatory effects of carotenoids could enhance immune response to tumorigenesis and cell communication to restrict expansion of tumor-initiated cells (Johnson 2002).

Phytonutrients may serve as antioxidants that enhance the immune response and cell-to-cell communication, alter estrogen metabolism, convert beta-carotene to vitamin A, promote apoptosis, repair DNA damage caused by smoking and other toxic exposures, and detoxify carcinogens through the activation of the cytochrome P450 and phase II enzyme systems (see frequently asked questions about phytonutrients, USDA, Beltsville Agricultural Research Center). In a double-blind, placebo-controlled study, researchers from the French Health and Medical Institute reported that by eating sufficient fruit and vegetables to maintain antioxidant vitamin and mineral levels, they could reduce the risk of digestive, respiratory, and skin cancers, and mortality by 31% in men. The researchers found a higher risk of cancer and heart disease among men with the lowest levels of beta-carotene. The lower the level of the nutrient, the higher was the risk of disease. This finding should support the value of a nutritious diet with regular consumption of fruits and vegetables rather than supplements (NutraIngredients.com).

The protective antioxidant potential of vegetables measures its ability to absorb damaging oxygen radicals. A recent report on antioxidants in vegetables (USDA 1999), by using oxygen radical absorbance capacity (ORAC) measurement, identified the vegetables with high ORAC values (micrograms per 100 g):

Garlic (*Allium sativum*): 2000
Kale (*Brassica oleracea* var. *acephala*): 1770
Spinach (*Spinacia oleracea*): 1260
Alfalfa (*Medicago sativa*) sprouts: 930
Broccoli (*Brassica oleracea* var. *italica*): 890
Beet (*Beta vulgaris*): 840
Onion (*Allium cepa*): 450
Corn (*Zea mays*): 400
Eggplant (*Solanum melongena*): 390
Pea (*Pisum sativum*): 390

Cabbage (*Brassica oleracea* var. *capitata*): 300
Potato (*Solanum tuberosum*): 300
Lettuce (*Lactuca sativa*): 250
Carrot (*Daucus carota*): 200
Green bean (*Phaseolus vulgaris*): 200
Tomato (*Lycopersicon esculentum*): 200
Celery (*Apium graveolens*): 100
Cucumber (*Cucumis sativus*): 100

Remedies containing plant materials from vegetables, especially cole crops, have long been used in folk medicine. Their effectiveness in the treatment of infectious disease has been substantiated by the discovery and characterization of antimicrobial phytochemicals from vegetables (Delaquis and Mazza 1995) and their role in the prevention of degenerative diseases. Several vegetables such as Jerusalem artichoke tubers, asparagus, tomatoes, and alliums are known to contain oligosaccharides. These compounds can improve intestinal microflora by suppressing the growth of harmful bacteria (Tomomatsu 1994) and reducing serum cholesterol and the anticonstipation effect (Yamashito et al. 1984).

Higher fruit and vegetable consumption has been associated with a lower risk of heart disease and other health conditions and continues to be an important part of a healthy diet (Smith-Warner 2001). Diets rich in fruits and vegetables may reduce the risk of ischemic stroke. Cruciferous vegetables such as broccoli and spinach seem to provide the greatest benefit. High blood pressure is a primary risk factor for heart disease and stroke. A diet rich in fruits, vegetables, and low-fat dairy products restricted in the amount of saturated and total fat can be a very effective tool for lowering blood pressure

In epidemiological studies, vegetables in the diet have been found to be protective against several chronic diseases, as compounds such as fiber and vitamin B_6 in the vegetables can reduce the risk of blood clots; potassium helps control blood pressure; and folate lowers levels of heart disease by promoting homocysteine, an important risk factor for heart disease. Epidemiological evidence suggests that flavonoid consumption in the diet is protective against heart disease (Vinson et al. 1998; Criqui and Ringel 1994) as well as possessing antibacterial, antiviral, anti-inflammatory, antiallergic, antithrombotic, and vasodilator activities (Cook and Samman 1996). The major components in flavonoids include kaempferol, quercetin, apigenin, luteolin, myricetin, isorhamnetin, (–)-epicatechin, (–)-epigallocatechin, and (+)-catechin (table 3). Many vegetables, especially dark green and cruciferous vegetables such as spinach, broccoli, and Brussels sprout contain chemical compounds that can prevent or ameliorate the course of various acute and chronic diseases. These compounds include quinine, digitalis, and other plant-derived compounds (S. Martin 2002). Anticancer compounds found in vegetables include lycopene in tomatoes; lutein and beta-carotene in carrots, pumpkin, and squash; and allyl sulfides in onions and garlic.

Flavonoids, such as anthocyanins, flavones, flavonols, isoflavonoids, and tannins, are a group of natural phenolic compounds in most fruits and vegetables. A diet high in flavonols might help reduce pancreatic cancer risk, especially in smokers (Kristal

2007). People who ate the largest amounts of flavonols has a 23% reduced risk of developing pancreatic cancer compared with those who ate the least, according to a research team led by Kolonel (2007) at the Cancer Research Center of Hawaii.

Flavonoids can inhibit allergic reactions by inhibiting the production of histamine (Berg and Daniel 1988). They may also affect immune function by inhibiting eicosanoid-mediated inflammation by inhibiting histamine-induced inflammation and by conserving vitamin C and other antioxidants (Welton et al. 1988). Flavonoids appear to influence a number of steps in both coagulation and fibrinolysis, inhibiting platelet adhesion and aggregation, most likely through inhibition of cAMP phosphodiesterase (Boik 1996). Several groups of compounds in cole crops, including the glucosinolates, isothiocyanates, dithiolthiones, indoles, sulfonates, and vitamins, have been reported to be capable of preventing or alleviating diseases and promoting health.

Flavonols are common in plant-based foods but are found in highest concentrations in vegetables and fruits such as onions, apples, berries, kale, and broccoli.

Cancer is the second leading cause of death in the United States, exceeded only by heart disease. Between 30% and 40% of all cases of cancer are preventable, through physical activity and maintenance of appropriate body weight and by feasible and appropriate diets, according to the American Institute for Cancer Research (AICR). Its diet guidelines for cancer prevention include a diet rich in a variety of plant-based foods, with plenty of vegetables and fruits (Ohr 2002).

There are several candidate compounds in specific vegetables that are associated with risk reduction of cancer occurrence. For example, cole crops in the genus *Brassica*, appear to protect against various cancers, especially lung cancer; onions (*Allium cepa*) and garlic (*Allium sativum*) appear to lower the risk of stomach cancer; tomato products (*Lycopersicum esculentum*), appear to lower the risk of prostate cancer. Lycopene, which is found almost exclusively in tomatoes, is the subject of a current National Cancer Institute program for prostate cancer prevention. Some studies have found associations between higher tomato intake and blood lycopene levels and reduced risk of lung, stomach, and other cancers.

New research is strengthening evidence that consumption of various vegetables and fruits may be some of the best health advice around. A large study of 500,000 American retirees has found that just one extra serving of fruit or vegetables a day may reduce the risk of developing head and neck cancer. Numerous studies have demonstrated that diet plays a role in cancer. Cancer experts now believe that up to two-thirds of all cancers come from lifestyle factors such as smoking, diet, and lack of exercise (Kristal 2007).

Carotenoids found in many fruits and vegetables with antioxidant property are chemopreventive agents. However, clinical trials have not found β-carotene to be cancer protective; indeed, in some cases, it has even had a negative effect. This suggests that other carotenoids or other substances in fruits and vegetables may be responsible for their anticancer effects (Hwang and Bowen 2002).

Vegetable consumption has been related to reduced risk of cancer and cardiovascular diseases in epidemiological studies (Block et al. 1992). By using in vitro technique for screening possible cancer-preventive agents, Wettasinghe et al. (2002) found that crude vegetable extracts triggered increases in protective proteins

— phase II enzymes. Among the vegetable extracts, sweet corn, kale, and beans showed the greatest effect on prevention of cancer. They concluded that antioxidant activities in commonly consumed vegetables can be used as dietary sources of cancer chemopreventive agents. Evidence is accumulating that nonnutrient compounds, including phytoestrogens, saponins, flavonoids, protease inhibitors, isoflavones, and lignans, may play a significant role in preventing cancer (Boik 1996). Wattenberg (1992) identified two basic mechanisms by which nonnutritive dietary constituents may inhibit carcinogenesis by blocking the action of carcinogens or tumor promoters and by suppressing the evaluation of initiated cells.

Strong antimutagenic activities in vitro were found for all cole vegetables except for Chinese cabbage, which had only weak antimutagenic activity. Other vegetables with strong antimutagenic activities were beets, chives, horseradish, onions, rhubarb, and spinach (Edenharder et al. 1994). Phytosterols are structurally similar to cholesterol. The most common phytosterols are β-sitosterol, campesterol, and stigmasterol. Epidemiologic and experimental studies suggest that dietary phytosterols may offer protection from the most common cancers, such as colon, breast, and prostate cancer (Awad and Fink 2000).

The exact link between fruits and vegetables and prostate cancer is still unclear. However, there have been promising studies that suggest that increased consumption of tomato-based products and other lycopene-containing foods may reduce the progression of prostate cancer. The cole vegetable crops such as broccoli, cabbage, Brussels sprout, cauliflower, mustard greens, turnips, and bok choy contain glucosinolates (Fenwick et al. 1983), which produce metabolic breakdown products that protect DNA against damage. The metabolic breakdown products, known as indoles and isothiocyanates, are therefore thought to protect against prostate cancer (Kristal 2002). Based on a multiethnic, case-control study, Kolonel et al. (2000) reported that there is strong evidence that *Brassica* consumption protects against prostate cancer. It was reported that increased consumption of fruits and vegetables among adults does not lower the risk of breast cancer for women (Smith-Warner 2001).

There have been numerous studies linking the vitamin folate with colon cancer risk. Folate is found in high amounts in dark leafy green vegetables (Harvard School of Public Health, http://www/hsph.harvard.edu/nutritionsource/fruit.html). Epidemiological investigations revealed that colon cancer occurs less frequently in individuals who regularly consume vegetables such as Brussels sprout, cabbage, and broccoli (Manousos et al. 1983).

1 Nutritional and Therapeutic Values of Vegetables

English Name	Scientific Name	Nutritional and Therapeutic Values
Adzuki bean	*Phaseolus angularis* *P. calcaratus*	The seeds are an important pulse crop, containing thiamine, riboflavin, niacin, and ascorbic acid. The beans are used as a diuretic and as a supportive, and are also used in treatment of abscesses, beriberi, dysentery, sores, and swelling (Perry 1980).
		The root is pulped and applied to abscesses; a decoction is used to disperse poison (Duke and Ayensu 1985).
		It has been reported that heat treatment (30-min cooking) causes significant declines in the apparent recovery of most of the essential amino acids except leucine and phenylalanine (Chau et al. 1999).
		The estrogenicity of the adzuki bean and its effect on progesterone receptor levels in human breast cancer MCF-7 cells have also been reported (Zhang and Zhao 2006).
		Adzuki bean is used to treat liver detoxification, jaundice, edema, and diarrhea. It contains fiber, folic acid, vitamins B1, B2, B3, and B6, zinc, potassium, phosphorus, manganese, iron, copper, and calcium.
		It has been reported that adzuki bean is a diuretic and may support organs and systems such as small intestines, urinary system, heart disorders, liver, and kidneys. Adzuki bean is also useful in assisting weight-loss endeavors (www.healingfoodreference.com).
Ailanthus	*Zanthoxylum ailanthoides*	An infusion of the leaves is ingested to treat chills and influenza. The fruits are used to treat indigestion, diarrhea, and sunstroke.
		The essential oil of the leaf contains methyl n-nonyl ketone, and the fruit contains isopimpinellin (Chiu 1955).
		Other compounds include alkaloids dictamnine, skimmianine, magnoflorine, and laurifoline, which were found in the wood and bark. Seeds and peel contain isopimpinellin (Y. Chang 2000).
		The stem and leaves of this plant have antioxidative and mutagenic properties (Chung et al. 2006).
		Root and stem bark are used as an anesthetic, analgesic, and anti-inflammatory. They also promote circulation and dispel stagnant blood. Ailanthus is used to treat rheumatism, bone pain, dermatitis, snake bite, and pyodermas (K. Lin 1998c).

English Name	Scientific Name	Nutritional and Therapeutic Values
		The bark, fruits, and seeds are used. Dried fruits yield 2.3% essential oil upon steam distillation. The chief content of the oil is linalool, while the other constituents include linalyl acetate, citral, geraniol, methyl cinnamate, limonene, and sabinene. The root bark contains spilanthol and an unidentified alkaloid identical with berberine (Chauhan 1999).
		Seeds and bark are used as an aromatic tonic in fever, dyspepsia, and cholera. Fruits, branches, and thorns are used as a remedy for toothache and are considered carminative, stomachic, and anthelmintic. The stem has exhibited hypoglycemic activity in preliminary trials. An extract of the fruits is reported to be useful in expelling roundworms (Chauhan 1999).
Alfalfa	*Medicago sativa*	Young leaves contain 6% protein, 2–3% saponin, glycine, glucose, sterol, and flavones. The plant is rich in vitamins A, C, and E. Aqueous extracts of the plant have antibacterial properties against mycobacteria (Duke 1981).
		Alfalfa is regarded as depurative, and the plant is cited in the Fen Tw'ao Kang Mu as useful in treating intestinal and kidney disorders (Perry 1980).
		Alfalfa is high in vitamins B, C, E, and K, and it can be used as a nutritional supplement. However, high doses of alfalfa may present some health risks (L-cavanine in the seeds may cause abnormal blood cell counts and spleen enlargement). Extracts from seeds, leaves, and roots may be helpful in lowering cholesterol levels (Colodny et al. 2001).
		Alfalfa is rich in chemical compounds beneficial to human health, including satiol, lucernol, tricia, formononetin, citrulline, canaline, dicoumarol, ononitol, vitamins A, C, D, E, and K, delphinidin, petunidin, malvidin, linalool, myrcene, limonene, homostachydrine, stachydrine, sialic acid, and vernin (N. Chiu and Chang 1995c).
		It has been reported that the aboveground parts of alfalfa can be steeped in hot water to make a drink for treating arthritis or ulcers (Marles et al. 2000).
		Alfalfa greens provide protein, fat, total carbohydrate, crude fiber, thiamine, riboflavin, niacin, vitamins A and C, and minerals. The leaves also contain tannins and coumestrol and several related compounds that have been reported to have an estrogenic effect (Marles et al. 2000).

English Name	Scientific Name	Nutritional and Therapeutic Values
Alfalfa sprout	*Medicago sativa*	Alfalfa is used as a diuretic for kidney, bladder, and prostate conditions, and for treatment of asthma, arthritis, diabetes, indigestion, and thrombocytopenic purpura. It is also used orally as a source of vitamins A, C, E, and K4 as well as the minerals calcium, potassium, phosphorous, and iron (Jellin et al. 2003).
		The alfalfa leaf contains saponins, which appear to decrease plasma cholesterol without creating a change in HDL levels. Constituents of alfalfa seem to decrease cholesterol absorption and increase excretion of neutral steroids and bile acids.
		Alfalfa contains manganese, which might be responsible for its hypoglycemic effect. It also contains medicagol, which appears to have antifungal properties (Newall et al. 1996).
		Alfalfa also contains coumestrol, genistein, biochanin A, and diadzein, which all seem to have estrogenic properties (Leung and Foster 1996).
		Isoflavonoids are commonly found in leguminous plants, especially alfalfa, where they play an important role in plant defense and have significant health benefits for animals and humans (Shao et al. 2007).
		The aboveground parts of alfalfa can be steeped in hot water to make a drink for treating arthritis or ulcers. The leaves and seeds are an excellent source of nutrients, particularly for vitamins C, D, E, and K (Dobelis 1986).
		Alfalfa sprouts contain phytoestrogens and are very popular among consumers. However, some have contended that the content of various antinutritional factors is sufficiently high that the consumption of both alfalfa and alfalfa sprouts should be limited (Tyler 1993).
		Certain saponins in alfalfa sprouts are alleged to have detrimental effects. On the other hand, these same saponins reduce levels of blood serum cholesterol in animals (Small 1980).
		Alfalfa contains acetone, adenine, aluminum, amylase, biochanin-A, butanone, calcium, campesterol, carbohydrates, β-carotene, citric acid, coumestrol, cytidine, daidzein, daphnoretin, fat, fiber, fructose, fumaric acid, genistein, hypoxanthine, inosine, inositol, iron, isocytosine, limonene, lutein, malic acid, malonic acid, manganese, medicagenic acid, 3(-methoxycoumestrol, 4-0-methyl coumestrol, 3-methylbutanol, 2-methylpropanol, molybdenum, myriston, oxalic acid, pectin, peroxidase, potassium, protein, quinic acid, saponin, sativol, selenium, silicon, β-sitosterol, sodium, soyasapogenols, α-spinasterol, L-stachydrine, sucrose, thiamine, α-tocopherol, triacontanol, trigonelline, tryptophan, xanthophylls, xylose, zeaxanthin, and zinc (Duke 2001).

English Name	Scientific Name	Nutritional and Therapeutic Values
		It can be eaten as a vegetable and may lower cancer risk. However, alfalfa sprouts may trigger lupus in sensitive individuals if there is a family history with lupus infection (Duke 2001).
		Alfalfa sprouts are a very good tonic, both for gaining health or retaining it. The pleasant tea made from the leaves is rejuvenating if taken every day. Alfalfa sprouts are listed as an appetizer, diuretic, tonic, and nutrient (Willard 1992).
Arrowhead	*Sagittaria sinensis*, *S. trifolia* var. *sinensis*	The arrowhead tubers should not be eaten raw. However, they can be dried and made into a powder that can be used as a gruel or added to cereal flours and used in making bread.
		Arrowhead (aboriginals call it "wapato") is a major source of food for the aboriginal community in British Columbia, Canada. Arrowhead is said to resemble the Irish potato in texture and appearance, but with a sweetish flavor reminiscent of chestnuts (Turner 2006).
		Arrowhead has nutritional and medicinal aspects (Simoons 1990). It has 16–23% starch and 4–7% protein. It is used to treat bug bites, snakebite, scrofulous ulcers, breast inflammation, and sore throat (Perry 1980).
		Arrowhead has been used as a discutient and as an antilactogogue (Bliss 1973). The tuber is discutient, galactofuge, and may induce premature birth (Duke and Ayensu 1985).
		The plant is antiscorbutic and diuretic.
		The leaf is used to treat a variety of skin problems.
		The fresh leaf can be washed and applied as a poultice to inflamed patches of skin that are associated with scrofula (Lamont 1977).
		The fresh leaf can be washed and applied as a poultice to inflamed patches of skin that are associated with scrofula (tuberculous lymphadenitis: an infection of the lymph glands by tuberculosis bacteria) (Marles et al. 2000).
		This herb contains d-raffinose, d-stachyose, d-verbascose, d-fructose, d-galactose, glucose, asparagine, and vitamin B.
		Bruised leaves are used to treat bug bites, foul sores, and scrofulous ulcers and are also used as an antilactogogue (T. Li 2002).

English Name	Scientific Name	Nutritional and Therapeutic Values
Asparagus	*Asparagus officinalis*	Asparagus contains flavonoids, amino acid derivatives, sulfur-containing acids, glycolic acid, tyrosine, vitamins, saponins, and essential oils.
		It also contains flutathione with antioxidant and anticarcinogenic properties (Bliss 1973; Duke and Ayensu 1985).
		Asparagine and 5-methoxy-methylfurfurol have been isolated from asparagus and used to relieve cough and phlegm (Y. Chang 2000).
		The plant also has diuretic and laxative properties (Leung 1980).
		It is used to treat parasitic diseases, cancer, neuritis, and rheumatism (Duke 1984).
		Asparagus contains glycolic acid, asparagome, essential oils, methanethiol, (+)-nyasol, asparagine, steroidal β-sitosterol, sarasapogenin, polysaccharide, diosgenin, and oleanene derivatives
		Asparagus is also diuretic and laxative.
		It can be used to treat cancer (antitumor and antioxidative activity), neuritis, rheumatism, and parasitic diseases (T. Li 2002).
		Root, stem, leaf, flower, fruit, and seeds contain asparagine, coumarin, sarasapogenin, glutathione, rutin, vitamin C, peptidase, quercetin, capsanthin, glucomannan, coniferin, and chelidonic acid.
		Goryanu is extracted from root, as are asparagosides a–h (Je 1999).
		Asparagus can be used to treat cough, nose cancer, leukemia, lung cancer, breast cancer, and lymphatic gland cancer (Je 1999).
		Asparagus is used along with copious fluid consumption as "irrigation therapy" to increase urine output.
		It is also used orally to treat urinary tract infections and other inflammatory conditions of the urinary tract; to prevent kidney; and to treat bladder stones, rheumatic joint pain and swelling, female hormone imbalances, and dryness in the lungs and throat (Jellin et al. 2003).
		Asparagus is used topically for cleansing the face, drying sores, and treating acne.
		In Chinese medicine, it is used orally as a laxative and as a treatment for neuritis, parasitic diseases, and cancer.

English Name	Scientific Name	Nutritional and Therapeutic Values
		The newly formed shoots, or spears, are eaten as a vegetable.
		The seed and root extracts of asparagus are used in alcoholic beverages (Jellin et al. 2003).
		The applicable parts of asparagus are the rhizome and root.
		Asparagus is rich in vitamin E (Brinker 1998).
		The asparagus root has diuretic effects in animal experiments (Blumenthal 1998).
		Asparagus also has hypotensive (Leung and Foster 1996), antibacterial, and antiviral effects in vitro (Peirce 1999).
		Fibers from the plant can have mutagen-adsorbing (cancer-preventing) activity (Leung and Foster 1996).
		The saponin constituents can irritate mucous membranes and can be cytotoxic (Jellin et al. 2003).
		It can also cause urinary tract irritation (Brinker 1998).
Asparagus lettuce	*Asparagus officinalis*	The effects of the ethanol extract and five partition fractions of the root of *Asparagus officinalis* were evaluated on insulin secretion together with exploration of other mechanisms of action .
		The findings reveal that constituents of *Asparagus officinalis* root extracts have wide-ranging stimulatory effects on physiological components and may provide new opportunities for diabetes therapy (Hannan et al. 2007).
		The plant contains alanine, α-aminodimethyl, butyrothetin, arginine, ascorbic acid, aspartic acid, α-carotene, β-carotene, fiber, fructose, glucose, glutamic acid, histidine, iron, isoleucine, jamogenin, kaempferol, lauric acid, linoleic acid, α-linolenic acid, lysine, magnesium, methionine, niacin, oleic acid, palmitic acid, palmitoleic acid, phenol, philothion, phosphorus, phytosterols, proline, quercetin, rhamnose, rutin, sarsapogenin, selenium, stearic acid, strontium, succinic acid, thiamine, threonine, tocopherol, tryptophan, tyrosine, valine, vanadium, 4-vinylguaiacol, 4-vinylphenol, zeaxanthin, zinc, and zirconium (Duke 2001).
Bay laurel	*Laurus nobilis*	Bay leaves contain protein, β-carotene, thiamine, riboflavin, niacin, and ascorbic acid.
		It also contains calcium, fiber, iron, riboflavin, pro-vitamin A, and vitamin C (Duke and Ayensu 1985).

English Name	Scientific Name	Nutritional and Therapeutic Values
		Bay leaves crushed with other ingredients have been used to treat pain from migraine headaches (E. Martin 1986).
		Bay laurel has been widely regarded in China as a folk cancer remedy.
		In the Far East, oil from the bark and leaves is applied to scabies (Perry and Metzger 1980).
		A series of research projects on plants used in Calabria in the folk plant medicine has been carried out over the past 20 years.
		The results indicate that *Laurus nobilis* has a galactagogue function (Passalacqua et al. 2007).
		Leaves are aromatic, narcotic, and stimulant and are used to treat amenorrhea, colic, and hysteria.
		It is carminative, diuretic, emmenagogue, and antiparasitic.
		This plant is widely regarded as a folk cancer remedy for such things as anal condylomata, cancer, indurations of liver and spleen, sclerosis and tumors of liver, parotid gland, stomach, testicles, and uterus, as well as tuberosities of the face (Duke and Ayensu 1985).
Bean (tao-tou)	*Canavalia gladiata* *C. ensiformis*	Bean contains canavanine, concanavalins A and B, canaline, and gibberellin.
		It is a tonic and is used as a bactericide and fungicide and as a treatment for stomachache (T. Li 2006).
		Roximate principles, minerals, and vitamins can be found in this plant
		It also has thiamine, riboflavin, and niacin.
		Vitamins B and K and tocopherol have been found in seeds (Patwardhan 1962).
		In China, the pods and seeds are used for their tonic, stomachic, and bechic properties, and they are also used to strengthen the kidneys (Perry 1980).
		It has been reported that glutamic acid, aspartic acids, isoleucine + leucine, tyrosine + phenylalanine, and lysine are the major amino acids of *Canavalia gladiata* seed proteins.
		The presence of certain antinutritional factors is also reported (Rajaram and Janardhanan 1992).
		Profiles of amino acids of total seed protein from bean detected in a study revealed that levels of valine, phenylalanine, tyrosine, isoleucine, and histidine are higher than the FAO/WHO (1991) reference pattern (Siddhuraju and Becker 2001).

English Name	Scientific Name	Nutritional and Therapeutic Values
Beet	*Beta vulgaris*	Beet contains arginine, betaine, histidine, isoleucine, leucine, phenylalanine, tyrosine, and tyrosinase (Jiangsu New Medical College 1979).
		It is recommended as a hemostatic, stomachic, and treatment for dysentery.
		Beet is used as a folk cancer remedy in Arabian, American, German, and Mexican medicine.
		In China, beet root is used as a tonic for women, and it is said to contain female sex hormones.
		Reported constituents are saponiside, phytosterol, fatty matter, betaine, leucine, tyrosine, isoleucine, arginine, histidine, phenylalanine, urease, and tyrosinase (Perry 1980).
		Exalate oxidase obtained from the stem of beet was covalently linked to polyethylene glycol, it exhibited decreased electrophoretic mobility, increased storage stability, higher thermal stability, and resistance to heavy metal inactivation and proteolytic digestion (Varalakshmi et al. 1995).
		Beet (Swiss chard) contains numerous active ingredients.
		It includes acetamide, aconitic acid, alanine, allantoin, aluminum, L-arabinose, abginine, ascorbic acid, barium, betaine, cadmium, caffeic acid, calcium, carbohydrates, β-carotene, chlorogenic acid, chromium, citric acid, copper, p-coumaric acid, cystine, daucic acid, farnesol, fat, ferulic acid, folacin, formaldehyde, glutamic acid, glycine, kaempferol, leucine, linoleic acid, α-linolenic acid, lithium, lysine, magnesium, manganese, mercury, molybdenum, niacin, nitrogen, ornithine, oxalic acid, oxycitronic acid, palmitic acid, pantothenic acid, pentosans, quercetin, raffinose, raphanol, riboflavin, salicylic acid, selenium, serine, β-sitosterol, stearic acid, strontium, thiamine, α-tocopherol, tricarballyl acid, vanillic acid, xylose, zinc, and zirconium (Duke 2001).
Betony	*Stachys sieboldii* *S. officinalis*	Betony is a comparatively new variety of vegetable of which the edible portion is the tuber.
		This species occurs wild in Northern China, where it is also cultivated.
		The tubers are eaten.
		The tuber steeped in wine is recommended as a treatment for influenza and colds (Perry 1980).
		It was used very widely in classical herbal medicine, but not in modern Western medicine.
		Powdered flowers were used as a laxative.
		An infusion of flowers, leaves, or root was used against fever.

English Name	Scientific Name	Nutritional and Therapeutic Values
		The leaf infusion was also used to treat headache, backache, migraine, toothache, eye problems, bronchitis, asthma, women's ailments, and wounds (Small 2006).
		Betony leaves contain 15% tannins, betaine, caffeic acid, and other compounds.
		The main alkaloids are betonicine and stachydrine (Duke and Ayensu 1985).
		The dietetic value resides especially in a carbonaceous substance, which reaches 16.6%; the nitrogenous ingredients amount to 3.2%; water forms 78.3% of the bulk (www.botanical.com/botanical/mgmh/a/artic067.html).
		It contains caffeic acid, chlorogenic acid, neochlorogenic acid, cryptochlorogenic acid, sesquiterpene lactones, cynaropicrin, dehydrocynaropicrin, grossheimin, and cynaratriol (Noble 2000).
		Betony has a cholagogic, hepatotoxic, and lipid-reducing effect. Cinnamic acid has a choleretic effect in rats (Noble 2000).
		One research study suggested that glycosides in betony may lower blood pressure.
		In normal usage, betony should not cause any notable side effect, but overdosing may result in excessive irritation of the stomach (Tyler 1993).
Bird-nest fern	*Asplenium nidus*	The plant has been reported to be depurative, sedative, deobstruent, pectoral, and vermifugal.
		The leaves are used as a diuretic and to treat dysuria and bladder complaints associated with beri-beri (Y. Chang 2000).
		Europeans use it to treat sclerosis of the spleen and cold impostumes of the uterus.
		Malayans apply pounded leaves to the feverish head and use the infusion to alleviate labor pains (Duke and Ayensu 1985).
		The bird-nest fern is nonpoisonous.
		The Malay used a decoction of the leaves to ease labor pain in childbirth and also to obtain a lotion to treat fever (Lee-Khoo Guan Fong, National Library Board, Singapore).
		It has been reported that bird-nest fern can be used to relieve inflammation and injuries (Y. Chang 2000).

English Name	Scientific Name	Nutritional and Therapeutic Values
		In ethnobotanical survey of reproductive behavior in Vanuatu and an extensive literature search have resulted in the selection of five plant species used for purposes relating to human reproduction in that country.
		Bird-nest fern (*Asplenium nidus*) is one of the five species selected.
		Preliminary screening was carried out to identify possible estrogenic activity in this plant as well as its effect on isolated rate uteri.
		Dysoxylum quadichaudianum presented the most interest due to its spasmolytic activity (Bourdy et al. 1996).
		Root of bird-nest fern is bitter and slightly poisonous.
		It contains filicic acid, tannin, essential oils, starch, resin, and sugar, and is anthelmintic, hemostatic, and an antidote (Keys 1976).
Bitter gourd	*Momordica charantia*	The bitter principle in the bitter gourd is due to the alkaloid momordicine (Cantwell et al. 1996).
		It contains momordic acid, gypsogenin, and α-eleostearic acid (Ye 1999).
		It acts as an antitumor agent and inhibits HIV-1 infection.
		Bitter gourd helps regulate blood sugar levels, as it contains gumarin, a polypeptide considered to be similar to bovine insulin.
		It is also rich in iron, β-carotene, calcium, potassium, and vitamins C, B1, B2, and B3.
		Bitter gourd is highly beneficial in the treatment of blood disorders such as boils, scabies, itching, ringworm, and fungal diseases (Abascal and Yarnell 2005).
		During the ripening process, there are more than 14 carotenoids, mainly cryptoxanthin (Rodriguez et al. 1976).
		It induces apoptosis in HL 60 human leukemia cells (Etoh et al. 2002) and has antitumor activity (Y. Xue et al. 1998).
		It has been reported that seed contains sterol, momordicine, elaterin, charantin, β-sitosterol, β-D-glucoside, and β-elaterin (T. Li 2006).

English Name	Scientific Name	Nutritional and Therapeutic Values
		There are components in bitter gourd that possess antiobesity properties, which may be helpful for weight control and glycemic control (Q. Chen and Li 2005).
		Fruits, roots, leaves, and flowers are used as an anti-inflammatory.
		Roots are used to treat amoebic dysentery.
		Fruits used to treat heat stoke, fever, pharyngitis, and ringworm infection (K. Lin 1998d).
		The bitter principle, for which the fruit is named, is due to the alkaloid momordicine. Bitter gourd is also important for various medicinal properties, with more recent attention focused on it as a hypoglycemic agent (Cantwell et al. 1996).
Black nightshade	*Solanum nigrum*	The plant is used to treat fever, flu, bronchitis, dysentery, and cancer.
		Although young shoots are eaten in the tropics as greens, its berries are toxic due to the presence of solamargine, solasonine, solavilline, solasodamine, tigogenin, and cornevin (Perry 1980; Y. Chang 2000).
		It contains solanine, solasonine, solamargine, solasodine, diosgenin, tigogenin, and vitamin A (N. Chiu and Chang 1995).
		Some Indian folk herbalists crush nightshade leaves, stir them into heavy cream, and pad the mixture on sunburn (Duke 1997).
		Ethanol extract of black nightshade showed remarkable hepatoprotective activity (Raju et al. 2003).
		Whole herb is used for antipyretic, anti-inflammatory, diuretic, antiswelling, colds and fever, sore throat, chronic bronchitis, urinary tract infection, acute nephritis, mastitis, and malignancies (K. Lin 1998c).
		Whole herb is used for colds and fever, sore throat, chronic bronchitis, urinary tract infection, acute nephritis, mastitis, malignancies. It is used externally to treat boils and pyoderms, impetigo, eczema, and snakebites (K. Lin 1998g).

English Name	Scientific Name	Nutritional and Therapeutic Values
		Leaf is a rich source of riboflavin, nicotinic acid, and vitamin C. It also contains β-carotene and citric acid. Fruits contain glucose and fructose, vitamin C, and β-carotene. Seeds contain around 17.5% protein (on dry-weight basis) and yield an oil. The immature green fruit contains four steroidal glycoalkaloids, solamargine, solasonine, and α- and β-solanigrine, and all of them yield solasodine as the aglycone. Dioxgenin is also present in leaves, stem, and fruits (Chauhan 1999).
		Black nightshade has antiseptic and antidysenteric properties and is given internally for neuralgia and gripe.
		An infusion of the plant is used as an enema for infants having abdominal upsets.
		It is a household remedy for anthrax pustules and is applied locally.
		Freshly prepared extract of the plant is effective in the treatment of cirrhosis of the liver and also serves as an antidote to opium poisoning.
		An alcoholic extract of the leaves is actively against *staphylococcus aureus* and *Escherichia coli*.
		Decoctions of the plant can be used for the treatment of ascites (Chauhan 1999).
		Black nightshade contains solanigrines, saponin, riboflavin, nicotinic acid, and vitamin C.
		It is antibacterial and diuretic.
		Black nightshade can be used to treat mastitis, cervicitis, chronic bronchitis, and dysentery (Huang 1999).
		It was also reported that black nightshade contain solanine, solasonine, solamargine, solasodine, diosgenin, tigogenin, and vitamins A and C (Rieger 2006). Solanum nigrum has been used in traditional folk medicine to treat different cancers.
		It is also used as a hepatoprotective and anti-inflammatory agent (H. Lin et al. 2007).
Bottle gourd	*Lagenaria siceraria* *L. leucantha* *L. vulgaris*	Leaves can be eaten as a vegetable. Sweet and green fruit is popular as a cooked vegetable. It is used to treat headache, with crushed leaves used as a topical application on the head (Y. Chang 2000).

English Name	Scientific Name	Nutritional and Therapeutic Values
		It has been reported that in male rats, a deficiency of dietary choline, one of the vitamin B's, is associated with infertility.
		It may also cause liver damage and is associated with the development of liver cancer.
		Whether choline can help heal the human liver is uncertain.
		The best source of choline is bottle gourd (1.6% on a dry-weight basis), which can be eaten the same as squash (Duke 1997).
		The fruit is antilithic, diuretic, emetic, and refrigerant.
		Rind of fruit is employed as a diuretic and is boiled in oil for rheumatism.
		In recent years, bottle gourd has been used to treat diabetes (Duke and Ayensu 1985).
		In China, the fruit pulp is considered to be cooling, diuretic, and antilithic.
		The seeds are used as a remedy for aching teeth and gum boils (Perry 1980).
		Fruit contains lagenaria D.
		It is used to treat anasarca ascites and beri-beri, and its antiswelling properties are useful in treating abdominal swelling and swelling of the feet (T. Li 2006).Preliminary phytochemical screening revealed the presence of flavonoids, sterols, cucurbitacins, saponins, polyphenolics, proteins, and carbohydrates in *Lagenaria siceraria*.
		The results obtained suggest marked antihyperlipidemic and hypolipidemic activity of the extracts (Ghule et al. 2006).
Broad bean	*Vicia faba*	Broad bean contains kaempferol, fumaric acid, D-glyceric acid, folinic acid, and plastoquinone (N. Chiu and Chang 1995b).
		Broad bean may be used to protect against prostate cancer (Kolonel et al. 2000).
		It is high in fiber, low in fat, and is rich in lecithin, a nutrient that helps cut cholesterol (Duke 1997).
		Saponins stimulate the immune system and decrease the growth of human epidermoid and cervical cancer cells in vitro (Messina and Barnes 1991; Naim et al. 1974).

English Name	Scientific Name	Nutritional and Therapeutic Values
		It is used to treat diarrhea, inflammation, bloody urine, and bleeding from the digestive system (Perry 1980).
		Anticancer metabolite and daidzein were found in the stems of *Vicia faba*.
		It has been reported that broad bean is an excellent food source for both genistein and daidzein (Kaufman et al. 1997).
		Broad bean contains alanine, arginine, arsenic, ascorbic acid, betulin, beta-carotene, ceraldone, chlorine, cholesterol, citric acid, p-coumaric acid, beta-cyanoalanine, ferulic acid, fiber, fumaric acid, gibberellin, glutamic acid, glyceric acid, p-hydroxybenzoic acid, gamma-hydroxycitrullin, d-hydroxylysine, kaempferol, leucine, linoleic acid, lysine, myristic acid, oleic acid, oxalic acid, palmitic acid, palmitoleic acid, phosphatides, quercetin, serine, stizolamine, thiamine, threonine, tryptophan, tyrosine, valine, vicine, and wyerone (Duke 2001).
Broccoli	*Brassica oleracea* var. *italica*	Broccoli contains folic acid (B. Lin and Lin 1999) and glucosinolates (Kristal 2002).
		Antioxidative and antimutagenic activities of polyphenols have been isolated from broccoli (Huifeny et al. 2001).
		The leaves are tonic and aid digestion.
		The boiled peel of the enlarged stem is used to cure dropsy and other swellings (Perry 1980).
		Broccoli has indole-3-carbinol that can combat breast cancer by converting a cancer-promoting estrogen into a more protective variety.
		Broccoli; especially sprouts, also has the phytochemical sulforaphane, a product of glucoraphanin, which is believed to aid in preventing some types of cancer (The Cancer Cure Foundation 2000, Newbury Park, California).
		Extracts from broccoli show significant antioxidant properties against lipid peroxidation.
		However, this antioxidant is not due to the glucosinolate content, which probably involves the hydroxylated phenol and polyphenol contents (Plumb et al. 1996).
		The antioxidative effect and protective potential against diabetes of the broccoli flower were investigated in vitro and in a diabetic rate model.

English Name	Scientific Name	Nutritional and Therapeutic Values
		This study demonstrated that the BuOH fraction has an antioxidative effect in vitro, and it protects against oxidative stress induced by diabotesin in an in vivo model (Cho et al. 2006).
		Studies indicate that people who are low in the antioxidant compound glutathione are more likely to have arthritis than those who have higher amounts (Duke 1997).
Brussels sprouts	*Brassica oleracea* var. *gemmifera*	The leaves are tonic and aid in digestion.
		The plant contains numerous phytochemical constituents (Duke and Ayensu 1985).
		The chemical component in Brussels sprout includes arginine, ascorbic acid, boron, caffeic acid, calcium, beta-carotene, citric acid, coumestrol, ferulic acid, fiber, histidine, iron, linoleic acid, lysine, niacin, oleic acid, quercetin, quinic acid, stearic acid, succinic acid, selenium, sodium, alpha-tocopherol, arachidonic acid, arginine, ascorbic acid, coumestrol, cystine, fumaric acid, indole-3-carboxylic acid, leucine, linoleic acid, malic acid, molybdenum, palmitic acid, palmitoleic acid, phytosterols, protein, riboflavin, butin, stearic acid, succinic acid, tryptophan, and valine (Duke 2001).
		Sprouts have always been eaten by vegetarians who tout their anticancer effects.
		The plant is protective against DNA damage, and it may reduce hardening of arteries (NewsTarget. com).
		Extracts from Brussels sprout show significant antioxidant properties against lipid peroxidation.
		However, this antioxidant is not due to the glucosinolate content, which probably involved the hydroxylated phenol and polyphenol contents (Plumb et al. 1996).
		It has been reported that consumption of Brassica vegetables is associated with a reduced risk of cancer of the alimentary tract in animal models and human populations.
		Brussels sprouts are rich in the glucosinolate sinigrin, and they have been used to explore the effect of naturally occurring glucosinolate breakdown products on cell-cycle progression and apoptosis in human colorectal carcinoma cells (HT29) (Smith et al. 2005).
Burdock	*Arctium lappa*	Seeds, stem, and root are considered to be alterative, depurative, disphoretic, and diuretic.

English Name	Scientific Name	Nutritional and Therapeutic Values
		The fruit contains arctin, arctigenin, matai-resinol, sesquilignins, stereoisomer, inulin, mucilage, pectin, lignans, and acetic, caffeic, chlorogenic, oleic, palmitic, propionic, stearic, and uglic acids (T. Li 2002).
		Arctigenin occurs in relatively high concentrations in Burdock seed, which has a long history of safe use in Chinese herbal medicine.
		Six in vitro studies have reported that arctigenine induced differentiation in or inhibited the proliferation of various cancer cell lines (Boik 2001).
		Seed extracts have shown antibacterial, antifungal, antifurunculous, antitumor, diuretic, estrogenic, and hypoglycemia activity (Duke and Ayensu 1985).
		Seeds should not be used in pregnancy, as this can cause spotting and even the rare case of miscarriage (Willard 1992).
		Burdock is used to treat for dermatitis, tumors, breast cancer, and nephritis.
		It is also diuretic, antibacterial, anti-inflammatory, and is used to relieve sore throat (T. Li 2002).
		It contains volatile oil, fatty oil, sucrose, resin, tannin, and large amounts of carbohydrate, specifically inulin.
		Active constituents include podophyllin-type lignan derivatives and guanidinobutyric acid.
		Burdock may have antipyretic, diuretic, and diaphoretic properties.
		It may inhibit HIV-1 infection, antagonize platelet-activating factor, prevent tumors, and affect the digestion of dietary fiber.
		Burdock is used orally to treat cancers, renal or urinary calculi, GI tract disorders, constipation, catarrh, fever, infection, gout, arthritis, and fluid retention.
		It is also used as a blood purifier, aphrodisiac, and diaphoretic (Carpenter 2001).
		Fruit contains arctin, arctigenin, sesquilignins, stereoisomer, inulin, lignans, mucilage, pectin, and acetic, butyric, caffeic, chlorogenic, lauric, linoleic, oleic, palmitic, propionic, stearic, and tiglic acids (Chauhan 1999; T. Li 2002).

English Name	Scientific Name	Nutritional and Therapeutic Values
		Burdock contains lappaol, arctigenin, arctin, isoarctigenin, matai-resinol, arctinone A and B, arctinol A, B, and C, lappaphen A and B, eremophilene, petasitolone, fukinanolide, β-eudesmol, and α-hydroxyeudesmol (Ye 1999).
		Burdock is used as a diuretic, blood purifier, antimicrobial, antipyretic, and to treat anorexia nervosa.
		It is used to treat rheumatism, gout, cystitis, and chronic skin conditions, including acne and psoriasis.
		Topically, burdock is used for dry skin and eczema.
		In folk medicine, burdock is used for treating colds, catarrh, cancers, and as an aphrodisiac.
		Historically, burdock has been used in the treatment of gout and syphilitic disorders (Jellin et al. 2003).
		The applicable part of burdock is the root.
		The leaf and flower have gram-positive and gram-negative antibacterial activity; the root is active against gram-negative bacteria (Newall et al. 1996). Arctiopiricin is active against gram-positive bacteria in vivo, and burdock has uterine stimulant activity in animals.
		The plant may have some antimutagenic and antitumor activity (Newall et al. 1996).
		A tincture of the seed applied topically is effective in curing psoriasis, inveterata, hemorrhoids, and chronic sores (Reid 1993).
Cabbage	*Brassica oleracea* var. *capitata*	Cabbage is rich in minerals, especially potassium and vitamins A, B6, and C (C. Xue 2001a).
		It is used as a tonic and aids digestion (Perry 1980; Wall et al. 1988).
		The Canadian cancer society recommends eating cabbage on a regular basis, as its high carotene content lessens the risk of cancer.
		The sulfur and histidine contained in cabbage reduce the growth of tumors and also detoxify and strengthen the immune system.
		It is also antidepressive and appetitive due to the rich vitamins and minerals.
		Cabbage is antidiarrhetic, antiscorbutic, and antiseptic.

English Name	Scientific Name	Nutritional and Therapeutic Values
		It has cosmetic properties and improves oily skin (TheWorldwideGourmet.com).
		Extracts from cabbage show significant antioxidant properties against lipid peroxidation.
		However, this antioxidant is not due to the glucosinolate content, which probably involves the hydroxylated phenol and polyphenol contents (Plumb et al. 1996).
		It contains aniline, arginine, ascorbic acid, aspartic acid, benzylamine, boron, butyl-glucosinolate, caffeic acid, calcium, carbohydrates, beta-carotene, citric acid, cyanidin, dehydrozascorbic acid, ethylamine, ferulic acid, fiber, fluorine, folacin, flucoiberin, glutamic acid, glycine, iron, isomenthol, kaempferol, leucine, alpha-linolenic acid, luten, lysine, magnesium, maleic acid, manganese, menthol, mevalonic acid, niacin, nitrogen, oleic acid, oxalate, palmitic acid, phosphorus, quercetin, quinic acid, selenium, threonine, tyrosine, vanadium, and zinc (Duke 2001).
		Cabbage is used to treat gastritis, gastric and duodenal ulcers, gastric pain, gastric hyperacidity, and Roemheld syndrome.
		Cabbage is used orally to treat asthma and morning sickness and to prevent osteoporosis.
		It is also used orally to prevent lung cancer, stomach cancer, colorectal cancer, breast cancer, and other cancers.
		Topically, cabbage leaves and its extracts are used to relieve swelling and to reduce breast engorgement (Jellin et al. 2003).
		When used topically for treating breast engorgement in lactating women, cabbage leaves seem to produce subjective relief similar to the standard practice of applying chilled gel-packs to the engorged breast (Roberts 1995).
		Both chilled and room temperature cabbage leaves seem to provide the same relief (Roberts et al. 1995).
		It is tonic and aids digestion (Perry 1980).
		A cabbage leaf extract applied as a cream has also been tried.
		The cabbage leaf extract cream seems to provide subjective relief, but not significantly better than a placebo cream (Roberts et al. 1998).

English Name	Scientific Name	Nutritional and Therapeutic Values
		The applicable part of cabbage is the leaf.
		Cabbage contains modest amounts of calcium and vitamins A, B, C, and E.
		It also contains other active constituents, including chlorogenic and caffeic acids and goitrin.
		These constituents seem to have antithyroid effects, possibly by inhibiting iodine uptake.
		Estrogen can be converted to either 16-alpha-hydroxyestrone or 2-alpha-hydroxyestrone (Michnovicz 1998).
Carrot	*Daucus carota* var. *sativus*	Carrot is rich in carotenoids. The main constituents are pyrrolidine, duacine, and daucosterine.
		Its essential oil has limonene, pinene, and cineole.
		The seeds contain tiglic acid, asaron, and bisabol (Mosig and Schramm 1955).
		It is used as a diuretic, to lower blood sugar, for prevention of cancer, and to treat diabetes, heart disease, dyspepsia, gout, and carcinomatous ulcers (Hartwell 1971; Duke 1985).
		It has been reported that very high consumption of carrots can give the skin an orange tone, particularly on the palms or hands and feet, but it is believed to be very difficult to consume too much beta-carotene, the precursor of vitamin A, by eating carrots, because the body does not convert the excess beta-carotene to vitamin A (Small 2006).
		Carrot has been reported to exert low antioxidant activity compared with other vegetables (Vinson et al. 1998).
		Extracts of carrot leaves and peel showed antioxidant activity toward oxidation of pure methyl lineolata at 40°C, while the carrot flesh was inactive (Kahkonen et al. 1999).
		It has been reported that carotenoid helps prevent cancer, cardiovascular disease, and cataracts.
		It may also reduce stroke risk by as much as 54% if consumed twice a month (Duke 1997).
		Carrot can be used to prevent cataracts and stroke, help in smoking cessation, and slow the aging process.
		Carrot is also used to treat amenorrhea, angina, asthma, diarrhea, high blood pressure, high cholesterol, liver and skin problems, and wrinkles (Duke 1997).

English Name	Scientific Name	Nutritional and Therapeutic Values
Cassava	*Manihot esculenta*	The paste of cassava is baked into a pancake-like bread, while the extracted juice is fermented into a strong liquor called kasiri.
		It is suggested that this plant be used carefully on account of the very high content of hydrocyanic acid.
		In Indonesia, the root mixed with several other plant parts is used to treat pain.
		A decoction of the bark is considered to be antirheumatic (Perry 1980).
		Cassava contains dextrin, mannitol, gutta-percha, hydrocyanic acid, and manihotin (N. Chiu and Chang 1995c).
		Root contains hydrocyanic acid and is used to dress ulcerous sores (Arthur and Cheung 1960).
		It contains alanine, arginine, ascorbic acid, aspartic acid, boron, calcium, beta-carotene, citrates, fiber, glutamic acid, histidine, iron, kilocalories, lauric acid, lysine, magnesium, niacin, oleic acid, oxalic acid, palmitic acid, phosphorus, potassium, proline, protein, riboflavin, serine, sodium, starch, stearic acid, succinates, sugars, sulfur, thiamin, threonine, tryptophan, tyrosine, valine, and zinc (Duke 2001).
		It has been reported that the cassava leaves with beta-carotene promotes growth and tissue weight in rats similar to that of the synthetic product.
		Beta-carotene from the leaf matrix may be bounded to protein complex or inside organelles, which impair carotenoid absorption.
		It is concluded that it aids in hepatic retinol recovery.
		It has been reported that beta-carotene in cassava leaf could maintain rat growth and avoid symptoms of vitamin A deficiency (Siqueira et al. 2006).
Cauliflower	*Brassica oleracea* var. *botrytis*	Cauliflower is rich in minerals, especially potassium, and vitamin C.
		It is used as a tonic and assists digestion (C. Xue 2001a).
		Curcumin and phenethyl isothiocyanate (PEITC) are abundant in cauliflower.
		Combination of these two compounds demonstrate significant cancer-preventive qualities in laboratory mice.

English Name	Scientific Name	Nutritional and Therapeutic Values
		It can also treat the established prostate cancers (Prof. Ah-Ng and Tony Kong, Dept. of Pharmaceutics, Rutgers University, New Brunswick, NJ) (www.sciencedaily.com).
		A new study conducted by a research team (Ah-Ng and Tony Kong) at Rutgers University has revealed that cauliflower, in particular, has natural ingredients that may reduce the risk of developing hereditary cancers (2006).
		Extracts from broccoli show significant antioxidant properties against lipid peroxidation.
		However, this antioxidant is not due to the glucosinolate content, which probably involved the hydroxylated phenol and polyphenol contents (Plumb et al. 1996).
		It contains alpha- and beta-amyrin, ascorbic acid, aspartic acid, caffeic acid, alpha- and beta-carotene, cinnamic acid, citric acid, fumaric acid, glucoerucin, glucoberin, glutamic acid, p-hydroxybenzoic acid, indole-3-carboxylic acid, linoleic acid, maleic acid, methanol, molybdenum, neoglucobrassicin, palmitic acid, pantothenic acid, phytosterols, quercetin, quinic acid, selenium, silicon, stigmasterol, succinic acid, threonine, alpha-tocopherol, tryptophan, and vanillic acid (Duke 2001).
Celery	*Apium graveolens* var. *dulce*	Celery contains volatile oil (terpenes limonene and b-selinene and phthalides), coumarins (seselin, osthenol, apigravin, celerin, umbelliferone), furanocoumarins (bergapten), flavonoids (apigenin, apiin), phenolic compounds, choline, ascorbate, and fatty acids.
		Celery shoots contain high calcium, fiber, riboflavin, and vitamin C (Duke and Ayensu 1985).
		Celery has been reported to demonstrate a number of functional properties, including antirheumatic, antispasmodic, diuretic, carminative, hypotensive, anti-inflammatory, sedative, nerve-stimulant, and urinary antiseptic (Malhotra 2006).
		It has been reported that celery has been successfully employed in curing rheumatoid arthritis (Guenther 1950).
		Celery seed was prescribed as an aphrodisiac, to expel gas from the alimentary canal, and to promote urination.
		Celery leaves contain thiamine, riboflavin, niacin, and ascorbic acid (Duke and Ayensu 1985).
		It also contains aplin and graveobiosides A and B.

English Name	Scientific Name	Nutritional and Therapeutic Values
		Celery seeds can be used to treat hypertension and hypercholesterolemia (T. Li 2002).
		Celery seed has a long history of use in traditional Chinese medicine as a treatment for dizziness and lowering high blood pressure.
		It was also reported that the juice significantly lowered total cholesterol and LDL levels in animals.
		It contains butylidenephthalide, a chemical that helps trigger menstrual flow.
		Celery contains calcium blockers and other plant chemicals such as apigenin, apiin, magnesium, and potassium that help prevent and treat arrhythmias, plus other compounds that help lower blood pressure and cholesterol.
		Celery seed extracts might help eliminate uric acid, which may avoid gout crises (Duke 1997).
Celery cabbage	*Brassica pekinensis* *B. petsai* *B. chinensis* var. *pekinensis*	Celery cabbage is now established as a crop in North America and among Asian populations. It has a depurative property. *Brassica chinensis* is stocked in Chinese pharmacies for medicinal use (Perry 1980).
		It contains phytoalexin and brassinin, which inhibit the development of DMBA-induced mammary lesions in vitro, and which inhibited tumor promotion in mice (Mehta et al. 1995).
		Chinese cabbage or celery cabbage contains arsenic, boron, cadmium, caffeic acid, calcium, cobalt, p-coumaric acid, ferulic acid, lithium, magnesium, mercury, molybdenum, phosphorus, potassium, selenium, sinapic acid, sulfur, alpha-tocopherol, and zinc (Duke 2001).
Celery seeds	*Apium graveolens* var. *dulce*	The volatile oil content of celery seeds averages 3% and consists primarily of 60% d-limonene, 10–20% selinene, sesquiterpene alcohols, sedanolide, and sedanonic anhydride (Simon et al. 1984).
		Ayurvedic physicians used celery seeds to treat people with colds, flu, water retention, poor digestion, various types of arthritis, and certain ailments of the liver and spleen.
		Recently, celery seeds have been used primarily as a diuretic to promote the excretion of urine and to treat urinary tract infections. (Information acquired from Univ. Maryland Medical Center, Center for Integrative Medicine. www.umm.edu/altmed/consHerbs/celeryseedsch.html.)
		The seeds are stimulant and digestive and serve as an antispasmodic for asthma and bronchitis (Perry 1980).

English Name	Scientific Name	Nutritional and Therapeutic Values
Chicory	*Cichorium intybus*	A bushy perennial herb with blue or lavender flowers.
		Chicory is grown and used as a salad green.
		Fresh chicory roots contain inulin and large amounts of vitamins A and C (Simon et al. 1984).
		It contains bitter compounds, choline, stearin, mannite, tartaric acid, tannin, and palmitic and linoleic acids.
		Young leaves contain tannin and glycoside (Morton 1981).
		Chicory has been used medicinally.
		A decoction of the roots is effective in treating jaundice, liver enlargements, gout, and rheumatic complaints.
		It stimulates urination, is a laxative and a tonic, and is used to treat warts, tumors, and cancer (Tyler 1993).
		Egyptian researchers have discovered that chicory root has two heart benefits. It slows a rapid heartbeat, and it also has a mild heart-stimulating effect, somewhat like the often-prescribed medication digitalis (Duke 1997).
		It contains acetophenone, arginine, ascorbic acid, caffeic acid, beta-carotene, cichoric acid, cichorin, ferulic acid, fiber, fructose, glucose, histidine, inositol, inulin, kaempferol, lactucin, lactucopicrin, linoleic acid, lysine, mannitol, niacin, oleic acid, pentin, quercetin, riboflavin, scopoletin, taraxasterol, thiamine, threonine, umbelliferone, valine, and vanillic acid (Duke 2001).
		The leaves of chicory can be eaten raw in salads or cooked as vegetable.
		The roots can be eaten raw, boiled, or roasted.
		It has been used as a coffee substitute. It is prepared like dandelion roots and sometimes commercially mixed with dandelion root coffee (Willard 1992).
Chili pepper	*Capsicum annuum* var. *longum*	The carotenoid capsanthin is the most important pigment of *Capsicum*.
		The pungent principle capsaicin is present on the placenta of the fruits, and is said to retain its pungency at dilutions of one part in one million (Purseglove et al. 1981).

English Name	Scientific Name	Nutritional and Therapeutic Values
		The main components, capsaicin, and dihydrocapsaicin are responsible for the inhibition against *Bacillus cereus*, *B. subtilis*, *Clostridium sporogenes*, *C. tetani*, and *Streptococcus pyogenes* (Cichewicz and Thorpe 1996).
		Chili pepper has been employed in a variety of folk remedies to treat asthma, inflamed gums, lumbago, neuralgia, pneumonia, rheumatism, sores, cancers, and tumors (Duke 1985).
		It contains acetylcholine, L-asparaginase, asparagine, aspartic acid, behenic, campesterol, capsaicin, capsanthin, capsianoside-A, alpha-carotene, beta-carotene, choline, chromium, cinnamic acid, citrostadienol, beta-cryptoxanthin, alpha-cryptoxanthin, cyclopentanol, cystine, funkioside, galactosamine, galactose, heneicosane, heptadecane, hexanoic acid, lanosterol, lanosterol, lithium, lupeol, lutein, margaric acid, molybdenum, myrcene, myristic acid, obtusifoliol, phenylalanine, proline, pyrrolidine, scopoletin, stearic acid, solanine, terpinolene, tetramethylpyrazine, tryptophan, valine, vanilloyl-glucose, xanthophyll, zeaxanthin, and zirconium (Duke 2001).
		In China, the leaves of the chili pepper are used to treat toothache, while the fruit is considered useful for stomach problems, rheumatism, and for increasing blood circulation (Perry and Metzger 1980).
Chinese artichoke	*Stachys sieboldii* *S. officinalis*	A perennial plant with white rhizomes.
		It stores large amounts of starches and sucrose.
		It is a comparatively new variety of vegetable, of which the edible portion is the tuber.
		This species occurs wild in Northern China, where it is also cultivated.
		The tuber steeped in wine is recommended as a treatment for influenza and cold (Perry 1980).
		The leaves contain 15% tannins, betaine, caffeic acid, and other compounds.
		The main alkaloids are betonicine and stachydrine (Duke and Ayensu 1985).
		The dietetic value resides especially in a carbonaceous substance, which reaches 16.6%; the nitrogenous ingredients amount to 3.2%, with water forming 78.3% of the bulk (www.botanical.com/botanical/mgmh/a/artic067.html).Medicinally, powdered flowers were used as a laxative, and the root was used against toothache, eye problems, bronchitis, asthma, women's ailments, and wounds (Small 2006).

English Name	Scientific Name	Nutritional and Therapeutic Values
		Leaves contain caffeic acid, chlorogenic acid, neochlorogenic acid, cryptochlorogenic acid, sesquiterpene lactones, cynaropicrin, dehydrocynaropicrin, grossheimin, and cynaratriol (Noble 2000).
		It has a cholagogic, hepatotoxic, and lipid-reducing effect.
		Cinnamic acid has a choleretic effect in rats (Noble 2000).
Chinese basil	*Perilla frutescens*	The plant is edible and medicinal.
		The leaves have a very pleasant sweet taste and are used as a spice, cooked as potherbs, or fried and combined with rice, vegetables, and soups.
		Although Chinese basil is widely consumed, this species has been shown to have poisonous constituents (Small 2006).
		Prolonged skin contact of basil may produce dermatitis (Kuebel and Tucker 1988).
		The volatile oils from *Perilla frutescens* contain several compounds, such as l-perillaldehyde, perilla ketone, egomaketone, and isoegomaketon (Kerr et al. 1986).
		Oil from dried leaves and inflorescences contains perillaldehyde and is used as a flavoring and antiseptic agent.
		The seed oil consists mainly of the polyunsaturated fatty acid and linolenic acid (J. I. Lee et al. 1989).
		Colored leaves of some forms of Perilla contain the anthocyanin perillanin chloride.
		The leaves are used for coloring plum preparation.
		Perilla is used as a sedative to treat spasms, uterine and head problems, and to increase perspiration (Panday 1990).
		Apigenin and luteolin are the major flavones in the seeds. The same flavones are in the leaves with nine flavone glycosides, chiefly the 3-p-coumarylglycoside-5-glucoside of cyanidin and the 7-caffeyl-glucosides of apigenin and luteolin.
		Five anthocyanins including cyanidin, 3,5-diglucoside, and cinnamic acid (Duke and Ayensu 1985).

English Name	Scientific Name	Nutritional and Therapeutic Values
		In Chinese medicine, it is employed alone or in combination with other herbs to treat cholera, colds, influenza, stomach problems, nausea, poisoning, asthma, bronchitis, chest pain, rheumatism, and other ailments (Duke and Ayensu 1985).
Chinese broccoli	*Brassica oleracea* var. *capitata* var. *gongylodes*	This flavorful broccoli is also called Chinese kale. The edible vegetable consists of a tender green flower stem with buds that become white flowers. The leaves and stems are light- to medium-green in color and are covered with a white haze due to cuticle and development (Larkcom 1991). It has a high content of vitamin A and contains appreciable amounts of thiamine and ascorbic acid. The leaf is digestive and tonic (Duke and Ayensu 1985). Chinese broccoli can be used as a medicinal plant, as it has cancer-preventive properties (Siegmund 1958; Beecher 1994). This vegetable is rich in an antioxidant compound, glutathione, which is used to prevent arthritis (Duke 1997). It contains alanine, aniline, arginine, arsenic, ascorbic acid, benzylamine, butenyl glucosinolate, butyl-glucosinolate, caffeic acid, calcium, beta-carotene, chlorogenic acid, citric acid, coumaric acid, crocetin, cystine, dehydroascorbic acid, dindolylmethane, dimethyl-amine, ferulic acid, fluorine, folacin, glucoiberin, kaempferol, linoleic acid, alpha-linolenic acid, lithium, lutein, lysine, malic acid, methionine, mevalonic acid, molybdenum, neochlorogenic acid, niacin, oleic acid, oxalic acid, palmitic acid, pantothenic acid, phenethylamine, phosphorus, phytosterols, progoitrin, quercetin, quinic acid, selenium, sinapic acid, stearic acid, succinic acid, thiamine, tryptophan, tyrosine, violaxanthin, zinc, and zirconium (Duke 2001).
Chinese cabbage	*Brassica chinensis*	Chinese cabbage is stocked in Chinese pharmacies for medicinal use. It is antiarthritic, antiscorbutic, and resolvent and is used for treatment of alcoholism, fevers, and intoxication (Duke and Ayensu 1985).

English Name	Scientific Name	Nutritional and Therapeutic Values
		Chinese cabbage contains alanine, arginine, ascorbic acid, calcium, carbohydrates, beta-carotene, cystine, fiber, glutamic acid, glycine, histidine, iron, isoleucine, kilocalories, leucine, linoleic acid, alpha-linolenic acid, lysine, methionine, niacin, oleic acid, palmitic acid, phenylalanine, proline, riboflavin, serine, stearic acid, thiamine, threonine, alpha-tocopherol, tryptophan, tyrosine, and valine (Duke 2001).
		Chinese cabbage or pak choi is a very popular tropical leaf vegetable.
		It has prominent white, fleshy petioles and upstanding glabrous leaves forming a loose rosette, as in a Swiss chard.
		Individual leaves or entire heads are harvested and used raw or cooked (Palada and Crossman 1999).
		Chinese cabbage is ranked in one of the top five vegetables in antioxidant activity assays (Easdown and Kalb 2004).
Chinese chive	*Allium tuberosum*	Chive is an allium grown for its leaves and not for its bulb.
	A. schoenoprasum	It has been considered a healthy food for its special spicy flavor.
		Chemically, chives are composed mainly of carbohydrates, proteins, and amino acids as well as many other vitamins and minerals.
		The unique spicy flavor comes mostly from volatile sulfur and glucosides.
		Thiosulfinates and sulfines were extracted from chive leaves, which contain n-propyl group (H. Chen 2006).
		Propenylcysteine sulfoxide is the most important soulful compound in chives.
		It has been used as a vermifuge, and it also has an antibiotic effect (Poulson 1990).
		Wild chives or onions (*Allium schoenoprasum*) have been known to cause digestive upset if consumed in excess (Marles 2000).
		These plants also have antibacterial activity.
		Chinese chive contains 2.1 mg/g fresh wt. of allicin.
		It is used as an intestinal tonic and to treat hematemesis and urethral ailments (Perry 1980; Duke and Wain 1981).

English Name	Scientific Name	Nutritional and Therapeutic Values
		The leaves are high in vitamin C and beta-carotene, 20–34% protein, 34–75% fat, and 54–67% carbohydrate (Duke and Ayensu 1985).
		It is reported that Chinese chive seed is useful in treatment of impotence, nocturnal ejaculation, and enuresis (K. Lin 1998f).
		It has been reported that the root of Chinese chive is used to relieve stomach discomfort (Y. Chang 2000).
		Chinese chives have a long history of cultivation for culinary and medicinal use (Cantwell et al. 1996).
Chinese kale	Brassica oleracea	The leaves are tonic and aid digestion (Perry and Metzger 1980).
		This crop is considered as one of the forgotten and future vegetable phytoceuticals (Goldman 2002).
		The leaves are cardiotonic and stomachic.
		Leaves have been used in the treatment of gout and rheumatism.
		The leaves can be used as a poultice to cleanse infected wounds (Chopra et al. 1986; Siegmund 1958).
Chinese leek	Allium tuberosum	A native of China and Japan, the plant is depurative, stimulant, and tonic.
		It contains beta-carotene, thiamine, riboflavin, niacin, and ascorbic acid.
		The seeds are said to be roborant, stomachic, carminative, and antidiarrhetic.
		The juice is useful against hemoptysis, hematuria, and hemorrhages (Perry 1980).
		The leaves are applied to bug bites, cuts, epistaxis, lacquer poisoning, and wounds (Perry 1980; Duke and Ayensu 1985).
		Chinese leek is rich in vitamins B1, B2, C, and carotene.
		It has been used as an herbal medicine in China, being considered effective for treatment of fatigue (Saito 1990).
		It has also been prescribed as an antidote for ingested poisons and as a way to control excessive bleeding (Harrington 1978).

English Name	Scientific Name	Nutritional and Therapeutic Values
		It is reported that Chinese leek seed is used in treatment of impotence, nocturnal ejaculation, and enuresis (K. Lin 1998f).
Chinese mahogany	*Toona sinensis*	The bark is taken to treat measles.
		It is astringent and depurative and is used to treat gonorrhea, menstrual troubles, and postpartum hemorrhage (Perry 1980).
		Mahogany contains toosendanin, sterol, catechol, carotene, and vitamins B and C (N. Chiu and Chang 1995c).
		It is well known in Taiwan that Chinese mahogany is a traditional Chinese medicine.
		It has been shown to exhibit an antioxidant effect.
		Toona sinensis extracts or gallic acid-induced HL-60 apoptotic cell death could be due to the generation of ROS (reactive oxygen species), especially H_2O_2.
		The data suggest that this plant exerts an antiproliferative action and growth inhibition on HL-60 cells, which is valuable for application in food and drug products (H. Yang et al. 2006).
Chinese mallow	*Malva verticillata* var. *crispa*	Leaves are eaten raw or cooked.
		It has a mild and very pleasant flavor that makes an excellent addition to salads.
		It has mucilaginous and demulcent properties useful in treating stomach and intestinal troubles.
		A decoction of this plant is suggested as an antidote for mineral poisonings.
		The root is antilithic, diuretic, thirst-relieving, and a treatment for foul ulcers (Perry 1980).
		It contains fiber, hemicellulose, cellulose, and lignin (Istam et al. 2004).
		It has diuretic properties and promotes lactation effects, and can be used to treat difficult urination, urethritis, swelling, insufficient lactation, and swollen and painful breasts (Reid 1993).
Chinese mustard	*Brassica rapa*	It has been reported that the decocted juice from the stems and leaves is used to treat cancer.
		Brassica rapa is antivinous, digestive, diuretic, emetic, laxative, refrigerant, and resolvent.
		It is also used to treat arthritis, chest colds, dysentery, fever, flu, hematochezia, mastitis, rheumatism, scurvy, skin ailments, sores, spasm, and warts (Duke and Ayensu 1985).

English Name	Scientific Name	Nutritional and Therapeutic Values
		Chinese mustard seeds are popular due to the low content of glucosinolates and saturated fatty acids and the high proportion of nutritionally desirable fatty acid (Jolliff and Snapp 1988).
		Brassica rapa contains alanine, allantoin, allantoic acid, arginine, arsenic, ascorbic acid, brassicasterol, campesterol, beta-carotene, fluorine, folacin, isoleucine, kilocalories, lycopene, linolenic acid, molybdenum, oleic acid, palmitic acid, palmitoleic acid, pantothenic acid, phenylalanine, riboflavin, silicon, stearic acid, thiamine, threonine, tryptophan, tyrosine, and valine (Duke 2001).
		Discovery of the first naturally occurring aromatic isothiocyanates and indole-3-isothiocyanates from *Brassica rapa* has been reported.
		Their first synthesis has antimicrobial activity and proposed biogenetic origin in canola plants (Pedras et al. 2007).
Chinese radish	*Raphanus sativus* var. *longipinnatus*	Radish leaves usually are medium green and lobed and have a rough texture. The leaves are popular in China and are used as a vegetable.
		It has a fair amount of vitamins B and C as well as pectin, phytin, iron, manganese, and copper (C. Xue 2001a).
		It is used to treat asthma, cough, diarrhea, dysentery, and malnutrition (Perry 1980).
		It contains ferulic acid, gentisic acid, raphanusin, erucic acid, glycerol, sinapate, raphanin, and sulforaphen (N. Chiu and Chang 1995a).
		The roots of Chinese radish stimulate the appetite and digestion, as well as have a tonic and laxative effect upon the intestines and indirectly stimulate the flow of bile.
		The plant is used in the treatment of intestinal parasites.
		The leaves are used for asthma and other chest complaints.
		The seeds are carminative, diuretic, expectorant, laxative, and stomachic (Bown 1995; Chevallier 1996).

English Name	Scientific Name	Nutritional and Therapeutic Values
		Seeds are used mainly for a productive cough and to treat indigestion, abdominal distention, constipation, dysentery, chronic bronchitis, and bad breath (K. Lin 1998g).
		It also contains erucic acid, glycerol sinapate, sinapine, raphanin, and sulforaphen.
		It is used to treat stomach cancer, diabetes, windpipe infection, constipation, blood pressure, and chronic cough (Ye 1999).
		Radish has been used in folk medicine as a natural drug against many toxicants.
		It is reported that radish extract is safe and can be overcome or, at least, can significantly diminish the zearalenone effect that is presented in corn and food mixtures for farm animals (Salah-Abbes et al. 2007).
Chinese spinach	*Amaranthus gangeticus*	A popular vegetable cultivated year-round and consumed as a leaf vegetable in many parts of the world.
	A. mangostanus	The plant is semi-upright with purple and green leaves oval in shape.
	A. mangosteens	The plant contains considerable potassium nitrate.
	A. tricolor	The root is used to treat rheumatism.
		It acts as an emmenagogue and as a diuretic in treating gonorrhea.
		It is sudorific and febrifuge in eruptive or very high fevers (Perry 1980).
		The leaves are said to be cooling, nonpoisonous, and remedial for dysentery and dropsy.
		Internally, the leaves are used to treat bronchitis or a chest cold.
		Chinese spinach is ranked among the top five vegetables in antioxidant activity assays (Easdown and Kalb 2004).
		It contains alanine, arginine, ascorbic acid, aspartic acid, calcium, carbohydrate, beta-carotene, copper, cystine, fat, fiber, folacin, glutamic acid, glycine, histidine, iron, isoleucine, leucine, lysine, magnesium, methionine, niacin, phenylalanine, phosphorus, potassium, proline, protein, riboflavin, rutin, serine, sodium, thiamine, threonine, tryptophan, tyrosine, valine, and zinc (Duke, 2001).
Chinese wolfberry	*Lycium chinese*	Root bark contains cinnamic acid, betaine, peptides, acyclic diterpene glycosides, polysaccharide, betaine, β-sitosterol, and kukoamines.

English Name	Scientific Name	Nutritional and Therapeutic Values
		It is reported to have properties to lower blood sugar and blood pressure (T. Li 2002).
		The red berry is a tonic for diabetes mellitus, pulmonary tuberculosis, and vertigo (Duke and Ayensu 1985).
		It contains physalin, carotene, and vitamins B1, B12, and C. Fruit, root bark, and leaves are used.
		It is a tonic to the liver and spleen.
		Chinese wolfberry improves eyesight.
		Fruits are used to treat oligospermia, knee and back pains, sexual neurasthenia, dizziness, and failing eyesight (K. Lin 1998g).
		Leaves, stem, and root are used.
		Leaves contains asteroid A and B, β-sitosterol, β-sitosterol glucoside, and anolide.
		It has an immunosuppressive effect.
		Root bark is used to treat fever, blood pressure, symptoms of the common cold, and diarrhea.
		Berry is used as a liver and kidney tonic (Noble 2000).
		Chinese wolfberry contains cinnamic and psyllic acid, betaine, β-sitosterol, linoleic and linolenic acids, kukoamine A, and lyciumins A and B.
		It is used internally for treatment of fever, hyperhidrosis, thirst, coughs, nose bleeds, pulpitis, diabetes, hypertension, and malaria.
		External uses include eczema and rheumatism (Ye 1999).
		Lycium barbarum fruits have been used as a traditional Chinese herbal medicine.
		An experiment found that the Lycium barbarum polysaccharides can be used in compensating the decline in TAOC, immune function, and the activities of antioxidant enzymes, thereby reducing the risks of lipid per oxidation accelerated by age-induced free radicals (X. Li et al. 2007).
		It is a tonic to kidneys, nourishes semen and the liver, and improves vision.
		It can be used to treat blurry vision, dizziness, and headaches (Reid 1993).

English Name	Scientific Name	Nutritional and Therapeutic Values
Chinese yam	*Dioscorea alata*	The root contains allantoin, arginine, d-abscisin, mannan, phytic acid, diosgenin, protein, glycosides, triterpene, glucosides, dioscorenin, dioscorecin, and diosbulbins A, B, and C (N. Chiu and Chang 1995d).
		It has properties for antitumor, sore throat, gullet cancer, swelling, food poisoning, goiter, hernia, purulence, inflammations, and helps dissolve phlegm (T. Li 2002).
		The tuber and axillary sprouts of Chinese yam have an acrid taste.
		Chinese yam has anti-inflammatory, anti-swelling, and expectorant properties.
		Its tuber is eaten during convalescence from phthisis and for kidney and spleen disorders.
		It is also used as a maturative poultice on boils (Perry 1980).
		Chinese yam is used for blood purifying and to treat hemostasis, goiter, tuberculous lymphadenitis, cancer of the gastrointestinal tract, hematemesis, hemoptysis, and uterine bleeding (K. Lin 1998b).
		Chinese yam (*Dioscorea alata*) has been used folklorically to treat menopausal symptoms in China for years.
		A study investigated the effects of yam ingestion on lipids, antioxidant status, and sex hormones in postmenopausal women.
		The results indicated that, although the exact mechanism is not clear, replacing two-thirds of staple food with yam for 30 days improves the status of sex hormones, lipids, and antioxidants.
		These effects might reduce the risk of breast cancer and cardiovascular diseases in postmenopausal women (W. Wu et al. 2005).
Chinese yam	*Dioscorea batatas*	Leaves and flowers are used as an anti-inflammatory, a laxative, and a parasiticide; they are used to treat headache, dizziness, constipation, infantile convulsion, malnutrition, and pertussis (K. Lin 1998c).
		The dried rhizomes (best collection season for medicinal use is when the plant is in dormant stage and the shoot portion is withered) contain 4.8–8% of diosgenin content, which is used in the partial synthesis of modern drugs like cortisone and other steroids.

English Name	Scientific Name	Nutritional and Therapeutic Values
		The main intermediate isolated from diosgenin is 16-DPA, which can be further synthesized to any desired steroid hormone used in various formulations, including oral contraceptive pills.
		It has been reported that the plant is one of the richest sources for the steroid sapogenin (Chauhan 1999).
		Cortisone has proved to be of great value in the treatment of a large variety of diseases, particularly in rheumatic diseases.
		Other diseases include ophthalmic disorders, allergic states, and idiopathic thrombocytopenic purpura (Chauhan 1999).
Common bracken	*Anisogonium esculentum* *Diplazium esculentum*	The plant is well known as vegetable fern.
		It is used as a stir-fry vegetable.
		It is used as an antifebrile and relieves depression.
		It can also be applied in a plaster to care for pimples and eruptions.
		It is added to ointments for skin diseases (Perry 1980).
		It showed antimicrobial properties with minimum inhibitory concentration and minimum lethal concentration values in the respective ranges of 100–800 g/ml.
		It also displayed cytotoxic activity against the HeLa cell line, with CD50 values in the range of 10–30 g/ml (Mackeen et al. 1997).
Coral flower	*Talinum paniculatum*	New young leaves and stems are used as a vegetable.
		The plant, including the root, is used to treat debilitation, weakness, and sweating.
		The leaves have cooling, emollient, antiscorbutic, alterative, vulnerary, and resolvent properties.
		The swollen root is used as an aphrodisiac (Perry 1980).
		Coral flower has antisifilitico, astringent, disputative, and vulneraria properties (R. Yang et al. 2005).
		Sitosterols were isolated from *Talinum paniculatum* (Komatsu et al. 1982).
		The whole plant is used to treat diarrhea, enuresis, and irregular menses.
		The coral flower contains sitosterols and sugar alcohols (K. Lin 1998a; T. Li 2006).

English Name	Scientific Name	Nutritional and Therapeutic Values
Coriander	*Coriandrum sativum*	The lacy foliage is "cilantro," a parsley-like garnish with a fresh fragrance.
		Coriander is used as an aromatic spice in Chinese cooking.
		This plant contains hypoglycemic, acetone, borneol, coriandrol, cymene, decanal, decanol, decylic aldehyde, dipentene, geraniol, limonene, linalool, malic acid, nonanal, oxalic acid, phellandrene, tannic acid, terpinene, and terpinolene.
		The leaves hasten the eruption of pox and measles.
		The plant is sedative.
		The fruit is anticatarrhal, antispasmodic, and a galactagogue (Duke and Ayensu 1985; Perry 1980).
		A form of the species used for its leaves is called Chinese parsley.
		Coriander is one of the world's most important spices.
		Seeds contain 0.3–1.7% essential oils, d-linalool, camphor, d-α-pinene, camphene, β-pinene, sabinene, myrcene, α-terpinene, γ-terpinene, and limonene (Small 2006).
		It is regarded as a tonic, a cough medicine, and a stomach curative (Small 2006).
		The whole herb or fruit of coriander can be used as a diaphoretic or stomachic, and it is used to promote eruption of rashes.
		The whole herb is used to treat incomplete eruption of measles and influenza without sweats.
		Fruits are used for indigestion, anorexia, stomachache, and distension (K. Lin 1998e).
		Coriander is used for dyspeptic complaints, loss of appetite, and complaints of the upper abdomen.
		It is also used to treat the pre-eruptive phase of chickenpox and measles, hemorrhoids, and rectal prolapse.
		It is used for digestive and gastric disorders, coughs, chest pains, bladder complaints, leprosy, rash, fever, and dysentery.
		It is used externally for headaches and oral and pharyngeal disorders (Noble 2000).
		Coriander is used for dyspepsia, loss of appetite, as a stomach function stimulant, spasmolytic, antiflatulent, bactericide, fungicide and for diarrhea.

English Name	Scientific Name	Nutritional and Therapeutic Values
		The seed/fruit is used.
		It is a rich source of vitamin C, calcium, magnesium, potassium, and iron (Blinker 1998).
		In North America, coriander seeds are commonly used in mixed pickling spices and in baking.
		It has a sweet, spicy aroma with a peppery flavor.
		Coriander is one of the world's most important spices, and is of great significance in international trade.
		The most abundant constituent is d-linalool.
		The seeds appear to be used not only as a condiment, but also as a stomachic, a carminative, a corrective, and a remedy for dyspepsia (Perry 1980).
		The main medicinal use of coriander is as a flavoring to mask the taste of certain medicines.
		It is also used to treat intestinal diseases.
		In Asia, the seeds are used as a general tonic to treat stomach problems and nausea, and the oil and other parts of the plant are used to treat a variety of ailments, including fever, measles, colds, hernia, and spasms.
		Coriander is rich in provitamins A and C.
		It also contains calcium, fiber, iron, phosphorus, and potassium (Small 2006).
		In Chinese medicine, it is used to treat measles, dysentery, hemorrhoids, and toothaches.
		The whole plant is used for stomachache, nausea, measles, and painful hernia (Jellin et al. 2003).
Corn	*Zea mays*	The leaves are used to improve passing urine, to release inflammation, and to treat gallstone, diabetes, and cancer (N. Chiu and Chang 1995b).
		Corn contains saponins, fatty acids, tannins, resin, maysin, essential oils, thiamine, and mucilage.
		Green corn silk is diuretic and is useful in treating dropsy, as are the undeveloped pistils of the flower and the fresh or dried stalks (Perry 1980).
		It is used for cystitis, urethritis, prostatitis, and urinary stones.
		Corn seed has volatile oil; common corn oil may be used as a carrier oil (T. Li 2000).

English Name	Scientific Name	Nutritional and Therapeutic Values
		It also contains abscisic acid, aconitic acid, adenosine, alanine, allantoin, aluminum, amino-adipic acid, delta-amino-levulinic acid, alpha-amylase, beta-amylase, alpha-amyrin, beta-amyrin, arachidic acid, arginine, astragalin, benzaldehyde, betaine, cryptoxanthin, caffeic acid, calcium, campesterol, carbohydrates, carvacrol, cellulose, chelidonic acid, choline, cobalt, alpha-copaene, beta-copaene, cryptoxanthin, cubebenol, cyanidin, cycloartenol, cytokinin, dihydrotosterol, ergosterol, ethanol, eugenol, geosmin, geranial, geraniol, globulin, alpha-glucoside, d-glucuronic acid, glutamic acid, glycolic acid, hydroxamic acid, indole, inositol, iron, isorhamnetin, kaempferol, kinetin, lactic acid, lanosterol, leucine, leucocyanidin, limonene, linalool, linoleic acid, maleic acid, malonic acid, menthol, mercury, methylamine, methyl phenylacetate, octadecadienoic acid, pelargonidin, peroxidase, phenylalanine, phosphatidyl glycerides, beta-pinene, alpha-pinene, quercetin, quinic acid, ricinoleic acid, salicylic acid, saponin, tricarballyl acid, uridine, uronic acid, vanillic acid, xanthotoxin, zeatin, zeaxanthin, beta-zein, alpha-zein, and zirconium (Duke 2001).
		The Chinese have used corn silk successfully to treat swelling caused by kidney disease, according to natural product pharmacist, Dr. Albert Leung (Duke 1997).
Cress	*Lepidium sativum*	Cress or garden cress is rich in vitamins A and C, iron, and calcium.
		Seed is frequently used medicinally in Asia (Morton 1976).
		It contains isothiocyanates with antibacterial properties (Zhao 1981).
		Cress is used to increase sexual power and acts as a diuretic and purgative.
		Seeds are used medicinally in Asia (Morton 1976).
		It is also used to treat pleurisy, dropsy, asthma, and coughing with nausea (Perry 1980).
		Cress is an expectorant, is used as a diuretic, reduces swelling, and is used as a sedative in asthma and bronchitis.
		It can be used to treat excess phlegm, coughs, asthma, facial paralysis, and water retention in the chest and abdomen (Reid 1993).
		The pungent taste of garden cress is due to the presence of glucosinolates (Small 2006).
		Garden cress is used for vitamin C deficiency, liver disease, asthma, hemorrhoids, and as an abortifacient.

English Name	Scientific Name	Nutritional and Therapeutic Values
		Seeds contain glucotropeolin for coughs, constipation, poor immunity, and as a diuretic (Noble 2000).
		Garden cress contains arachidic acid, ascorbic acid, behenic acid, carbohydrates, beta-carotene, cellulose, erucic acid, fiber, gadoleic acid, iron, linoleic acid, miacin, palmitic acid, riboflavin, sinapic acid, beta-sitosterol, stearic acid, thiamine, alpha-tocopherol, uric acid, and d-sylose (Duke 2001).
		Cress also contains strophanthidine, evomonoside, helveticoside, evobioside, glucosimolates, benzyl isothiocyanate, allyl isothiocyanate, 3-butenyl isothiocyanate, and linolenic, linoleic, oleic, sinapic, paolinitic, and steraric acids.
		Seeds contain sinalbin, fat, protein, and sucrose (Ye 1999).
Cucumber	*Cucumis sativus*	The flower buds of the cucumber contain a bitter principle that causes nausea and vomiting.
		The seeds are used as a digestive, and they contain myristic acid, phosphates, galactane, lysine, citrulline, tryptophan, cystine, and histidine.
		The fruit is a stomachic and contains urease, peptidase, protease, and vitamins A, B, and C.
		Cucumber can be used to treat skin problems, swelling, and wrinkles (Duke 1997).
		Cucumber is mentioned as cooling and diuretic.
		A cucumber soup relieves retention of urine.
		A salve made from cucumbers is recommended for skin disorders, scalds, and to treat beri-beri.
		Juice from the crushed leaves is used as an emetic in acute indigestion of children (Perry 1980).
		It contains arginine, caffeic and chlorogenic acids, cucurbitacins, isoquercitrin, and mannose.
		It is diuretic, purgative, and resolvent (Jiangsu New Medical College 1979).
		Fruit, vine, and leaves are used for anti-inflammatory and diuretic purposes, and they promote salivary secretion and thirst quenching. They can be used to treat heat and thirst, sore throat, sore eye, high blood pressure, and burns and scalds (K. Lin 1998e).
		Fruits, vines, and leaves are used for sore throat, sore eye, high blood pressure, burns, and scalds.

English Name	Scientific Name	Nutritional and Therapeutic Values
		Juice is extracted from fresh cucumber for topical application (K. Lin 1998f).
		It contains cucurbitacins A, B, C, and D, oleic acid, linoleic acid, palmitic acid, and stearic acid (N. Chiu and Chang 1995d).
Dandelion	*Taraxacum officinale*	The bitter resin in the roots and shoots contains taraxacin, taraxerin, taraxerol, taraxasterol, inulin, gluten, gum, potash, choline, levulin, and putin (Simon et al. 1984).
		Root extracts were once used extensively as a diuretic, and are still sometimes so employed.
		Dandelion juice, expressed from the roots, used to be sold by druggists.
		The flowers have been used in folk medicine to treat jaundice and other liver ailments.
		Dandelion has also served as a tonic (Small 2006).
		Dandelion has been used for hundreds of years.
		The juiciness of the dandelion, suggestive of water retention, was interpreted as indicating usefulness as a diuretic.
		Other ailments treated in the past include fever, insomnia, rheumatism, eczema and other skin diseases, constipation, warts, cancers, and tumors.
		Taraxacin and taraxasterol are active ingredients of the dandelion roots.
		The dried plant contains 2.8% tannins (Small and Catling 1999).
		The bitter taste of dandelions is due to 11,13-dihydrotaraxine acid-1-O-β-D-glucopyranoside and several other awesomely named chemicals (Kuusi et al. 1985).
		The leaves are high in vitamin A and an excellent source for B complex and vitamin C.
		They can be cooked like spinach (Willard 1992).
		It contains a bitter crystalline principle, taraxacin, and a crystalline substance, taraxacerine.
		It also contains the phytosterols taraxasterol and homotaraxasterol as well as saponin.
		The milky sap contains ceryl alcohol, lactuce-rolltaraxacin, and choline.
		The root yields inulin, tannin, and some etheral oil; the leaves contain vitamins A and C, and the flowers contain xanthophyll (Chauhan 1999).

English Name	Scientific Name	Nutritional and Therapeutic Values
		Root is diuretic, tonic, laxative, cholagogue, antirheumatic, and aperient.
		The tender leaves are used as a salad when harvested early in spring.
		The plant has a slight inulin content and is used as a bitter for loss of appetite and stomach upsets.
		The chemical component promotes the secretion of gall and is a useful remedy for chronic disorders of kidney and liver.
		It has been in use for gallstones, cholecystitis, jaundice, atonic dyspepsia with constipation, muscular rheumatism, and oligurea (Chauhan 1999).
		Dandelion above ground parts are used for loss of appetite and dyspepsia, flatulence, and feelings of fullness.
		They are also used as a laxative, promoter of healthy circulation, skin toner, blood vessel cleanser and strengthener, for rheumatism, arthritic joints, and as a tonic (Jellin et al. 2003).
		The entire dandelion plant is used for gallstones, bile stimulation, muscle aches, low urine output, indigestion, constipation, flatulence, as a tonic, and, in anti-smoking preparations.
		In Chinese medicine, the entire plant is used for treating breast cancer.
		Traditionally, dandelion plant has been used orally for diabetes, rheumatic conditions, heartburn, bruises, gout, stiff joints, eczema, and cancer (Jellin et al. 2003).
		For food uses, dandelion leaves are added to salads.
		The roasted root and extract are used as coffee substitutes.
		In food manufacturing, dandelion plant is a flavoring component for foods as well as beverages (Jellin et al. 2003).
Dasheen	*Colocasia esculenta*	Leaves and stalk are used for bug bites and other poisons.
		In China, the seeds, leaves, and stalks are used in medicine.
		The seeds, although considered somewhat poisonous, are recommended as a remedy for indigestion, flatulence, and disorders of parturient women (Perry 1980).

English Name	Scientific Name	Nutritional and Therapeutic Values
		Stem is used to treat snakebites and the tubers are used as a poultice for bug bites, swellings, and rheumatism (Duke and Ayensu 1985).
		It has been reported that *Colocasia esculenta* may have novel tumor-specific anticancer activities (Brown et al. 2005).
		See also the entry for "taro."
Daylily	*Hemerocallis fulva*	Flowers, leaves, and root are edible.
	H. longituba	Cooked leaves and young shoots are excellent, sweet-tasting vegetables.
		The flowers can be dried and used as a thickener in soups.
		The edible dried flowers are used for cooking and considered to be depurative (Perry 1980).
		The rhizome and roots are diuretic and are used for treating dropsy, dasyure, lithiasis, jaundice, piles, and tumors of the breast (Y. Chang 2000).
		Daylily contains colchicine, tre-halase, asparagine, friedelin, β-sitosterol, chrysophanol, rhein, obtusifolin, z-methoxy-obtusifolin, hemerocallin, and vitamins A, B, and C (N. Chiu and Chang 1995a).
		Roots are used for anti-inflammatory, diuretic, blood purifying, hemostasis, cystitis, oliguria, hematuria, epistaxis, melena, hemoptysis, hepatitis, jaundice, mastitis, parotitis, and cervical lymphadenitis (K. Lin 1998c).
Ducks tongue grass	*Monochoria vaginalis*	Flower is edible and is used for cholera, stomachache, and sunstroke (Duke and Ayensu 1985).
		The whole plant provides a medication to treat diseases of the digestive organs, asthma, and toothache (Perry 1980).
		It contains trigonelline to treat throat pain, intestine infection, dysentery, cough, and windpipe infection (N. Chiu and Chang 1995a).
Edamame, vegetable soybean	*Glycine max*	Edamame is highly nutritious and rich in phytochemicals and is considered to be a nutraceutical or a functional food crop (Messina 2001; Mentreddy et al. 2002).

English Name	Scientific Name	Nutritional and Therapeutic Values
		Fresh vegetable soybean contains protein (35–38 g/100 g dry wt.) and monounsaturated fatty acid (5–7% fresh wt.) (Johnson et al. 1999), and isoflavones (78–220 g/g dry wt.) and tocopherols (84/128 g/g dry wt.) (Mohamed et al. 2001).
		It has been reported that isoflavones have antiproliferative effects on human cancer cell lines established from the gastrointestinal tract (Yanagihara et al. 1993).
		Vegetable soybean is rich in ascorbic acid and contains 60% more Ca and twice the P and K, and similar quantities of Fe, vitamins B1 and B2 compared with green peas (Warner and Mounts 1990; Masuda 1991; Wei et al. 1995; S. Martin 2002; Messina 2001; Naim et al. 1974).
		Polyphenolic antioxidants were found in the form of isoflavones, chlorogenic acid isomers, caffeic acid, and ferulic acid (Pratt and Birac 1979).
Eggplant	*Solanum melongena*	Eggplant has high contents of potassium and phosphate (C. Xue 2001a).
		Leaves are used for internal hemorrhages; fruit is an antidote for poisonous mushrooms; root is an astringent for bladder flux, enterrhagia, and hematuria (Bliss 1973).
		Eggplant has been reported to be a treatment for rheumatism, cardiovascular illnesses, obesity, high cholesterol, and constipation.
		It is also a digestive aid, diuretic, sedative, and calmative, with the ability to relieve colic, reduce stomach ulcers, and serve as a stimulant for the liver and intestines (*The Wordwide Gourmet* 2007).
		It contains solanine, solasonins, solamargine, solasodine, diosgenin, and tigogenin (N. Chiu and Chang 1995a).
		Eggplant infusion had a modest and transitory effect, which was not different from that obtained with standard orientation for dyslipidemia patients (Guimaraes et al. 2000).
		Root is used as an anti-inflammatory and to promote circulation.
		Leaves have anti-inflammatory properties and can be used to reduce swelling and to treat rheumatoid arthritis, chronic bronchitis, and hematuria melaena (K. Lin 1998g).
		Eggplant yields carpesteral and glucoalkaloid, solasodine, solasonine, and solanocarpine; upon hydrolysis, solanine yields an alkaloid, solanidine.

English Name	Scientific Name	Nutritional and Therapeutic Values
		It is used in treatment of cough, asthma, chest pain, and certain kinds of fevers.
		It is diuretic and is considered to be useful in control of stones in bladders.
		Antibacterial property in fruits and shoots has also been shown experimentally.
		It is also used in bronchitis, muscular pains, enlargement of liver and spleen.
		Antifertility properties are also found (Chauhan 1999).
		It contains solanine, trigonelline, choline, arginine glucoside, caffeic acid, solasodine, imidazolylethyl amine, adenine, peroxidase, stachydrine, nasunin, shisonin, delphinidin-3-monoglycoside, and delphinidin-3,5,diglucoside (N. Chiu and Chang 1995f).
		Eggplant is ranked among the top five vegetables in antioxidant activity assays (Easdown and Kalb 2004).
Endive	*Cichorium endivia*	Endive leaves are dissected and curly, and escarole leaves are flat and broad.
		Both are rather bitter-tasting salad greens popular in Europe and in trendy American restaurants.
		Four compounds have been isolated from the root of Cichorium intybus: α-amyrin, taraxerone, baurenyl acetate, and β-sitosterol (Du et al. 1998).
Fennel	*Foeniculum vulgare*	All parts of fennel have a sweet licorice fragrance reminiscent of anise, tarragon, and chervil.
		It contains anethole, d-fenchone, and fenicularin.
		The leaves and stalks of fennel can be eaten as a vegetable.
		It is used to treat ailment of cold excess, hernias and pains in groin, drooping testicle, pain and cold in abdomen, nausea, and vomiting (Reid 1993).
		The ripe fruit is used for abdominal and hernia pain, backache, bed-wetting, cholera, cold, colic, dysmenorrhea, dyspepsia, gastroenteritis, hernia, and nausea.
		The roots are purgative and the leaves are diuretic.
		The leaves contain about 3% protein, some β-carotene, thiamine, riboflavin, niacin, and ascorbic acid (Duke and Ayensu 1985).
		A tea made from its crushed seeds is used to treat indigestion and cramps (Dobelis 1986).

English Name	Scientific Name	Nutritional and Therapeutic Values
		The seeds produce an essential oil consisting mainly of anethole, mucilage, traces of tannin, limarase, fenchone, phellandrene, limonene, dipentene, camphene, pinene, methyl chavicol, anisic acid, thymohydroquinone, anicetone, and vitamin A (Perry 1980; Duke and Ayensu 1985; Y. Chang 2000).
		Fennel seeds and oil are currently employed in Chinese medicine to treat a variety of ailments.
		In Western medicine today, fennel is considered useful in treatment of diseases of the chest, spleen, and kidney (Tyler 1993).
		Fennel has anethole, d-fenchone, vitamin A, and fenicularin.
		It is used to treat stomach pain, hernia pain, and menstruation pain (Y. Chang 2000).
		Fennel contains compounds including alanine, anisaldehyde, anisic acid, arginine, ascorbic acid, benzoic acid, caffeic acid, beta-carotene, ceryl-alcohol, choline, 1,8-cineole, cinnamic acid, citric acid, coumaric acid, fenchone, fiber, fumaric acid, gentisic acid, glutamic acid, glycolic acid, isoleucine, kaempferol, limonene, linalool, linoleic acid, pectin, palmitic acid, alpha-phellandrene, beta-phellandrene, phenylalanine, beta-pinene, proline, psoralen, quercetin, quinic acid, riboflavin, sabinene, scoparone, selenium, beta-sitosterol, stigmasterol, syringic acid, tartaric acid, alpha-terpinene, threonine, valine, and xanthotoxin (Duke 2001).
		The ripe fruit, official in many pharmacopeias, is widely used as a stimulant, a stomachic, an expectorant, a carminative, and a flavoring agent.
		The roots are purgative and the leaves are diuretic.
		In China, the whole plant may be used to make a decoction said to be antiemetic, useful for hernia, and to improve vision (Perry 1980).
Fenugreek	*Trigonella foenum-graecum*	Fenugreek fodder has been used to promote animal health for millennia.
		It has been used to treat a variety of human diseases, including sore throats, swelling glands, diabetes, ulcers, cancer, and ailments like digestive disorder, fever, and bronchitis (Small 2006).
		The fixed oil content is about 7% in fenugreek, which is responsible for the odor and flavor.
		The fatty acids in fixed oil are mainly linoleic, oleic, and palmitic acids (Lewis 1984).

English Name	Scientific Name	Nutritional and Therapeutic Values
		There are two alkaloids, trigonelline and choline (Farrell 1985).
		Seed is a source of the steroid sapogenin diosgenin and a good source of protein, ascorbic acid, niacin, and potassium (Simon et al. 1984).
		It is one of the better sources of choline, which may prevent liver cancer (Duke 1999).
		Fenugreek is generally considered to be safe and well tolerated, although side effects from its use have been reported and include diarrhea, dizziness, and flatulence.
		It should not be consumed by persons allergic to chickpeas or by pregnant women (Basch et al. 2003).
		Fenugreek contains acetylcholine, alanine, gamma-aminobutyric acid, arabinose, ascorbic acid, aspartic acid, behenic acid, beta-carotene, chromium, chlorine, coumarin, hypoglycemic, cyanocobalamin, diosgenin, folacin, folic acid, fructose, galactinol, galactomannan, alpha-galactosidase, gentianine, glutamic acid, glycine, homo-orientin, isoleucine, kaempferol, lecithan, leucine, lignin, luteolin, lysine, beta-mannanan, methionine, niacin, nicotinic acid, oleic acid, quercetin, selenine, selenium, stearic acid, trigonelline, trigofoenosides, trigoforin, trigonellosides, tyrosine, valine, vicenin, xanthophyll, xylose, yamogenin, and zinc (Duke 2001).
Garden cress	*Lepidium sativum*	Cress or garden cress is rich in vitamins A and C, iron, and calcium.
		Seeds are frequently used medicinally in Asia (Morton 1976).
		It contains isothiocyanates with antibacterial property (Zhao 1981).
		Garden cress is used to increase sexual power and acts as a diuretic and purgative.
		Seeds are used medicinally in Asia (Morton 1976).
		It is also used to treat pleurisy, dropsy, asthma, and coughing with nausea (Perry 1980).
		The pungent taste of garden cress is due to the presence of glucosinolates (Small 2006).
		Garden cress is used for vitamin C deficiency, liver disease, asthma, hemorrhoids, and as an abortifacient.
		Seeds contain glucotropeolin for coughs, constipation, poor immunity, and as a diuretic (Noble 2000).

English Name	Scientific Name	Nutritional and Therapeutic Values
		Garden cress contains arachidic acid, ascorbic acid, behenic acid, carbohydrates, beta-carotene, cellulose, erucic acid, fiber, gadoleic acid, iron, linoleic acid, miacin, palmitic acid, riboflavin, sinapic acid, beta-sitosterol, stearic acid, thiamine, alpha-tocopherol, uric acid, and d-sylose (Duke 2001).
		Cress also contains strophanthidine, evomonoside, helveticoside, evobioside, glucosimolates, benzyl isothiocyanate, allyl isothiocyanate, 3-butenyl isothiocyanate, and linolenic, linoleic, oleic, sinapic, paolinitic, and steraric acids.
		Seeds contain sinalbin, fat, protein, and sucrose (Ye 1999).
Garden pea	*Pisum sativum*	Garden pea is high in protein, minerals, and vitamins A and C (C. Xue 2001a).
		Garden pea is contraceptive, fungistatic, and spermicidal.
		It is used to treat diabetes, fever, flu, nausea, and urinary problems (Bliss 1973).
		Garden pea contains vitamins A, B, and C, lecithin, cholesterin, betaine, trigonelline, choline, adenine, lysine, erepsin, leucine, arginine, tryptophan, phytin, vernin, asparagine, glutamine, alantoinase, urea, pepsin, trypsin, amylase, maltase, catalase, lipase, nuclease, phytagglutinin, abscisic acid, and gibberellin A (N. Chiu and Chang 1995a).
		Garden pea is one of the better sources for choline, which may prevent liver cancer (Duke 1999).
		Garden pea also contains abscisic acid, alanine, arachidic acid, arginine, ascorbic acid, betaine, cadmium, caffeic acid, calcium, carbohydrates, beta-carotene, cephalin, choline, citric acid, coumestrol, beta-cryptoxanthin, cyanidin, delphinidin, fiber, gibberellins, glutamic acid, histidine, inositol, iodine, iron, isoleucine, kaempferol, kilocalories, lecithin, leucine, lutein, malic acid, methionine, mevalonic acid, palmitic acid, pantothenic acid, proline, quercetin, quercitrin, stearic acid, stigmasterol, succinic acid, thiamine, trigonelline, valine, xanthophyll, xenognosin, and zinc (Duke 2001).
		Peas are considered cooling and are recommended for feverish conditions, to increase flesh, and to treat diabetes (Perry 1980).
Garland chrysanthemum	*Chrysanthemum coronarium*	It is a commonly eaten vegetable in the orient where it is known as "shungikee" in Japan and "kortongho" in China.

English Name	Scientific Name	Nutritional and Therapeutic Values
		Chrysanthemum is an edible flower commonly encountered in gardens and around homes.
		Although the leaves have been termed poisonous, the tender shoots are consumed as a vegetable.
		The leaves contain protein, fat, carbohydrate, fiber, and minerals.
		It also has thiamine, riboflavin, niacin, ascorbic acid, and adenine (Duke and Ayensu 1985).
		It contains pyrethrins I and II, cinerins I and II, stachydrine, choline, pyrethrol, pyrethrosin, and β-cyclopyrethrosin (N. Chiu and Chang 1995d).
		It also contains pyrethrins, cinerins, palmitic and linoleic acids, and sesquiterpene lactones.
		It is used externally as a contact insecticide (T. Li 2002).
		The bark of chrysanthemum is purgative.
		It is used in the treatment of syphilis.
		Leaves are aromatic, bitter, and stomachic (Chopra et al. 1982).
		Garland chrysanthemum is bitter, with an acrid taste.
		It is antipyretic, antibiotic, anti-inflammatory, blood purifying, and hypertensive.
		It is also used for prevention of colds, influenza, epidemic encephalitis, mastitis, hypertension, hepatitis, and dysentery.
		It is externally useful in treating furunculosis, snakebites, and traumatic injury by applying mashed fresh herb topically.
Garlic	*Allium sativum*	It contains allicin, a major flavoring ingredient.
		Allicin and disulfide compounds are antibacterial against both gram-positive and gram-negative pathogens (Tyler 1993).
		In China, garlic is used to treat abscesses, boils, cancer, diarrhea, diphtheria, typhoid, hepatitis, ringworm, vaginitis, and other ailments (Small 2006).
		Garlic has allyl sulfur compounds, including S-allylcysteine, a water-soluble sulfur-containing amino acid, allistatin, and glucominol (Huang 1999; Song and Milner 2001).

English Name	Scientific Name	Nutritional and Therapeutic Values
		In Chinese medicine, garlic continues to be used to treat abscesses, boils, cancer, diarrhea, diphtheria, typhoid, hepatitis, ringworm, vaginitis, and other ailments (Duke and Ayensu 1985).
		Garlic intake in China results in relatively low risk of gastric cancer (You et al. 1998).
		On the other hand, it has been reported that synergistic interactions will be required for garlic to produce an anticancer effect in humans (Boik 2001).
		The allicin content (3.5 mg/g fresh wt.) is responsible for antioxidant, antilipemic, antimicrobial, anti-inflammatory activities, and is used to prevent cancer (Prasad et al. 1995).
		Garlic may well have helped to cure many diseases because it is a potent antiseptic.
		Recent research has further revealed that garlic contains vitamins A, B1, B2, and C (Dobelis 1986).
		Garlic contains allyl methyl sulfide, diallyl sulfide, 6-methyl-1-thio-2,4-cyclohexadiene, dimethyl sulfide, divinyl sulfide, dimethyl disulfide, allyl methyl disulfide, dithiocydopentene, 5-methyl-1,2-dithio-3-cydopentene, allyl propyl disulfide, dimethyl trisulfide, allyl methyl trisulfide, diallyl tetrasulfide, methyl propyl trisulfide, allyl methyl pentasulfide, sulfur dioxide, 2-hydroxypropylene, cymene, trans-ajoene, cis-ajoene, citral, geraniol, and linalool (Je 1999).
Ginger	*Zingiber officinale*	The pungency of ginger root comes from the chemicals zingerone, shogaol, and gingerol.
		The flavor is mainly due to cineol, borneol, geraniol, linalool, zingiberene, and farnasene (Purseglove et al. 1981).
		Ginger has a long history of use as a medicinal plant.
		It is useful in preventing the effects of seasickness and motion sickness (Tyler 1993, Eernst and Pitler 2000).
		In China, it has been used to treat bleeding, chest congestion, cholera, colds, diarrhea, nausea, stomachache, baldness, cancer, rheumatism, snakebite, and toothache (Duke and Ayensu 1985).
		Ginger can be used to treat gastric duodenal ulcer bleeding, pulmonary tuberculosis, hemoptysis, bronchitis, and hematuria melaena (K. Lin 1998g).
		Ginger is known to have antioxidant activity.

English Name	Scientific Name	Nutritional and Therapeutic Values
		The nonvolatile fraction of dichloromethane extract of dried ginger was purified to yield more than 30 compounds (Kikuzaki et al. 1994).
		Ginger contains essential oils, zingiberol, zingiberene, phellandrene, camphene, citral, linalool, methylheptenone, nonylaldehyde, d-borneol, and gingerol (Vimala 1999).
		Ginger has anti-inflammatory properties, preventing cataracts, heart disease, migraines, and stroke.
		Ginger can be used to treat amenorrhea, angina, ankylosing spondylitis, arthritis, athlete's foot, body odor, bunions, bursitis, colds, cough, dandruff, depression, dizziness, morning sickness, motion sickness, nausea, sore throat, swelling, tendinitis, ulcers, and gingivitis (Duke 1997).
		An experiment was conducted for the use of ginger-free phenolic (GRFP) and ginger-hydrolyzed phenolic (GRHP) fractions of ginger as potent inhibitors of Helicobacter pylori growth.
		It was found that GRFD and GRHP may have potential as inexpensive multistep blockers against ulcer (Siddaraju and Dharmesh 2007).
		Ginger is ranked among the top five vegetables in antioxidant activity assays (Easdown and Kalb 2004).
		Ginger contains numerous compounds, including heptanol, 1,3,4-trimethyltricycloheptane, tricyclene, α-pinene, β-fenchene, β-pinene, 5-hepten-2-one-6-methyl, myrcene, octanal, thujene, menthene, 1,3,4-trimethyl-2-orybicylcho, nonylalcohol, 2-nonanone, Δ3-menthene, citral, sareole, geraniol, methyl eugenol, 1,1,5-dimethyl-4-hex-enyl-4-methyl cenzent, nerolidol, farnesol, nerol, n-heptane, n-octane, n-nonone, acetaldehyde, propionaldehyde, n-butyl aldehyde, isocaleraldehyde, acetone, methyl isobutyl ketone, glyoxal, methylglyoxal, n-propanol, secbutanol, tert-butanol, n-honanol, diethyl sulfide, methyl allyl sulfide, methyl acetate, ethyl acetate, ethyl propionate, camphene, sabinene, limonene, phellanerene, 1,8-cineole, terpinolene, linalool, preillal, camphor, isoborneol, borneol, terpinen-4-ol, terpineol, neral, geraniol, citronellyl acetate, cubebene, geranyl, bornyl acetate, geranyl acetate, elemene, caryophyllene, alloaromadenerene, zingiberene, bisabolene, santalol, nerolidol, farnesol, elemol, eadesmol, cis-β-sesquiphellandrol, trans-S-sesquiphellandrol, 2-caraneol, 3-caraneol, 2-borneol, β-cedreene, and zingerone (Duke 2001).
Globe artichoke	*Cynara scolymus*	Globe artichoke contains caffeic, glycolic, and glyceric acids as well as cynarin, inulin, cyanropierin, and cynaratriol.

English Name	Scientific Name	Nutritional and Therapeutic Values
		It is reported to have stimulant, choleretic, and diuretic properties (Leung and Foster 1996).
		It has been reported that the volume of nonalcoholic drinks consumed and the duration of sleep were similar during interventions using artichoke extract and placebo.
		Based on the results of the experiment, it is concluded that artichoke extract is not effective in preventing the signs and symptoms of alcohol-induced hangover (Pittler et al. 2003).
Goa bean	Psophocarpus tetragonolobus	Goa bean is a nutritious plant.
		The leaves, flowers, pods, green seeds, dried seeds, and tuberous roots are all edible.
		The leaves are boiled to make a decoction applied as a lotion to smallpox.
		The root is used as a poultice to treat vertigo.
		The pods and edible tubers are considered roborant.
		Leaves and seeds are eaten to cure skin sores and ulcers (Perry 1980).
Gourd	Lagenaria vulgaris L. leucantha L. siceraria	The fruit is antilithic, diuretic, emetic, and refrigerant.
		Rind of fruit is employed as a diuretic and is boiled in oil for treatment of rheumatism.
		In recent years, gourd has been used to treat diabetes (Duke and Ayensu 1985).
		Fruit contains Lagenaria D.
		It is used to treat anasarca ascites and beri-beri.
		It also has antiswelling properties and is used to treat abdominal swelling and swelling feet (T. Li 2006).
Green onion	Allium cepa var. aggregatum	It has bacchic, emmenagogue, and diuretic properties.
		The fresh juice has been found to contain a hypoglycemic agent.
		It is regarded as alterative, resolvent, and vulnerary.
		It is used to treat chest colds, shortness of breath, headache, stomach and intestinal trouble (Perry 1980).

English Name	Scientific Name	Nutritional and Therapeutic Values
		Onion contains throb, methyl disulfide, allyl disulfide, trisulfide, thiosulfinates, citrate, malate, and O-coumaric, caffeic, ferulic, sinapic, p-coumaric, and protocatechuic acids, polysaccharide A and B, quercetin, thymine, kaempferol, and carotenes (N. Chiu and Chang 1995a).
Gynura	*Gynura formosana*	It is well known as a purple passion plant.
		It has chocolate-like brown foliage made by prominent green veins.
		The juice from leaves and root of this plant is used as an antihemorrhagic and is applied externally to wounds and snake bites (Perry 1980).
		This folk medicinal plant has recently become a popular vegetable in Taiwan.
		The free-radical scavenging activities of a 70% aqueous acetone extract from this plant were evaluated.
		The results indicated that the free-radical scavenging activity may improve the economic value of this plant and assist in its development as a health food (Hou et al. 2004).
		Gynura contains flavonoids.
		It can be used to improve blood circulation and stop bleeding.
		It is a detoxicant and relieves swelling and cough with blood (T. Li 2002).
Hairy melon	*Benincasa hispida* var. *chieh-gua*	The fruit is fuzzy when young.
		At maturity, the fruit loses its hairs and develops a waxy coating, giving rise to the name "wax gourd." Hairy melons are used as a stir-fry vegetable or to make winter melon soup.
		Raw or cooked fruit is used as a vegetable and in pickles, curries, and preserves.
		The fruit can be eaten when it is young.
		The fruit contains 22-deoxocucur bitacin D (Y. Chang 2000).
		It also contains 0.02 mg/100 g edible portion of vitamin A, 0.07 mg of thiamine, 0.05 mg of riboflavin, 0.20 mg of niacin, and 69 mg of vitamin C (Wills et al. 1984).
		It is antilithic, diuretic, emetic, refrigerant, and antibiotic and is used to treat diabetes (Bliss 1973).
		Hairy melon contains ascorbic, palmitic, stearic, and linoleic acids as well as thiamine.

English Name	Scientific Name	Nutritional and Therapeutic Values
		It has diuretic and laxative properties.
		It is also used to treat diabetes, dropsy, and rhinitis (Duke and Ayensu 1985).
		Hairy melon or wax gourd contains ascorbic acid, calcium, carbohydrates, beta-carotene, fiber, ison, isomultiflorenyl acetate, kilocalories, linoleic acid, lysine, methionine, niacin, oleic acid, oxalic acid, palmitic acid, phosphorus, potassium, protein, pufa, riboflavin, sodium, stearic acid, thiamine, and tryptophan (Duke 2001).
		In China, the seeds, rind, pulp, and juice are all regarded as medicinal, each part being mentioned as diuretic.
		In addition, the seeds are considered to have mildly laxative, febrifuge, nutritive, demulcent, and tonic properties.
		It has been used as a remedy for hemorrhoids, intestinal inflammation, and urinary and kidney diseases.
		The ash of the seed has been prescribed to treat gonorrhea.
		The ash of the rind is administered in cases of painful wounds.
		The pulp is cooling and demulcent (Perry 1980).
Horseradish	*Armoracia rusticana*	Intact horseradish root does not exhibit much aroma, but upon cutting, shredding, and especially grating, a pungent and lachrymatory, very strong odor is released.
		The root is high in potassium and vitamins B and C, calcium, phosphorus, and iron.
		It will stimulate appetite and aid digestion.
		It is laxative, diaphoretic, diuretic, rubefacient, and antiseptic.
		The root contains essential oils and has antibacterial and antifungal properties (Foster 1993).
		The principal flavor ingredients are allyl and 2-phenethyl isothiocyanate (Mazza 1984).
		Horseradish was used to cure a wide variety of illnesses including: asthma, coughs, colic, toothache, ulcers, venereal disease, cancer, worms, chilblains, and rheumatism (Small 2006).

English Name	Scientific Name	Nutritional and Therapeutic Values
		Horseradish contains alloxurbasen, allyl isothiocyanate, aluminum, amylase, arginine, arsenic, ascorbic acid, ash, asparagine, bioside, boron, bromine, butylisothiocyanate, cadmium, carbohydrates, chromium, cobalt, copper, fat, fiber, fluorine, fructose, gentisic acid, glucocochlearin, glucoconringin, glucoputranjivin, glucose, 3-O-β-D-glucosyl-β-D-quercetin-xyloside, p-hydroxy-benzoic acid, inverstase, iron, isopropylisothiocyanate, kaempferol, limonene, lipase, magnesium, mercury, molybdenum, myrosin, niacin, nickel, nitrogen, peroxidase, phenylethyl isothiocyanate, phosphatase, phosphorus, quercetin, raphanin, riboflavin, rubidium, rutoside, selenium, silicon, sinapic acid, sinapin, sinigrin, sodium, sulfur, tannin, thiamine, vanillic acid, and zinc (Duke 2001).
		Horseradish is used for urinary tract infection, urinary stones, edematous conditions, cough, and bronchitis.
		Topically, horseradish is used for inflamed joints or tissues and minor muscle aches.
		Traditionally, horseradish has been used for expelling afterbirth, treating gout, rheumatism, gallbladder disorders, sciatica pain, relief of colic, increasing urination, and intestinal worms in children (Jellin et al. 2003).
		The applicable part of horseradish is the root.
		Researchers state horseradish has antimicrobial efficacy against gram-negative and gram-positive bacteria.
		It also has antispasmodic properties.
		Horseradish shows evidence that it can stimulate local blood flow, and it might be carcinostatic (Blumenthal 1998; Gruenwald 1998).
		The toxic mustard oil constituents of horseradish are extremely irritating to mucous membranes (Blumenthal 1998) and the urinary tract (Brinker 1998).
		Consuming large amounts of horseradish orally can cause gastrointestinal upset, bloody vomiting, and diarrhea (2), as well as irritation of mucous membranes and the urinary tract (19).
		Horseradish and other members of the cabbage and mustard family are associated with depressed thyroid function.

English Name	Scientific Name	Nutritional and Therapeutic Values
		Topically, skin contact with fresh horseradish can cause irritation or allergic reaction (Jellin et al. 2003).
		In foods, horseradish is normally used as a flavoring agent.
Hyacinth bean (lablab)	*Dolichos lablab*	In Asia and Africa, lablab is grown for food.
		Lablab bean is an excellent nitrogen fixer and is sometimes grown as a cover crop or for livestock fodder.
		Flower is used for leucorrhea and menorrhagia, and it is antivinous, alexiteric, and carminative.
		Juice from pods is used for inflamed ears and throats.
		Seed is a tonic to the viscera.
		Plant is decocted to treat alcoholic intoxication, cholera, diarrhea, globefish poisoning, gonorrhea, leucorrhea, nausea, and thirst (Duke and Ayensu 1985).
		Seeds and their hulls are used for stomachic and to treat diarrhea from heat and loose stools.
		It promotes absorption and relieves summer heat, impaired digestion, anorexia, nausea, and vomiting.
		It treats leucorrhea and chronic nephritis (K. Lin 1998e).
		Seeds are a rich source of urea.
		They also contain lectins, phytagglutinin, globulin, coumestrol, and psoralidin.
		The seeds are considered anthelmintic, antilithic, astringent, diaphoretic, diuretic, emmenagogue, expectorant, febrifuge, ophthalmic, and tonic (Chauhan 1999).
		Seeds contain protein, fat, carbohydrate, phytin, calcium, phosphate, iron, vitamins A, B, and C, and hemagglutinins A and B.
		It is used to treat liver cancer, tumor, and stomach cancer (Ye 1999).

English Name	Scientific Name	Nutritional and Therapeutic Values
		Hyacinth bean and others were cooked under pressure or in a microwave oven and were analyzed for nutrient composition. Raw bean was served as control. It was found that cooking methods did not affect the nutrient composition of legumes. However, thiamine decreased in cooked samples. Cooking altered the dietary fiber content of some legumes (Khatoon and Prakash 2004).
Indian lettuce	*Lactuca indica*	The whole herb including roots is used as an anti-inflammatory for treatment of tonsillitis, mastitis, cervicitis, furunculosis, and hammerhead with bleeding (K. Lin 1998g).
		Indian lettuce is used to treat headache and pain caused by inflammation (Y. Chang 2000). It contains pectic compounds, oxalic, malic, and citric acids, ceryl alcohol, ergosterol, and vitamin E. It is used for anodyne, lactagogue, genital swelling, hemorrhoids, and lumbago (T. Li 2002).
		Lactuca indica is used as a folk medicine in anti-inflammatory, antibacterial, antidiabetic, and other medications in Asia.
		A study was conducted to evaluate the antiproliferative effect of ethanol extracts of *Lactuca indica* on human leukemic HL-60 cell lines and its active components. The results showed that it exhibited strong cytotoxic effects against HL-60 cells; moreover, it could induce typical DNA fragmentation in a concentration- and time-dependent manner as determined by electrophoresis and tunnel assays (Y. Chen et al. 2007).
		It has been reported that *Lactuca indica* also induced apoptosis in HL-60 cells, which is associated with the loss of mitochondrial membrane potential. Among the four active phenolic compounds, quercetin was found to be the most effective in inhibition against cell viability and in alteration of mitochondrial function. It is suggested that the induction of apoptosis by *Lactuca indica* might offer a pivotal mechanism for its chemopreventive action (Y. Chen et al. 2007).
Japanese honeywort, Mitsuba	*Cryptotaenia canadensis* var. *japonica* *C. japonica*	Young leaves, stems, and flowers — raw or cooked — are used as a potherb or added to salads. It has a flavor like celery.
		Japanese honeywort is a member of the carrot family. It is like celery but is a much smaller plant (Yamaguchi 1990).
		Mitsuba has a very distinct, pungent flavor, reminiscent of celery, but described as a blend of parsley, celery, and angelica (Larkcom 1984).

English Name	Scientific Name	Nutritional and Therapeutic Values
		It has isomesityl oxide, mesityl oxide, methyl isobutyl ketone, trans-beta-ocimene, and terpinolene (Duke and Ayensu 1985).
		The whole plant is taken as a remedy for colds, rheumatism, and tubercular glands. It also regulates menstruation and stops diarrhea (Perry 1980).
		Japanese honeywort is an important and widely employed medicinal plant in China. Mitsuba is an important and widely employed medicinal herb in China, used to treat cold, diarrhea, rheumatism, painful menstruation, and certain glandular conditions (Perry and Metzger 1980).
		It contains cryptotaenen, kiganen, kiganol, petroselic acid, isomesityl oxide, mesityl oxide, methyl isobutyl, ketone, trans-beta-ocimene, and terpinolene.
		It is used for diarrhea, dysmenorrhea, rheumatism, and tubercular glands (T. Li 2002).
Kidney bean	*Phaseolus vulgaris*	It is used homeopathically as a diuretic, for bladder ailments, gout, renitis, rheumatism, anticancer, and reduced blood sugar level. Green pods contain a compound that reduces the blood sugar level. Phaseolin is fungicidal.
		Seeds were used to treat leukemia (Duke and Ayensu 1985).
		It contains adenine, arginine, histidine, choline, globulins A and B, lysine, tryptophan, cystine, phasedunatin, amide, humine, and trigonenine (N. Chiu and Chang 1995d).
		It has been reported that kidney bean has strong antioxidant activity. Tocopherol contents ranged from 13 to 152 ppm in the extracts, and those with the highest antioxidant activity also had the highest tocopherol concentrations (Tsuda et al. 1993).
		Kidney bean is used for urinary tract infection, kidney or bladder stones, and the promotion of urine flow.
		In herbal tea combinations, bean is used for kidney and bladder problems.
		In folk medicine, bean is used as a diuretic and for treatment of diabetes (Jellin et al. 2003). The applicable part is the bean pod without seeds.
		Bean pods demonstrate a weak diuretic effect in animals and humans. The chromium salts found in bean pods play a role in its antidiabetic properties (Gruenwald 1998).

English Name	Scientific Name	Nutritional and Therapeutic Values
Konjac	*Amorphophallus konjac* *A. rivieri*	The plant can be made into a popular Asian jelly fruit snack.
		The tubers are poisonous, although they can be eaten after washing and prolonged boiling. The mashed tubers can be used as a poultice to relieve constipation (Perry 1980).
		The plant contains leviduline, levidulinase, and mannose.
		The flower is used to treat aching bones and eye inflammation. The root is used to treat cancer, rodent bites, and ulcers (Duke and Ayensu 1985).
		It is also used to treat aching bones, eye inflammation, cancer, ulcers, and snakebite (T. Li 2002).
		The effect of oral intake of ceramide on atopic dermatitis was studied. Ceramide is a main component of the intercellular lipids that is responsible for cell cohesion at the top layer of the epidermis, the stratum corneum (Kimata 2006).
		The results indicated that oral intake of konjac ceramide improved skin symptoms and reduced allergic responses with concomitant skewing of the cytokine pattern toward the Th-1 type. Konjac contains glucomannan, which is obtained from the root.
		A polysaccharide composed of D-glucose and D-mannose is a prominent component of coniferous tree with physiological effects and therapeutic uses (Kimata 2006).
Kudzu	*Pueraria lobata* *P. montana*	Kudzu root possesses a high content of flavonoid derivatives called puerarin. The root contains compounds with potent antioxidant activity (Guerra et al. 2000). It contains isoflavonoid glycoside with a hypotensive effect. It also contains tectoridin, daidzein, daidzin, and puerarin. It is useful in treatment of angina pectoris and migraine, and has antipyretic, antispasmodic, and hypoglycemic activities (Gao and Liu 1979; Q. Fang 1980; Y. Chang 2000).
		Root is used as an antipyretic. It promotes salivation and measles rash eruption. Stem and leaves have anti-inflammatory function. Flowers relieve drunkenness and thirst (K. Lin 1998d). It has been reported that kudzu may help heavy or binge drinkers reduce their alcohol consumption (Lukas et al. 2005).

English Name	Scientific Name	Nutritional and Therapeutic Values
		Kudzu tubers contain vitamin B1, sucrose, glucose, and fructose. The roots are demulcent and refrigerant and are used as a cataplasm on swollen joints and as a lactagogue (Anonymous 1980). The tubers are aphrodisiac, cardiac, emetic, expectorant, and febrifuge and are used to treat heart weakness and rheumatism (Chauhan 1999).

It has calcium, carbohydrates, carotene, p-coumaric acid, daidzein, fiber, genistein, irisolidone, kilocalories, magnesium, phosphorus, potassium, protein, puerarin, quercetin, riboflavin, robinin, silica, starch, and tectoridin (Duke 2001).

Kudzu is used for headache, upset stomach, dizziness and vomiting caused by an alcohol hangover. In Chinese medicine, it is used orally for managing alcoholism and drunkenness, myalgia, measles, dysentery, gastritis, fever, diarrhea, thirst, cold, flu, and neck stiffness, and it also serves as a diaphoretic (Jellin et al. 2003).

The applicable parts of kudzu are the root and flower.

Isoflavone constituents (daidzin, daidzein, and puerarin) and their derivatives are thought to be reversible inhibitors of alcohol and aldehyde dehydrogenase (Jellin et al. 2003). However, recent studies dispute this finding (R. Lin 1998). Puerarin demonstrates hypoglycemic, hypocholesterolemic, antiarrhythmic, antipyretic, and antioxidant activity (Leung and Foster 1996).

Kudzu extract, daidzein and daidzin, decreases alcohol consumption and peak blood alcohol levels, and shortens alcohol-induced sleep in alcohol-craving animals (R. Lin 1998).

Decreased peak blood alcohol levels might be due to delayed gastric emptying. Preliminary evidence suggests that puerarin might decrease heat rate, plasma renin activity, capillary permeability, and platelet aggregation (Leung and Foster 1996).

It has been reported that the leaves and vines can be used as protein-rich forage (Sasek and Strain 1988).

Kudzu root extracts dilate coronary and cerebral blood vessels and increase myocardial and cerebral blood flow; decrease vascular resistance, myocardial oxygen demand, and lactic acid production in anaerobic myocardial tissues; and increase the bollo oxygen supply (Leung and Foster 1996).

Studies are needed to investigate the effect of kudzu in humans.

English Name	Scientific Name	Nutritional and Therapeutic Values
Lamb's quarter	*Chenopodium album*	It is a good source of calcium, iron, carotene, riboflavin, and ascorbic acid. The average oil content is about 2% on a dry-weight basis. Ascaridole is the active principle in the oil and predominates. Mature seeds contain d-camphor, methyl salicylate, and numerous other compounds (Perry and Metzger 1980).
		In folk medicine, it is used to treat asthma, malaria, and various nervous diseases, but the main use has been as a vermifuge (Small 2006). The entire plant can be boiled and used as a crude green dye (Willard 1992).
		The leaves can be eaten raw or cooked as a vegetable. A decoction of the plant can be taken internally or applied externally as a wash to treat painful limbs. They should be consumed only in moderation because they contain soluble oxalates that can bind to and reduce the body's levels of calcium when eaten in large quantities and may cause photosensitization (Marles et al. 2000).
		It has been reported that lamb's quarter can relieve toothache and stomach pain (Y. Chang 2000).
		Lamb's quarter contains alanine, arginine, ascaridole, ascorbic acid, betaine, campesterol, carbohydrates, beta-carotene, chenopodine, cystine, beta-ecdysterone, ferulic acid, glycine, isoleucine, leucine, lysine, molybdenum, niacin, octacosanyl acetate, oleanoic acid, oxalic acid, polypodine-B, proline, serine, stigmasterol, thiamine, trigonelline, tyrosine, valine, vanillic acid, xanthotoxin, and zinc (Duke 2001).
Leaf celery	*Apium graveolens* var. *dulce*	Celery also contains volatile oil (terpenes, limonene, b-selinene, phthalides), coumarins (seselin, osthenol, apigravin, celerin, umbelliferone), furanocoumarins (bergapten), flavonoids (apigenin, apiin), phenolic compounds, choline, ascorbate, and fatty acids.
		Celery shoots contain high calcium, fiber, riboflavin, and vitamin C (Duke and Ayensu 1985). Therapeutic values include mild diuretic, spasmolytic, carminative, anti-inflammatory, antirheumatic, sedative, hypotensive, and urinary antiseptic.
		Celery seed has been prescribed as an aphrodisiac, to expel gas from the alimentary canal, and to promote urination. Celery leaves contain thiamine, riboflavin, niacin, and ascorbic acid (Duke and Ayensu 1985).
Lettuce	*Lactuca sativa*	Lettuce is used in folk medicine to treat asthma, bronchitis, burns, cancer, fever, insomnia, sclerosis, sores, and swellings (Hartwell 1971).

English Name	Scientific Name	Nutritional and Therapeutic Values
		Lettuce seeds are a remedy for liver disorders and lumbago, with galactagogue, anodyne, and diuretic properties. The plant has tonic, carminative, antidotal, aperient, and thirst-quenching properties (Perry 1980). In China, the seeds are used in treating swelling of the genitals and to make hair grow on scar tissue. The plant has tonic, carminative, antidotal, aperient, and thirst-quenching properties (Perry 1980).
		It contains alanine, arginine, arsenic, ascorbic acid, delta-5-avenasterol, cadmium, caffeic acid, beta-carotene, chlorine, p-coumaric acid, ergosterol, ferulic acid, folic acid, glutamic acid, glycine, histidine, isoleucine, kaempferol, beta-lactucerol, lactucin, lactucopicrin, lanthanum, alpha-linolenic acid, lysine, molybdenum, oleic acid, oxalic acid, palmitic acid, palmitoleic acid, pantothenic acid, proline, quercetin, selenium, sitosterol, stearic acid, stigmasterol, tryptophan, tyrosine, valine, and vitamins B6, E, G, and K (Duke 2001).
Lily bulb	*Lilium tigrinum*	Hybrids of lily are important export products in the cut-flower industry. The bulb is edible, and the bulb scales are used as a tonic or remedy for pulmonary diseases. It has also been recommended for gynecologic disorders (Perry 1980).
		Lily has alkaloids and polysaccharides, and its main constituent is colchicine (Huang 1999).
		Bulblets are antitussive and are used for intestinal disorders, cough, dysuria, edema, fever, neuroses, swellings, and weakness. Flowers mixed with oil are used for bruises, cuts, eczema, and vesicular eruptions (Bliss 1973).
		It is used for increasing leukocyte count, to improve digestion, and to treat neurasthenia and insomnia (Huang 1999).
Lima bean	*Phaseolus lunatus* *P. limensis*	Lima bean is a great source of folate, iron, and potassium. Leaves and stem contain phaseolunatin, are high in carbohydrates and protein, and are fair in iron content but deficient in calcium. The cultivated bean has white seeds.
		It contains cyanogenetic glycoside, which, on contact with water, becomes hydrocyanic acid through the action of the enzyme linamarase (Perry 1980).
		Eighty-five samples from fifteen different legume seed lines were classified into four groups and examined by measurements of their net protein utilization by rats.

English Name	Scientific Name	Nutritional and Therapeutic Values
		The seeds of lima bean (*Phaseolus lunatus*) did not support proper growth of the rats, although the animals survived the 10-day experimental period (Grant et al. 1983).
		It contains alanine, amygdalin, aroinine, ascorbic acid, barium, calcium, carbohydrates, beta-carotene, chromium, cystine, fat, fiber, glutamic acid, glutamyl-5-methylcystene, glycine, iron, isoleucine, kilocalories, lead, leucine, lignin, linoleic acid, alpha-linoleic acid, lysine, magnesium, manganese, S-methylcysteine, molybdenum, myristic acid, niacin, oleic acid, palmitic acid, pantothenic acid, phaseolunatin, phenylalanine, phosphorus, potassium, proline, protein, riboflavin, serine, sodium, stearic acid, strontium, thiamine, threonine, titanium, tryptophan, tyrosine, valine, vanadium, zinc, and zirconium (Duke 2001).
Lotus	*Nelumbo nucifera*	The flowers, seeds, young leaves, and rhizomes are all edible. Traditionally, lotus roots are considered as a very healthy food in China. Every part of the lotus plant is used in medicine: the stem relieves congestion in chest due to "damp-heat" excess; the peduncle is used for stomachaches, to calm the fetus, and to treat leukorrhea. The seeds are used for insomnia, spermatorrhea, and diarrhea. The stamens are a preventive for premature ejaculation (Reid 1993).
		Lotus has been grown in the Imperial Valley of California and may be successfully grown in the southeastern United States (Yamaguchi 1990).
		It is used for diarrhea, dysentery, and dyspepsia. Extracts show antitumor activity due to its liriodenine, nuciferine, quercetin, etc., contents (Jiangsu New Medical College 1979).
		Lotus contains quercetin, luteolin, isoquercitrin, kaempferol, nelumbine, raffinose, liensinine, isoliensinine, neferine, nuciferine, nornuciferine, pronuciferine, lotusine, galuteolin, heparin, rutin, roemerine, asparagine, anonaine, gluconic acid, and oxoushinsunine (N. Chiu and Chang 1995a).
		It also contains stachyose, fructose, sucrose, protein, and vitamin C. Lotus also has phospho-glucose isomerase, 5-adenosine monophosphate, asparagine, and altheine (Ye 1999).
		Lotus is used as a salad vegetable and has relatively low nutrient density. However, it contains calcium, iron, zinc, tannins, phytic acid, and provitamin carotenoids (Ogle et al. 2001).
		It has been reported that lotus flowers are used as an astringent for bleeding. Orally, lotus seed is used for digestive disorders and diarrhea. However, there is insufficient reliable information available about the effectiveness of lotus flowers and seeds (Jellin et al. 2003).

English Name	Scientific Name	Nutritional and Therapeutic Values
Luffa	*Luffa aculangula*	Luffa contains 0.06 and 18 mg/100 g of vitamins A and C, respectively (Wills et al. 1984). Luffa is antirheumatic and used for meridians. It also has analgesic and hemostatic properties.
		Luffa can be used to treat rheumatic pains in joints and aches in the chest and rib cage and to treat painful breast tumors (Reid 1993).
		It also contains cucurbitacin B, rotenone, and two antitumor compounds, apigenin-7-glucoside and luteolin-7-glucoside. It has antitumor, antidotal, purgative, and expectorant properties and is used to treat ophthalmia, inflammation, paralysis, stomachache, and thyroid cancer (Perry 1980; Duke and Wain 1981; Hsu 1982).
		Luffa contains such compounds as aegyptinin-A, ascorbic acid, beta-carotene, cucurbitacin B, fiber, iron, gypsogenin-lactone, kilocalories, linoleic acid, luffamarin, oleanolic acid, oleic acid, palmitic acid, riboflavin, alpha-spinasterol, stearic acid, and thiamine (Duke 2001).
Malabar spinach	*Anredera cordifolia*	Malabar spinach is tonic. It reduces swelling and hematoma (K. Lin 1998g). It contains 3-hydroxy-30-horoleana-12, 18-dien-29-oate, larreagenin, ethyl ester, and ursolic acid. Malabar spinach is used to treat boils (T. Li 2002).
		Extracts of one of six ethnobotanically selected medicinal plants, *Anredera cordifolia* is used traditionally to treat sexually transmitted diseases were investigated for antibacterial activity using the agar dilution were also investigated for cytotoxicity. The results of the antimicrobial screening support the ethnomedicinal uses of this plant to some extent (Tshikalange et al. 2005).
Mint	*Mentha arvensis*	Menthol is used in cough drops, lozenges, and inhalers to relieve cough and sore throat. The leaf is used as a carminative, disphoretic, stimulant, and a stomachic. It is a classical remedy for stomach cancer (Duke and Ayensu 1985).
		It is used in China as an anesthetic, antispasmodic, antiseptic, aromatic, carminative, diaphoretic, and stimulant. It is also used to treat cancer, cramps, diarrhea, and dyspepsia (Duke and Ayensu, 1985).
		Mint has an acrid taste. It is used as an aromatic, antipyretic, diaphoretic, stomachic, and antipruritic. It is used to soothe the throat and serves as an antiswelling agent. It is also used to relieve colds and fever, sore throat, pharyngitis, and cough and to treat early-stage measles, dyspepsia, abdominal distention, and pruritus of skin (K. Lin 1998b).

English Name	Scientific Name	Nutritional and Therapeutic Values
		The leaves are used to make mint tea, which can be drunk to treat a cough or cold, congestion, fever, chills, or menstrual cramps, to soothe teething babies' gums, or as a tonic to treat tiredness or fatigue. It is also used as a sleep aid to treat children's diarrhea, as a digestive aid to treat headache and high blood pressure, as part of compound medicines for treating cancer or diabetes or pain, and as a wash for sores.
		The whole fresh plant can be boiled and the steam inhaled to clear the nasal passages. The flowers can be part of a mixture applied topically to gums to reduce infection or relieve a toothache (Marles et al. 2000).
		Mint leaves can be used as a stomach tonic, for colic or gripe relief, and as a sedative due to their content of essential oils, in which carvone dominates other monoterpenes and some sesquiterpenes and their derivatives, plus bioactive flavonoids (Bisset and Wichtl 1994).
		It also has diaphoretic, carminative, stomachic, and stimulant effects (Reid 1993).
		It contains menthol, menthone, menthyl acetate, camphene, pinene, limonene, isomenthone, menthenone, azulen, isoraifolin, luteolin-7-glucoside, menthoside, rosmarinic acid, and isoraifolin (Ye 1999).
Mitsuba, Japanese honeywort	*Cryptotaenia canadensis* var. *japonica* *C. japonica*	Japanese honeywort is a member of the carrot family. It is like celery but is a much smaller plant (Yamaguchi 1990).
		Mitsuba has a very distinct, pungent flavor, reminiscent of celery, but described as a blend of parsley, celery, and angelica (Larkcom 1984).
		It has isomesityl oxide, mesityl oxide, methyl isobutyl ketone, trans-beta-ocimene, and terpinolene (Duke and Ayensu 1985).
		The whole plant is taken as a remedy for colds, rheumatism, and tubercular glands. It also regulates menstruation and stops diarrhea (Perry 1980).
		Japanese honeywort is an important and widely employed medicinal plant in China. Mitsuba is an important and widely employed medicinal herb in China, used to treat cold, diarrhea, rheumatism, painful menstruation, and certain glandular conditions (Perry and Metzger 1980).

English Name	Scientific Name	Nutritional and Therapeutic Values
Moso bamboo	*Phyllostachys pubescens* P. bambusoides	It contains cryptotaenen, kiganen, kiganol, petroselic acid, isomesityl oxide, mesityl oxide, methyl isobutyl, ketone, trans-beta-ocimene, and terpinolene. It is used for diarrhea, dysmenorrhea, rheumatism, and tubercular glands (T. Li 2002).
		Moso bamboo is edible when harvested during an early young age. New shoots are used to treat hematuria (Duke and Ayensu 1985). The leaves are used as an herbal medicine for inflammation of the joints of the body. It has antipyretic properties.
		The culm sheaths are used as a remedy for vomiting and sour stomach (Perry 1980).
		Bamboo leaves are used specifically for the heart and small intestine. It has antipyretic, diuretic, and antispasmodic effects. The fresh leaves are more effective for heat excess symptoms in the stomach and heart, but the dried leaves are better for diuretic purposes (Reid 1993).
Mu-erh	*Auricularia auricula-judae*	This parasitic tree fungus contains mannan, glucuronic acid, lecithin, cephalin, and ergosterol.
		It promotes the blood circulation and treats hemorrhoids (N. Chiu and Chang 1995).
		Nutritionally, mu-erh is a valuable source of health food that is low in calories and rich in carbohydrates, essential amino acids, fiber, vitamins, and minerals. It has also been used in medicine for centuries in the Orient.
		It has recently been recognized as a potential health food for improving the immune system (Lakhanpal and Monika 2005).
		It has hemostatic properties that are nourishing to the blood that promote circulation. It is used to treat cough, hemoptysis, hematemesis, epistaxis, uterine bleeding, hypertension, and constipation (K. Lin 1998e).
Mung bean	*Phaseolus sureus*	Mung bean has shown a hepatoprotective effect on APAP-induced hepatotoxicity (P. Wu et al. 2001).
		Mung bean hulls inhibit lipid peroxidation and nonlipid oxidative damage (Duh et al. 1999). The beans contain verbascose, stachyose, raffinose, sucrose, fructose, and glucose (Udayasekhara and Belavady 1978).
		Mung beans are also known as green beans (*Phaseolus radiatus*).
		Beans are used to prevent heat stroke and to treat summer thirst and food poisoning. Externally, green beans are ground into powders, blended, and applied to lesions.

English Name	Scientific Name	Nutritional and Therapeutic Values
		Juice extracted or soup made from fresh green bean sprouts is effective against arthritis and alcohol intoxication (K. Lin 1998e).
		The effects of a commercial product of mung bean nuclease were studied on the proliferation of ML-2 human tumor cells. The aspermatogenic, embryotoxic, immunogenic, immunosuppressive activity, and therapeutic efficiency were also studied in thymic mice bearing human melanoma tumor. Significant antitumor activity was detected on human melanoma tumor after intratumoral or intraperitoneal administration into mice (Soucek et al. 2006).
Mung bean sprout	*Phaseolus sureus*	Mung bean sprout is produced by germinating mung bean seeds.
		It contains verbascose, stachyose, raffinose, sucrose, fructose, and glucose (Udayasekhara and Belavady 1978).
Muskmelon	*Cucumis melo*	Seeds contains citrulline, cystine, galactane, histidine, lysine, and tryptophan.
		Fruit contains peptidase, protease, and vitamins A, B, and C.
		It is an expectorant, used for jaundice, and a stomachic (Hartwell 1971; Perry 1980).Muskmelon has a compound, cucurbitacin C, that is used to treat tumors. It also contains vitamin G, cucurbitacins A, B, C, and D, and oleic, linoleic, palmitic, and stearic acids (N. Chiu and Chang 1995d).
		Soluble dietary fiber in fruit was composed of a large amount of uronic acids, while the composition of insoluble noncellulose polysaccharides varied among fresh fruits in Taiwan (S. Chang et al. 1998).
		The fruit is used to treat headache and malaria (Y. Chang, 2000). Unripe fruit contains elaterin and meletexin as sell as cucurbitacins B, D, and E.
		Muskmelon contains acetaldehyde, adenosine, beta-myrin, arachidic acid, ascorbic acid, avenasterol, behenic acid, benzaldehyde, boron, caffeic acid, campesterol, capric acid, caproic acid, caprylic acid, chromium, cinnamic acetate, citric acid, clerosterol, codisterol, cucurbitacins B and E, eugenol-methyl-ether, euphol, fiber, pantothenic acid, pentadecanoic acid, phytosterols, riboflavin, stigmasterol, strontium, taraxerol, thiamine, tirucallol, titanium, tridecanoic acid, trigonelline, vitamin B6, zinc, and zirconium (Duke 2001).

English Name	Scientific Name	Nutritional and Therapeutic Values
Mustard cabbage	*Brassica juncea* var. *sareptona*	Chinese mustard has the highest calcium bioavailability (Weaver et al. 1997) and is used in Chinese medicine (Duke and Ayensu 1985). The leaves are boiled in soups to treat bladder inflammation, and a broth is consumed to stop hemorrhage. Seeds are employed to treat abscesses, colds, rheumatism, and stomach disorders (Perry 1980). Seed oils are used to treat eruptions, ulcers, and tumors (Tyler 1994; Small 2006).
		Water or moisture activates the enzyme myrosinase, causing the glycoside sinigrin to yield allyl and 3-butenyl isothiocyanates, glucose, and potassium hydrogen sulfate (Lewis 1984). These isothiocyanates are very pungent, having an irritating odor and a sharply acrid flavor.
		Note: A case of acute mustard seed toxicosis in cattle was reported in Saskatchewan, Canada (Kernaleguen et al. 1989).
Night-blooming cereus	*Hylocereus undatus*	The fruit is popular eaten chilled. It is used to flavor drinks and pastries. Unopened flower buds are cooked and eaten as vegetables.
		It contains hentriacontane, beta-sitosterol, minerals, and vitamins. The flower boiled with meat into a soup is given to relieve bronchitis, cough, and pain in the respiratory system (Duke and Ayensu 1985; Perry 1980).
		Aqueous extracts of leaves, rind, fruit pulp, and flowers were studied for their wound-healing properties. Application of Hylocereus undatus produced increases in hydroxyproline, tensile strength. On the other hand, *H. undatus* has no hypoglycemic activity (Perez et al. 2005).
		Flowers and fleshy stem are used. Flowers are anti-inflammatory, nourishing to the lungs, and antitussive. They are used to treat bronchitis, tuberculous, lymphadenitis, pulmonary disease, and tuberculosis. Stems are used to promote circulation and are anti-inflammatory (K. Lin 1998d).
		Aqueous extracts of leaves, rind, fruit pulp, and flowers of *H. undatus* were studied for their wound-healing properties. In streptozotocin diabetic rats, where healing is delayed, topical applications of *H. undatus* produced increases in hydroxyproline, tensile strength, total proteins, DNA collagen content, and better epithelization, thereby facilitating healing. *H. undatus* had no hypoglycemic activity (Perez et al. 2005).
Oil vegetable	*Brassica chinensis* var. *utilis*	Oil vegetable contains β-carotene equivalent, thiamine, riboflavin, niacin, and ascorbic acid (Duke and Atchley 1984).

English Name	Scientific Name	Nutritional and Therapeutic Values
		It is antiarthritic, antiscorbutic, and resolvent and is used to treat alcoholism, fevers, and intoxication (Perry 1980).
		Brassica chinensis has a preventive effect on PHIP-initiated carcinogenesis in cats, and the mechanism is likely to involve the induction of detoxification enzymes (Wen et al. 1999).
Okra	Hibiscus esculentus	Okra contains saponin, saponaretin, and vitexin.
	H. syriacus	The leaf is high in calcium, fiber, niacin, and vitamins A and C.
		Leaves are used for their stomachic, diuretic, and expectorant properties. Stem, bark, and root are used to treat diarrhea, dysentery, dysmenorrhea, itching, and painful skin diseases.
		A root bark decoction is used to treat dermatophytosis. The decoction is a vermifuge and is hemostatic, antiphlogistic, and emollient. The decoction is used to treat amebic dysentery and colitis and is applied externally to piles. It is also used to treat ascariasis, dysentery, dyspepsia, enterorrhagia, leucorrhea, and nausea.
		The fresh fruits contain saponin, saponaretin, and vitexin (Duke and Ayensu 1985).
		In Taiwan, the seeds are employed as a laxative and tonic and to stimulate urination (Anonymous).
Onion	Allium cepa var. aggregatum	Onion has bacchic, emmenagogue, and diuretic properties. The fresh juice has been found to contain a hypoglycemic agent. It is regarded as alterative, resolvent, and vulnerary. It is used to treat chest colds, shortness of breath, headache, and stomach and intestinal troubles (Perry 1980).
	A. chinese	Onion contains throb, methyl disulfide, allyl disulfide, trisulfide, thiosulfinates, citrate, malate, polysaccharides A and B, quercetin, thymine, kaempferol, carotenes, and 0-coumaric, caffeic, ferulic, sinapic, p-coumaric, and protocate chuic acids (N. Chiu and Chang 1995a).
		It has been reported that when quercetin is used with a carcinogen, it can increase the carcinogen's effects. In this situation, quercetin acts as a tumor-promoting agent (Boik 2001).
		Onion has been used medicinally for centuries as an external antiseptic. It may be helpful in allaying intestinal gas pains; in reducing hypertension, high blood sugar, and the cholesterol and fat content of the blood; and in relieving pain and inflammation. It is used both raw and cooked (Dobelis 1986).

English Name	Scientific Name	Nutritional and Therapeutic Values
Oriental pickling melon	*Cucumis melo* var. *conomon*	The flower buds contain a bitter principle that causes nausea and vomiting. Seeds contain citrulline, cystine, galactane, histidine, lysine, myristic acid, and tryptophan.
		Fruit contains peptidase, protease, and vitamins A, B, and C.
		Root contains melonemetine, elaterin, melotoxin, and the plant contains the antitumor cucurbitacin B occur. Stalks contain stigmasterol and spinasterol, which is used in China for alimentary cancers (Duke and Ayensu 1985).
Parsley	*Apium petroselinum*	The parsley plant possesses a small quantity of a pleasant volatile oil from leaves. The root is an agreeable aromatic, relaxant, and mild stimulant. Its chief power is expended upon the kidney.
		It contains up to 22% protein. It is high in vitamins A and C, fiber, calcium, iron, magnesium, potassium and riboflavin, niacin, thiamine, and phosphorus. The seeds and leaves have been used medicinally to treat indigestion, jaundice, menstrual problems, gallstones, coughs, asthma, and dropsy (Foster 1993).
		Parsley is used in the diet to treat osteoporosis. It can be used to concoct a beneficial, palliative, nutritional drink. It is a rich source of zinc, especially in the root (Foster 1993).
		It contains apiol, myristicin, 1-allyl-2,3,4,5-tetramethoxy benzole, α-β-pinene, α-β-phellandrene, bergapten, oxypeucedanin, isopimpinellin, psoralen, xanthotoxin, imperatorin, and apiin (Noble 2000).
		Parsley root mainly contains volatile oils, including erispumapiole, myristicin, terpinolene, tuberosum apiols, and α-β-pinene. It is used to treat infection of the urinary tract and kidney, bladder stones, gastrointestinal disorders, jaundice, and kidney and bladder inflammation. It is a diuretic and an emmenagogue. The fruit has been used to treat menstrual disturbances as well as disorders of the gastrointestinal tract, the kidneys, and the lower urinary tract (Noble 2000).
		Parsley leaf and root are used as a breath freshener, for urinary tract infections, and kidney or bladder stones. Topically, parsley is used for cracked or chapped skin, bruises, tumors, insect bites, lice, parasites, and to stimulate hair growth.

English Name	Scientific Name	Nutritional and Therapeutic Values
		Traditionally, parsley has been used to treat gastrointestinal disorders, constipation, jaundice, flatulence, indigestion, colic, bronchitic cough, asthma, general edema, rheumatism, anemia, hypotension, and diseases of the prostate, liver, and spleen. It is also used to promote menstrual flow and as an aphrodisiac. In foods and beverages, parsley is widely used as a garnish, condiment, food, and flavoring (Jellin et al. 2003).
		Parsley leaf and root contain volatile oils, carotene, and vitamins B1, B2, and C. The volatile oil contains apiole, myristicin, and photosensitizing furanocoumarins. It has antiflatulent, antispasmodic, antirheumatic, expectorant, antimicrobial, and aquaretic effects (Robbers and Tyler 1999).
		Aquaretics increase urine volume but not sodium excretion. The constituent apiole appears to be associated with antispasmodic, vasodilator, and menstrual-flow-stimulant effects. Apiole can also increase smooth muscle contractibility in the bladder and intestines (Leung and Foster 1996). Both the apiol and myristicin constituents are believed to have aquaretic and uterine stimulant effects. The mechanism of aquaresis is that parsley irritates the kidney epithelium, which increases renal blood flow and glomerular filtration rate (Robbers and Tyler 1999).
		Apiole and myristicin have a structure similar to safrole, which is considered carcinogenic and hepatotoxic (Jellin et al. 2003).
Parsnip	*Peucedanum sativum* *Pustinaca sativa*	Parsnip has phytosterol as well as butyric, acetic, propionic, palmitic, stearic, oleic, and linoleic acids (Roi 1955).
		It is antitussive and a stimulant.
		It is used to treat apoplexy, arthritis, asthma, bronchitis, cold, dropsy, fever, headache, and rheumatism (Bliss 1973).
		It contains anomalin, coumarin, and peuformosin (N. Chiu and Chang 1995d).
		Intestinal function was improved with fiber diets.
		In rats, blood glucose levels tended to be reduced.
		Serum and HDL cholesterol levels were not affected.

English Name	Scientific Name	Nutritional and Therapeutic Values
		The weights of the heart, spleen, and liver were significantly decreased by parsnip (Mongeau et al. 1990).
		Parsnip contains scopolin, skimmin, apiosylskimmin, peucedanol, furocoumarins, nodakenin, nodakenetin, psoralen, 5-methoxypsoralen, rutarin, isorutarin, apterin, rutaretin, marmesinin, decuroside, pyranocoumarins, decursin, decursidin, praeruptorin, angeloyloxy, isovaleryloxy, qianhucoumarin, peucedanocoumarin, limonene, chavicol methyl ether, spongesterol, β-sitosterol, β-sitosterol-3-O-D-glucoside, mannitol, and galactitol (Ye 1999).
		Parsnip leaves are used for digestive and kidney disorders. They contain the furocoumarins angelicin, bergapten, xanthotoxin, and psoralen. Furocoumarins are phototoxic and mutagenic; photosensitizing is responsible for adverse dermatological reaction (Foster and Tyler 1999).
		Parsnip roots are used to treat kidney complaints and fever, and they have analgesic and diuretic properties. The root contains the furocoumarins angelicin, bergapten, xanthotoxin, and psoralen (Jellin et al. 2003).
Pea	*Pisum sativum*	Pea contains vitamins A, B, and C, lecithin, cholesterin, betaine, trigonelline, choline, adenine, lysine, erepsin, leucine, arginine, tryptophan, phytin, vernin, asparagine, glutamine, alantoinase, urea, pepsin, trypsin, amylase, maltase, catalase, lipase, nuclease, phytagglutinin, abscisic acid, and gibberellin A (N. Chiu and Chang 1995a).
		It is one of the better sources for choline, which may prevent liver cancer (Duke 1999).
		Seed is contraceptive, ecbolic, fungistatic, and spermicidal.
		It is prescribed for diabetes, fever, flux, lack of lactation, nausea, and urinary problems.
		It has been reported that pea oil, given once a month to women, showed promise of preventing pregnancy by interfering with the working of progesterone.
		The drug moxylohydroquinone reduced spermatozoa in males by ca. 50%, with the count reverting to normal in about four days. Experimental results suggest a hypoglycemic effect. Fresh green peas contain crude fiber, ash, calcium, phosphate, iron, potassium and beta-carotene equivalent, thiamine, riboflavin, niacin, and ascorbic acid (Duke and Ayensu 1985).

English Name	Scientific Name	Nutritional and Therapeutic Values
		Peas are considered cooling and are recommended for feverish conditions, to increase flesh, and to treat diabetes (Perry 1980).
Pepper	*Capsicum annuum* var. *longum*	The carotenoid capsanthin is the most important pigment of *Capsicum*.
		The pungent principle capsaicin is present on the placenta of the fruits and is said to retain its pungency at dilutions of one part per million (Purseglove et al. 1981). Chili pepper has been employed in a variety of folk remedies to treat asthma, inflamed gums, lumbago, neuralgia, pneumonia, rheumatism, sores, cancers, and tumors (Duke 1985).
		The main component, capsaicin, and dihydrocapsaicin are responsible for the inhibition against *Bacillus cereus*, *B. subtilis*, *Clostridium sporogenes*, *C. tetani*, and *Streptococcus pyogenes* (Cichewicz and Thorpe 1996).
		The chemistry of the components contributes to color and pungency.
		The carotenoid capsanthin is the most important pigment of Capsicum. There are seven closely related capsaicinoids, often collectively termed capsaicin. Capsicum peppers do not contain volatile oils, but they do have a distinctive aroma that is particularly pleasing in the sweet varieties.
		Chili pepper has been employed in a variety of folk remedies to treat such conditions as asthma, lumbago, neuralgia, pneumonia, rheumatism, sores, cancers, and tumors.
		In China, the leaves are used to treat toothache, while the fruit is considered useful for stomach disorder, rheumatism, and for increasing circulation of the blood (Small 2006).
Perilla	*Perilla frutescens*	The seeds contain flavones such as apigenin and luteolin. Leaves have nine flavone glycosides, such as the 3-p-coumarylglycoside-5-glucoside of cyanidin and the 7-caffeyl-glucosides of apigenin and luteolin. Five anthocyanins.
		Leaves are emollient, stomachic, tonic, antiseptic, antitussive, and diaphoretic (Duke and Ayensu 1985).
		In Asia, perilla is used as a sedative to treat spasms as well as uterine and head problems.
		It can be used to increase perspiration and to treat cholera, colds, influenza, stomach problems, nausea, poison, asthma, bronchitis, chest pain, and rheumatism (Small 2006).

English Name	Scientific Name	Nutritional and Therapeutic Values
		Perilla has been used by traditional herbalists in Asia for centuries to help manage hay fever and allergy symptoms and cough and colds, and to reduce the incidence of influenza and other similar conditions (health.nutralife.co.nz).
		Leaves, stems, and seeds are used. Leaves have diaphoretic and stomachic properties and are used to dispel chills. Seeds have antiasthmatic and antitussive properties and are used to liquefy sputum (K. Lin 1998c).
		It contains caffeic acid, beta-carotene, cyanidin-3,5-diglucoside, fiber, glucose, iron, linalool, luteolin, niacin, phenylpropanoids, alpha-pinene, protocatechuic acid, riboflavin, rosmarinic acid, scutellerein, thiamine, and zinc (Duke 2001).
Pigeon pea	*Cajanus cajan*	Pigeon peas are a popular food in developing tropical countries. The green seeds and pods are nutritious and wholesome and are served as a vegetable.
		The seeds are said to be bechic, astringent, and diuretic.
		The crushed leaves are applied to herpes and other itching skin eruptions (Perry 1980).
		It has a diuretic property and is used to stop bleeding and to treat digestion, dysentery, mouth infection, cough, and windpipe and tonsil infections (N. Chiu and Chang, 1995a).
		Eighty-five legume seeds were examined by measurements of their net protein utilization by rats and by hemagglutination tests with erythrocytes from a number of different animal species. Pigeon pea had low reactivity with all cells and was nontoxic (Grant et al. 1983).
		The aim of investigating new indigenous vegetable crops is to address the issues of malnutrition and community development and to establish entrepreneurs to address these issues. Indigenous edible seed and leafy vegetables have been investigated for purposes of commercialization. Pigeon pea has been described as a source of protein, iron, calcium, vitamin A, and amino acids (Reinten and Coetzee 2002).
Prickly pear cactus	*Opuntia dillenii*	The plant contains α-pyrone, 4-ethexyl-6-hydroxymethyl, 1-α-pyrone, 1-hepstanecanol, vanillic acid, and arabinogalactan. It is antitoxic and is used to treat stomachache, sore throat, cough, diarrhea, and hernia (T. Li 2006).

English Name	Scientific Name	Nutritional and Therapeutic Values
		The hypoglycemic properties of *Opuntia dillenii* polysaccharides were tested on mice with streptozotocin-induced diabetes. The polysaccharides from this plant showed hypoglycemic properties (Tao et al. 2005).

The antihyperglycemic effect of the fruit juice of *Opuntia dillenii* was studied in alloxan-induced diabetic rats through acute and long-term experiments (Ahmed et al. 2005a). Flavonoids were isolated with anti-inflammatory properties (Ahmed 2005a). *Opuntia dillenii* flowers are used in folk medicine as an antidiabetic and as an anti-inflammatory (Ahmed et al. 2005b).

Oral administration of the phylloclade extract of *Opuntia dillenii* to male rats caused a significant decrease in the weights of testes, epididymides, seminal vesicle, and ventral prostate (R. S. Gupta et al. 2002).

Root, stem, and fruits are edible. It has antipyretic, antitoxic, analgesic, antitussive, and antidiarrheal properties and is used to reduce swelling and hematoma. Prickly pear cactus is used to treat gastric and duodenal ulcers, acute dysentery, and cough. It is used externally to treat epidemic parotitis, mastitis, pyoderma, snakebites, and burns (K. Lin 1998a). In foods, the prickly pear juice is used in jellies and candies. Prickly pear cactus also contains isorhamnetin and quercetin (Ye 1999).

Prickly pear cactus is used to treat diabetes, hypercholesterolemia, and obesity, and as an antiviral agent. It is also used for colitis, diarrhea, and benign prostatic hypertrophy (Jellin et al. 2003).

The applicable parts of this plant are the leaves and stems. It is often consumed as part of the diet. Ingesting 500 g of prickly pear cactus provides 14 g carbohydrate, 8 g protein, 1 g lipids, 19 g cellulose (fibrous polysaccharide), 455 g water, and 99 g kilocalories (Rayburn et al. 1998).

Some species can lower blood glucose and lipid levels (Anonymous 2000). This effect is often attributed to the high fibrous polysaccharide content, including pectin (Opticantha 2000). Fiber can slow carbohydrate absorption and decrease lipid absorption from the gut. However, some researchers suspect prickly pear might also have an insulin-sensitizing effect (Gelenberg et al. 1990). |

English Name	Scientific Name	Nutritional and Therapeutic Values
		There is also some evidence that the pectin component can alter the liver metabolism of cholesterol and affect cholesterol levels (Fernandez et al. 1994). Boiled stems seem to be more effective for reducing blood glucose levels than raw stems (Frati-Munari 1989). There is some preliminary evidence that prickly pear has antiviral activity against the herpes simplex virus (HSV), respiratory syncytial virus (RSV), and human immunodeficiency virus (HIV) (Ahmad et al. 1996).
		The fruit of the prickly pear as well as the pulp of the cacti can be eaten. A poultice of the pulp can be used for wounds, bruises, and warts. The pulp can be used as a lung remedy (Willard 1992).
Pumpkin	*Cucurbita pepo*	Pumpkin contains β-carotene equivalent, thiamine, riboflavin, niacin, and ascorbic acid. The seeds are used to treat hypertrophy of the prostate (Osman et al. 1979).
		The chemical composition in pumpkin contains sterol, sesquiterpenes, terpenoids, and squalene acids. It is used to treat hyperplasia and the prostate (Bombardelli and Morazzoni 1997).
		Seeds contain cucurbitine, linoleic acid, oleata, oleic acid, octadecanoic acid, stearic acid, carotene, and vitamins A1, B1, B2, and C (Ye 1999).
		Seeds are recognized as an anthelmintic (Dobelis 1986).
		Pumpkin is used to treat dysuria secondary to benign prostatic hyperplasia (BPH), bladder irritation, intestinal worms, and pyelonephritis. Pumpkin is used in an herbal combination to treat symptoms of BPH. Roasted pumpkins seeds are considered to be a snack food (Jellin et al. 2003).
		The applicable part of pumpkin is the seed.
		Pumpkin seeds are rich in carotenoids, including lutein, carotene, and beta-carotene (515). The seed oil is rich in unsaturated fatty acids, including linoleic, oleic, palmitic, and stearic acids. The oil is also rich in vitamin E, including both gamma-tocopherol and alpha-tocopherol (Younis et al. 2000).
		Pumpkin seed oil can exhibit a diuretic effect that can relieve bladder discomfort, causing the perception of reduced prostate gland swelling without reducing the gland size. The phytosterol constituents are also believed to affect urine flow. Another constituent, cucurbitin, has anthelmintic effects. The concentration of cucurbitin varies significantly among *Cucurbita* species (Foster and Tyler 1999).

English Name	Scientific Name	Nutritional and Therapeutic Values
Purslane	*Portulaca oleracea*	Purslane is an Australian native plant with succulent leaves that are oval shaped and about 25 mm long. Its juicy leaves are used in salads and cooked as a substitute for spinach. The plant is suggested as having cooling, emollient, antiscorbutic, alterative, vulnerary, antibacterial, antifungal, antiviral, hypoglycemic, sedative, and resolvent properties.
		The seeds contain fatty acids, including palmitic, stearic, behenic, oleic, linoleic, and linolenic acids. It also contains beta-sitosterol (Duke and Ayensu 1985) as well as portulal, betacyanin, betanin, and betanidin (N. Chiu and Chang 1995b).
		Purslane is sour tasting. It has antipyretic, diuretic, and antitoxic properties and is used to treat dysentery, acute enteritis, acute appendicitis, mastitis, and hemorrhoidal bleeding. It is used externally for furunculosis and eczema (K. Lin 1998a).
		Portulaca oleracea is a weed in both temperate and tropical regions. Recently, in tropical regions, it is being used as a vegetable. The fresh leaves are best for all therapeutic purposes.
		The plant contains tannin, phosphates, magnesium, iron, aluminum, manganese, calcium, potassium, sodium, and urea (Perry 1980).
		It is antipyretic, antidote, refrigerant, antidysenteric, and antiphlogistic. Purslane can be used to treat amoebic dysentery, hemorrhoids, and abscesses due to heat excess (Reid 1993).
		Purslane has been used medicinally in the form of an infusion for stomachache, excess menstrual flow, and high blood pressure. The seed has been used for removing worms in children and as a palliative for hemorrhoids. The juice, with some added honey, can be used as a cough syrup (Willard 1992).
Red bean	*Phaseolus calcaratus* *P. angularis*	Two lectins — an N-acetylgalactosamine-binding lectin, lectin-I, which reacts specifically with human erythrocytes of blood group A, and a galactose-binding lectin, lectin II, which is specific for human blood group B erythrocytes — have been isolated and purified from *Phaseolus calcaratus* (Datta et al. 1988).
		It contains α- and β-globulin, fatic acid, starch, triterpenoid saponin, vitamins B1 and B2, thiamine, riboflavin, nicotinic acid, protein, fat, carbohydrate, and fiber (Ye 1999).

English Name	Scientific Name	Nutritional and Therapeutic Values
		In an experiment, the hypocholesterolemic effect of the protein concentrates prepared from *Phaseolus angularis*, *Phaseolus calcaratus*, and *Dolichos lablab* seeds relative to that of casein were studied in hamsters. As compared with casein, the three legume protein concentrates produced significantly lower (p < .05) levels of triglyceride and total and low-density lipoprotein cholesterol in the blood serum as well as lower liver total lipids and cholesterol contents. It is concluded that, in general, the protein concentrates of *P. calcaratus* and *D. lablab* seemed to be more potent at lowering raised serum cholesterol levels than that of *P. angularis* (Chau et al. 1998).
		The antilipid peroxidation activity, free-radical scavenger activity, and antisuperoxide formation of hot-water extracts of legumes (HWEL), such as mung bean (*Phaseolus radiatus*), adzuki bean (*Phaseolus aureus*), black bean (*Glycine max*), and red bean (*Phaseolus calcaratus*) were evaluated to test antioxidant activity. The results showed that all HWELs exhibited remarkable inhibition of FeCl2–ascorbic acid-induced lipid peroxidation of mouse-liver homogenate. All extracts showed antilipid peroxidation activities (C. Lin et al. 2001).
Rhubarb	*Rheum rhaponticum*	Rhubarb contains anthraquinones, chrysophanol, emodin, physcion, aloe-emodin, rhein, chrysophenol, rheum tannic acid, gallic acid, calechin, blanthraquinonyl, and sennoside (T. Li 2002).
		Four anthraquinones — aloe-emodin, emodin, chrysophenol, anthocyanins, and physcion — have been extracted from rhubarb (Y. Li et al. 2000; Vaccari et al. 1981).
		Experiments with ALI model rats suggest that rhubarb could reduce edema of the lung tissue and decrease red blood cell exudation, neutrophil infiltration, and plasma protein exudation in the alveoli (C. Li et al. 2001).
		It also may prevent intestinal bacterial translocation (X. Chen and Ran 1996), lower blood pressure and cholesterol levels (T. Li 2002), and serve as an anticancer agent..
		Rhubarb is a laxative. It has been used for stomach and bowel problems in infants and to treat sores. Rhubarb stalks contain calcium, potassium, and vitamins A and C (Marshall 1988).
		Rhubarb contains cinnamic acid, gallic acid, emodin, rhein, enthrones, catechin, anthraquinone compounds, tannins, and calcium oxalate (Noble 2000).

English Name	Scientific Name	Nutritional and Therapeutic Values
		Chinese rhubarb, a native of western China and Tibet, is apparently the chief source of medicinal rhubarb drugs, obtained from the roots. Rhubarb has been used to treat stomach and bowel problems in infants and to treat sores. Rhubarb stalks are low in vitamins and minerals, but contain significant amounts of calcium, potassium, and vitamins A and C (Small 2006).
Scallion	*Allium chinese* *A. fistulosum*	The bulb of this plant can be eaten raw or cooked. The bulb has a strong onion flavor. Flowers and young seedpods are used as a garnish on salads. A paste of fresh scallion with honey is used as an ointment for abscesses and infections (Reid 1993).
		This plant has antiseptic, diuretic, lactagogue, stomachic, vermifuge, and vulnerary properties. It is used to impede intestinal parasites. Pounded bulb is a decongestant and allays inflammation of stuffy nose. Compounds include sulfides, thiolanes, alcohols, aldehydes, ketones, and furanones (Duke and Ayensu 1985).
		It contains allicin, allyl sulfide, vitamins C, B1, and B2, palmitic, stearic, arachidic, oleic, and linoleic acids, pectin, fructose oligosaccharides, and protopectin (N. Chiu and Chang 1995b).
		Scallion has diaphoretic, diuretic, and anti-inflammatory functions and is used to treat intestinal obstruction from Ascaris. It is also used to treat colds, headache, and nasal stuffiness (K. Lin 1998d).
		Allium chinese contains allicin, allistatin, glucominol, neo-allicin, steroidal saponins, polysaccharides, furostanol saponins, proto-isoerubosides, and diallyl sulfide. It is antibacterial, antimutagenic, anticarcinogenesis, carminative, antiarrhythmic, hypotensive, and has a vessel-protective effect. It is used to lower plasma cholesterol and low-density lipoproteins and to prevent thrombosis (T. Li 2002).
		Allium chinese also contains essential oils, dimethyl disulfide, 2,4-dimethyl thiophene, allyl methyl disulfide, dimethyl trisulfide, methyl allyl trisulfide, propyl allyl trisulfide, methyl propyl disulfide, n-propyl, allyl disulfide, palmitic acid, and octadeca-9-12-decanoic acid (Je 1999).
Shan-Chiai-Ts'ai	*Rorippa indica*	The plant contains hirsutin, arabin, camelinin, and three novel w-methyl sulfonylalkyl isothiocyanates. The leaves are antihyperglycemic and antitussive (Yamane et al. 1992), and it is antihyperglycemic and antitussive.

English Name	Scientific Name	Nutritional and Therapeutic Values
		Rorippa indica has α-phenylethylisothiocyanate, gluconasturin, rorifone, and rorifamide. It has been reported that this plant can stop vomiting of blood, relieve stomachache, and relieve pain caused by the nervous system and by menstruation (T. Li 2002).
Shepherd's purse	*Capsella bursa-pastoris* var. *auriculata*	It is hemostatic, antipyretic, anti-inflammatory, and diuretic. It is used for blood purifying and to cure inflammation of the eyes and hematuria secondary to renal tuberculosis (K. Lin 1998b).
		Shepherd's purse is also used to treat hemoptysis from pulmonary tuberculosis, nephritic edema, urolithiasis, chyharia, uterine bleeding, menorrhagia, colds and fever, enteritis, hypertension, and sore eyes (K. Lin 1998b).
		Shepherd's purse is listed as being astringent, diuretic, antiscorbutic, styptic, and a vasoconstrictor. It also acts as a stimulant and as a moderate tonic for catarrh of the urinary tract; it is also helpful for both kidney and bladder.
		An infusion of the dried leaf is an effective blood coagulant and is used internally and externally. It also acts on the circulatory system to equalize blood pressure and menstrual flow and to treat other menstrual problems (Willard 1992).
Slender amaranth	*Amaranthus viridis*	Fresh leaves and shoots are an excellent source of vitamin B. Decoction of entire plant is used to stop dysentery and inflammation. The plant is emollient and vermifuge (Duke and Ayensu 1985).
		Amaranthus viridis was found to be an excellent source of protein. Its amino acid composition compared favorably with that of the WHO protein standard. It also contains considerable amounts of the two fatty acids (linoleic and α-linolenic acids) that are essential in humans as well as a number of minerals including iron, magnesium, calcium, and zinc (Sena et al. 2004).
		It contains alanine, arginine, ascorbic acid, aspartic acid, calcium, carbohydrate, beta-carotene, copper, cystine, fat, fiber, folacin, glutamic acid, glycine, histidine, iron, isoleucine, leucine, lysine, magnesium, methionine, niacin, phenylalanine, phosphorus, potassium, proline, protein, riboflavin, rutin, serine, sodium, thiamine, threonine, tryptophan, tyrosine, valine, and zinc (Duke 2001).
		Juice or tea made from amaranth can be used to wash hives and to treat eczema and psoriasis (Duke 1997).

English Name	Scientific Name	Nutritional and Therapeutic Values
		The root is used to treat rheumatism. It acts as an emmenagogue and as a diuretic in treating gonorrhea. It is sudorific and febrifuge in eruptive or very high fevers. The leaves are said to be cooling, nonpoisonous, and remedial for dysentery, dropsy, and malnutrition. The plant is used as a diuretic and a galactagogue. Internally, the leaves are used to treat bronchitis or a cold in the chest. The plant contains considerable potassium nitrate (Perry 1980).
Snake gourd	*Trichosanthes anguina*	Snake gourd contains kaempferitrin, choline, trichosanic acid, r-guanidinobutyric acid, and diaminopropionic acid (Y. Chang 2000).
		The plant is used as a purgative and a vermifuge. The inner pulp of the fruit is made into a syrup to treat cough (Perry 1980). It is also used to treat throat infection, cough, and windpipe inflammation (Y. Chang 2000).
		Root is anti-inflammatory and analgesic and is used to dispel stagnant blood and to treat, snakebite, sore throat, oligomenorrhea, gastric pain, wound pain, postoperative pain, boils, and pyodermas (K. Lin 1998d).
		Snake gourd contains ascorbic acid, ash, calcium, carbohydrate, beta-carotene, chlorine, chondrillasterol, copper, alpha-eleostearic acid, fat, fiber, iodine, iron, linoleic acid, magnesium, niacin, oleic acid, oxalic acid, palmitic acid, phosphorus, potassium, protein, punicic acid, riboflavin, sodium, stearic acid, sulfur, and thiamine (Duke 2001).
		Snake gourd is an expectorant and is used to dilate bronchial tubes. It is also an emollient and has laxative effects. It is used to treat coughs due to excess heat in lungs, heavy yellow phlegm, lung tumors, pains in chest and rib cage, and constipation (Reid 1993).
		It contains nonanoic, capric, lanric, myristic, pentadecanoic, palmitoleic, palmitic, linoleic, linolenic, and stearic acids. It also contains Δ7-stigmastenol, β-spinasterol, Δ7-stigmastenol-β-D-gincopyranoside, cerotic, montanic, and melissic acids, heptacosane, nonacosane, hentriacontane, trichosanic acid, campesterol, 7-campesterol, sitosterol, stigmasterol, 7-stigmasterol, 5,25-stigmastadienol, 7-stigmastenol, α-spinasterol, 7,24-stigmastadienol, 7,25-stigmastatrienol, stigmastanol, trichkirin, vanillic acid, tricin, and 11-methoxy-noryangonin (Ye 1999).

English Name	Scientific Name	Nutritional and Therapeutic Values
Soybean	*Glycine max*	Soybean health claims on food labels have been approved by the U.S. Food and Drug Administration for more than 30 years. Soy concentrates and aqueous extracts of soybeans contain isoflavones and phenolic acids as the main antioxidants.
		Black soybean is fermented soybean with medicinal values. It has carminative, sedative, and antipyretic effects. It is used to treat colds, fevers, and headaches due to "wind-heat" injury, oppression in chest, and insomnia (Reid 1993).
		Organic solvent extracts contain tocopherols, sterols, phospholipids, and other flavonoids, while protein hydrolysates contain antioxidant amino acids and peptides.
		Isoflavones are the predominant flavonoid in soybean and have been promoted for their estrogenic activity. The glucoside form of isoflavones represents 99% of the total isoflavones in soybeans (Naim et al. 1974).
		Seeds are recommended as carminative, and with other drugs are employed to treat a large number of illnesses. The seeds are regarded as tonic, diuretic, febrifuge, and antidote. They are said to assist the flow of digestive juices, to increase the assimilation of high-protein foods, and to be a source of riboflavin, thiamine, niacin, pentothenic acid, and choline. The raw soybeans contain a toxic principle with hemolytic activity (Perry 1980). It has been reported that the use of soybean products and soybean isoflavones by postmenopausal women may be beneficial for bone and cardiovascular health and in reducing hot flashes (Cassidy et al. 2006; Ryan-Borchers et al. 2006).
Soybean sprout	*Glycine max*	Sprouts are a valuable food because of their generally high content of vitamins, minerals, carbohydrates, and proteins. However, some leguminous seed sprouts, such as soybean, contain toxins that may be harmful if large amounts are consumed raw (Small 2006).
Spinach	*Spinacia oleracea*	Spinach contains chlorophylls a and b, ecdysteroids, protoporphyrin, coproporphyrin I, xanthophyll epoxide, and oxalic, citronic, malic, and folic acids (Bathory et al. 1982).
		It is regarded as carminative and laxative. A drug "spinacin" stimulates digestive secretions (Kariyone and Kimura 1949; Perry 1980).
		Spinach is ranked among the top five vegetables in antioxidant activity assays (Easdown and Kalb 2004).

English Name	Scientific Name	Nutritional and Therapeutic Values
		It has been reported that nutritional approaches can help prevent stroke. Studies at Tufts University in Boston and at the University of Alabama in Birmingham have demonstrated that the folate in spinach can help prevent both heart disease and stroke, compared with people who consumed little folate. Folate is not plentiful in plants; however, it was demonstrated that spinach contains this important compound (Duke 1997).
		Spinach contains acetylcholine, n-acetylhistamine, alanine, ascorbic acid, aspartic acid, boron, cadmium, calcium, carbohydrates, beta-carotene, cephalin, chlorine, cholesterol, p-coumaric acid, ferulic acid, fiber, fluorine, folic acid, glutamic acid, glutathione, glycine, 6-(hydroxymethyl)-lumazine, 3-hydroxytyramine, iron, isoleucine, kaempferol, lecithin, linoleic acid, alpha-linolenic acid, magnesium, myristic acid, oleic acid, oxalic acid, palmitic acid, palmitoleic acid, phosphatidylglycerol, protein, quercetin, riboflavin, selenium, spinasaponins, alpha-tocopherol, trimethyl histamine, tyrosine, valine, and zinc (Duke 2001).
Sunflower	*Helianthus annuus*	Sunflower contains β-carotene equivalent, thiamine, riboflavin, niacin, and ascorbic acid. It is used for dysuria (Perry 1980).
		A chemical (S-adenosyl-methionine) from sunflower has been shown to have pain-relieving and anti-inflammatory properties similar to those found in the over-the-counter medication ibuprofen (Duke 1997).
		Flower head is used as a hypotensive and an analgesic.
		Root and stem pulp are used for their anti-inflammatory, diuretic, antitussive, and analgesic properties.
		Leaves are used for their anti-inflammatory, analgesic, and antimalarial properties. Seeds are anti-dysentery, tonic to body fluids, and promote eruption of measles rash (K. Lin 1998f).
		The antioxidants of seed oil include phenolic acids, tocopherols, and sterols, while purple-hulled varieties contain significant concentrations of anthocyanins (Garden 1989).
		Sunflower oil is used internally to alleviate constipation. It is used externally as a massage oil for poorly healing wounds and in the treatment of skin lesions, psoriasis, and rheumatism (Noble 2000).

English Name	Scientific Name	Nutritional and Therapeutic Values
		It contains linolenic acid, oleic acid, palmitic acid, and arachic acid. It is used internally to relieve constipation and externally on cuts and bruises. Sunflower seed contains essential oils, including alpha-tocopherol and linolenic, oleic, myristic, palmitic, palmitoleic, margaric, stearic, arachidic, linoleic, and eicosenic acids (T. Li 2000).
Sweet basil	*Ocimum basilicum*	The leaves are oval and slightly toothed. The flowers are white or purple. The essential oil, leaves, seeds, flowers, and roots are used as medicine.
		Sweet basil contains eucalyptol, estragol, ocimene, α-pinene, 1,8-cineole, eucalyptole, linalool, limonene, methylchavicol, eugenol, methyl ether, anethole, and methyl chavicol (Y. Chang 2000).
		Decoction of leaves is used to treat fever, asthma, earache, and ringworm, and it is considered to be digestive and tonic. Seeds are used to remove film and opacity from eyes. Infusion of plant is used to treat cepalalgia, gout, and halitosis (Duke and Ayensu 1985).
		Five chemical types of basil have been recognized (Lawrence 1992). These are geraniol, eugenol, linalool, camphor, and methyl cinnamate. It also contains the carcinogens astragal and safrole. Basil has been used in folk medicine to treat alcoholism, boredom, childbirth, cholera, colic, constipation, cough, cramps, whooping cough, and sore throat (Rinzler 1990).
		Whole herb is used.
		It promotes absorption, dispels stagnant blood, and has diaphoretic, diuretic, and analgesic properties. Sweet basil can be used to treat colds, headache, gastric pain, abdominal distention, indigestion, ententes, diarrhea, irregular menses, and rheumatoid arthritis. It is used externally to treat snake and insect bites, eczema, and dermatitis (K. Lin 1998c).
Sweet corn	*Zea mays* var. *rugosa*	Both carotenoids and tocopherols can be found in corn kernel tissue. These compounds are associated with the prevention of degenerative diseases (Grams et al. 1970; Kurilich and Juvik 1999).
		Corn silks are used as a diuretic in dropsy and to treat sugar diabetes (Perry 1980).
		The Chinese have used corn silk successfully to treat swelling caused by kidney disease, according to pharmacognosists (Duke 1997).

English Name	Scientific Name	Nutritional and Therapeutic Values
		It contains cryptoxanthin, vitamin K3, α-tocopherolquinone, gibberellic acid, dihydro-B-sitosteryl ferulate, C39H60O, 6,7-dimethoxy-2-benzozolinone, 6-methoxy-benzozolinone, benzoxazin, and malate dehydrogenase (Ye 1999).
		The green corn silk is diuretic and is useful in treating dropsy, either renal or cardiac, as are the undeveloped pistils of the flower and the fresh or dried stalks. A decoction of a hard cob of corn is drunk to treat menorrhagia and nosebleed. Corn hulls used with pomegranate peel are a remedy for diarrhea in children, strangury, and gravel.
		The root is used as a remedy for blennorrhea. A ball made of roasted corn seeds with *Combretum trifoliatum* fruits and palm sugar is chewed to treat angina. A decoction of the pith of the cob is drunk to relieve stomachache (Perry 1980).
		Corn silk contains galactan, xylan, and dextrose. The seeds contain much sugar, zeaxanthin, protein, inosite, hexaphosphoric acid, maizenic acid, resins, and fixed oil (Perry 1980).
Sweet potato	*Ipomoea batatas*	A tuberous-rooted perennial, usually grown as an annual. The top is herbaceous, with the stems forming a running vine, usually prostrate and slender with milky juice.
		The plant is herbaceous, an aquatic annual with hollow stems and ovate to elliptic shaped leaves. It has a creeping growth habit but may grow erect in water (Yamaguchi 1990).
		The plant contains antioxidative components, including chlorogenic acid, isochlorogenic acids, and caffeic acid. The effective antioxidant activity is mainly based on the synergistic effect of phenolic compounds with amino acids (Hayase and Kato 1984).
		In folk medicine, it is used as a remedy for mouth and throat tumors, asthma, burns, diarrhea, fever, nausea, and stomach disorder. It is alterative, aphrodisiac, astringent, bactericide, demulcent, laxative, and tonic (Duke and Wain 1981).
		It is tonic, increasing salivary secretion, and hemostatic.
		Tubers are used for gastric and duodenal ulcer bleeding and constipation.
		Leaves and vines are used to treat massive uterine bleeding, boils and abscesses, mastitis, burns and scalds, and sprains (K. Lin 1998f).
		Sweet potato leaf contributed almost one-third to overall antioxidant activity intake from vegetables.

English Name	Scientific Name	Nutritional and Therapeutic Values
Sweet potato vine	*Ipomoea batatas*	The leaves are eaten as a cooked leafy vegetable in many countries.
		The leaves contain anthocyanins and phenolic acids and have shown antimutagenic properties (Easdown and Kalb 2004).
		The plant is herbaceous, an aquatic annual with hollow stems and ovate to elliptic shaped leaves. It has a creeping growth habit but may grow erect in water (Yamaguchi 1990).
		In folk medicine, it is used as a remedy for mouth and throat tumors, asthma, burns, diarrhea, fever, nausea, and stomach disorder. It is alterative, aphrodisiac, astringent, bactericide, demulcent, laxative, and tonic (Duke 1981).
		It contain alanine, arginine, ascorbic acid, boron, batatic acid, caffeic acid, carbohydrates, beta-carotene, zeta-carotene, carotenoids, chlorine, chlorogenic acid, cystine, glutamic acid, glycine, histidine, iodine, isoquercitrin, kilocalories, leucine, linoleic acid, oxalic acid, palmitic acid, pantothenic acid, pectin, peonidin, phosphorus, phytin, phytoene, phytosterols, thilamin, threonine, tocopherol, tryptophan, uronic acid, and vitamin B6 (Duke 2001).
Sword bean	*Canavalia ensiformis* *C. gladiata*	The seed meal contains a thermolabile toxin, causing hemorrhage of the stomach mucosa. It contains several globulins, including canavalin and concanavalins A and B. The meal contains a crystalline diamino acid, canavanine. Canavanine is bactericidal and fungicidal (Duke and Ayensu 1985).
		It contains canavanine, concanavalins A and B, canaline, and lymphoblast (N. Chiu and Chang 1995a).
		Sword bean contains canavalia gibberellins I and II, concanavalin A, and canaline. Unripe seeds contain canavalia gibberellin A21, C19H22O6, and canavanine (Je 1999).
Table beet (Swiss chard)	*Beta vulgaris*	It is also known as Swiss chard. Appearance of the leaf of beet is similar to spinach, but leaf beet is larger. Leaf shape is an ovoid figure or even long-ovoid figure, and the leaves are lustrous.
		It contains arginine, betaine, histidine, isoleucine, leucine, phenylalanine, tyrosine, and tyrosinase (Jiangsu New Medical College 1979).
		It is used to treat dysentery and is a folk cancer remedy in Arabian, American, German, and Mexican medicine (Perry 1980).

English Name	Scientific Name	Nutritional and Therapeutic Values
		Oxalate oxidase obtained from the stem of beet was covalently linked to polyethylene glycol. It exhibited decreased electrophoretic mobility, increased storage stability, higher thermal stability, and resistance to heavy metal inactivation and proteolytic digestion (Varalakshmi et al. 1995).
		Beet (Swiss chard) contains numerous active ingredients. These include acetamide, aconitic acid, alanine, allantoin, aluminum, L-arabinose, abginine, ascorbic acid, barium, betaine, cadmium, caffeic acid, calcium, carbohydrates, β-carotene, chlorogenic acid, chromium, citric acid, copper, p-coumaric acid, cystine, daucic acid, farnesol, fat, ferulic acid, folacin, formaldehyde, glutamic acid, glycine, kaempferol, leucine, linoleic acid, α-linolenic acid, lithium, lysine, magnesium, manganese, mercury, molybdenum, niacin, nitrogen, ornithine, oxalic acid, oxycitronic acid, palmitic acid, pantothenic acid, pentosans, quercetin, raffinose, raphanol, riboflavin, salicylic acid, selenium, serine, β-sitosterol, stearic acid, strontium, thiamine, α-tocopherol, tricarballyl acid, vanillic acid, xylose, zinc, and zirconium (Duke 2001).
Taiwan velvet plant	Gynura formosana G. procumbens G. segetum	Root is hemostatic and vulnerary and is used to treat bleeding, bruises, furunculosis, hemorrhage, snakebite, and wounds. Whole plant decocted or crushed in white wine is used as a remedy for amenorrhea, epistaxis, hematemesis, hemoptysis, mastitis, and traumatic injuries (Duke and Ayensu 1985).
		Whole herb is used.
		It is slightly toxic. Taiwan velvet plant has functions of anti-inflammatory, antiswelling, blood purifying, and dispelling of stagnant blood. It is used to treat bronchitis, pulmonary tuberculosis, pertussis, sore eye, toothache, rheumatoid arthritis, and uterine bleeding. It is used externally to treat traumatic injury, fractures, bleeding wounds, mastitis, boils, and burn scalds (K. Lin 1998c).
Tao-tou	Canavalia gladiata	The young pods and beans are used as vegetables in tropical Asia.
		It contains canavanine, concanavalins A and B, canaline, and gibberellin. It is a tonic, used as bactericidal and fungicidal. It is also used to treat stomachache (T. Li 2006).
		Proximate principles, minerals, and vitamins can be found in this plant. It also has thiamine, riboflavin, and niacin. Vitamins B and K and tocopherol have been found in seeds (Patwardhan 1962).

English Name	Scientific Name	Nutritional and Therapeutic Values
		It has been reported that glutamic acid, aspartic acids, isoleucine + leucine, tyrosine + phenylalanine, and lysine are the major amino acids of *Canavalia gladiata* seed proteins. The presence of certain antinutritional factors is also reported (Rajaram and Janardhanan 1992).
Taro	*Colocasia antiquorum* var. *esculenta*	Taro's main constituent is sapotoxin. It is rich in protein, starch, and minerals.
		It is used as a poultice for bug bites, snakebite, swellings, and rheumatism (Perry 1980; Bliss 1973).
		Dried Colocasia leaf powder fed to rats resulted in a significant increase in total lipids, total cholesterol, and triglyceride levels in the cholesterol-fed rats.
		Liver cholesterol showed a slight reduction.
		It was concluded that Colocasia leaves had an aggravating effect on serum and tissue lipids in cholesterol-fed rats (Mani et al. 2005).
		A potential medicinal use of the cooked, mashed corm of taro (poi) is as a probiotic because it contains the predominant lactic acid bacteria. It is used as a remedy for diarrhea, gastroenteritis, irritable bowel syndrome, inflammatory bowel disease, cancer, depressed immune function, and inadequate lactase digestion (Brown and Valiere 2004).
Thousand-veined mustard	*Brassica juncea* var. *multiseps*	The plant contains behenic acid, benzyl isothiocyanate, eicosenoic and erucic acids, mustard oil, myrocin, sinapic acid, sinapine, and sinigrin (Jiangsu New Medical College 1979).
		It is antitumor and is used to relieve bladder inflammation and to stop hemorrhage (Perry 1980).
Tomato	*Lycopersicon esculentum*	The tomato plant contains protein, fat, carbohydrate, minerals such as calcium, phosphorus, and iron, carotene, thiamine, nicotinic acid, riboflavin, and ascorbic acid (Duke and Ayensu 1995).
		It also contains vitamins A and C, adenine, carotenoids, lycopene, tomatine, tomatidine, solanine, solanidine, and trigonelline. Carotenoids in tomatoes can reduce risks of breast cancer and prostate cancer and infection by certain viruses, can help in lowering blood pressure, and can be used to treat cloistral (Y. Chang 2000; Wagner 2002).
		Tomato is ranked among the top five vegetables in antioxidant activity assays (Easdown and Kalb 2004).
Turnip	*Brassica rapa* var. *rapa*	Turnip greens are considered valuable in the diet, primarily because of the content of minerals, calcium, and iron, and vitamins A, B, and C.

English Name	Scientific Name	Nutritional and Therapeutic Values
		In folk medicine, it is used for its antivinous, digestive, diuretic, emetic, laxative, refrigerant, and resolvent properties. Turnip is also used as a remedy for arthritis, colds, dysentery, hematochezia, mastitis, rheumatism, scurvy, skin ailments, sores, spasms, and warts (Duke and Ayensu 1985). It is also used as a remedy for arthritis, chest colds, fever, and flu (Duke and Wain 1981).
		Leaves contain protein, fat, carbohydrate, fiber, thiamine, and riboflavin. Roots contain ascorbic acid (Duke and Ayensu 1985).
Vegetable soybean	*Glycine max*	Vegetable soybean is highly nutritious and rich in phytochemicals and is considered to be a nutraceutical or a functional food crop (Messina 2001; Mentreddy et al. 2002).
		Fresh vegetable soybean contains protein (35–38 g/100 g dry wt.), monounsaturated fatty acid (5–7% fresh wt.) (Johnson et al. 1999), isoflavones (78–220 g/g dry wt.), and tocopherols (84–128 g/g dry wt.) (Mohamed et al. 2001).
		Vegetable soybean is rich in ascorbic acid and contains 60% more calcium, twice the phosphorus and potassium, and similar quantities of iron and vitamins B1 and B2 as green peas (Warner and Mounts 1990; Masuda 1991; Wei et al. 1995; S. Martin 2002; Messina 2001; Naim et al. 1974).
		Polyphenolic antioxidants were found to be isoflavones, chlorogenic acid isomers, caffeic acid, and ferulic acid (Pratt and Birac 1979).
Vegetable sponge	*Luffa cylindrica*	Fruits can be eaten, but the vine is most commonly grown for the fibrous matter, which is used as a sponge.
		It contains cucurbitacin B, vitamins B1 and C, xylan, mannagalactan, and rotenone. Two antitumor compounds, apigenin-7-glucoside and luteolin-7-glucoside, are the characteristic flavonoids of the leaves and flowers. Juice is used as a remedy for orchitis and skin diseases. Crushed fruit is used to treat abscesses, carbuncles, heat rash, and swellings. Fresh fruit is a tonic to the genitals (Duke and Ayensu 1985; Y. Chang 2000).
Wasabi	*Wasabia japonica*	Fresh wasabi is a highly prized culinary ingredient used mainly in restaurants and sushi bars.
		Its rhizome is used in Japan as a condiment like the root of common horseradish.
		It has a distinct flavor and pungency, derived from its singrin content, that is superior to common horseradish (Facciola 1990).

English Name	Scientific Name	Nutritional and Therapeutic Values
		The rhizome of this plant is applied as a remedy for neuralgic pain.
		It is also an effective antiseptic and a fragrant appetizer.
		It is eaten as a diuretic, and the juice is drunk as an antidote for fish poison.
		The root and stem contain allyl sinapic oil (Perry 1980).
		There have been two reports in the United States of serious adverse reactions to wasabi, involving paleness, confusion, profuse sweating, and collapse after eating a large serving. Both reports suggested that the response may be serious for those with weakened blood vessels in the heart or brain (Rinzler 1990).
Water bamboo shoot	*Zizania latifolia*	A perennial aquatic grass with a swollen stem base infected with the smut fungus. It is eaten as a vegetable by the Chinese. Young inflorescences can be cooked and used as a vegetable.
		Water bamboo is a very popular vegetable in China. The edible portion is the succulent stem after the husks are removed.
		The swollen stem is sliced and eaten cooked. Generally, it lacks nutrients (Yamaguchi 1990). Enlarged stems of water bamboo are harvested, the upper leaves cut off, and only the stem with husk-like wrapper leaves is sent to market.
		The edible portion is the succulent stem after the husks are removed (Yamaguchi 1990)It has low vitamin contents but is high in phosphate (36 mg/100 g) and carbohydrate (5.5 g/100 g) (Yamaguchi 1990).
		It is valued for its diuretic, febrifuge, and thirst-relieving properties (Perry 1980).
Water celery	*Oenanthe javanica*	A major vegetable in many parts of the Orient. The leaves are used as a seasoning in soups. The flavor is reminiscent of carrots or parsley. The best time to harvest is when the young shoots sprout from the root.
		The whole herb has anti-inflammatory, diuretic, and hypotensive properties. It is used as a remedy for colds, fever, tonsilitis, hypertension, diarrhea, and vomiting. The herb is used externally in treatment of parotitis, mastitis, and traumatic injury.
		Freshly mashed herb can be used as a poultice (K. Lin 1998e).

English Name	Scientific Name	Nutritional and Therapeutic Values
Water chestnut	*Eleocharis dulcis* *E. plantaginea*	Water chestnut is a popular ingredient in Western-style Chinese dishes. In China, they are most often eaten raw, sometimes sweetened. If eaten uncooked, the surface of the plants can transmit fascioliasis. Expressed juice of the tuber is bactericidal. It contains β-carotene, ascorbic acid, carbohydrate, puchiin, and albuminoids. It is used for abdominal pain, amenorrhea, anemia, inflammation, and malnutrition (Hartwell 1977).
Watercress	*Roripa nasturtium-aquaticum* *Nasturtium officinale*	The older leaves of watercress are compounds, with each leaf consisting of 3 to 11 smooth or wavy-edged, oval, or lance-shaped leaflets growing from a central stalk. Watercress is eaten as an antiscorbutic because of its high vitamin C content (Dobelis 1986).Folk medicinal uses for watercress include treatment of anemia, boils, liver disorders, tumors, and warts (Simon et al. 1984), as well as asthma, baldness, bronchitis, eczema, flu, goiter, hepatitis, impotence, polyps, scabies, scurvy, and tuberculosis (Duke 1984).Watercress is an extremely nutritious herb. It is a good dietary source of the vitamins A, B2, C, D, and E, nicotinamide, protein, and the minerals calcium, iodine, iron, manganese, and phosphorus (Chadwick 1985; Simon et al. 1984). It contains almost twice as much vitamin A as broccoli, and 100 g of raw stems and leaves has more calcium than half a glass of milk and as much vitamin C as an orange (Halpin 1978). Watercress contains phenethyl isothiocyanate. Watercress is used as a remedy for inflammation of the respiratory tract mucous membrane. Watercress is used topically as a remedy for arthritis, rheumatoid arthritis, earache, eczema, scabies, and warts. In folk medicine, watercress is used orally as a spring tonic, an appetite stimulant, and to improve digestion. It is also used orally to treat coughs, bronchitis, alopecia, cancer, flu, goiter, polyps, scurvy, tuberculosis, and gland tumors. It is used as an abortifacient, aphrodisiac, bactericide, laxative, restorative, stimulant, and anthelmintic (Jellin et al. 2003). For food uses, watercress is widely used in leaf salads and as a culinary spice.

English Name	Scientific Name	Nutritional and Therapeutic Values
		The applicable parts of watercress are the aboveground parts. It is thought to have antibiotic and diuretic activity (Gruenwald 1998). The leaves contain mustard oil, vitamin C, beta-carotene, and vitamin K (Brinker 1998).
Water dropwort	*Oenanthe stolonifera* *O. javanica*	Water dropwort contains Bis (2-ethyl butyl) phthalate, n-butyl-2-ethyl butyl phthalate, diethyl phthalate, myrcene, α-pinene, and terpinolene (Jiangsu New Medical College 1979).
		It is used as a remedy for cholera, cold, dysuria, fever, influenza, jaundice, and metrorrhagia and is considered to be antivinous and hemostatic (Perry 1980).
		Water dropwort contains α-pinene, myrcene, terpinolene, and diethyl phthalate (N. Chiu and Chang 1995a).
Water spinach	*Ipomoea aquatica*	Water spinach is a semiaquatic tropical plant grown as a leaf vegetable. Common names include water spinach and swamp cabbage.
		It grows in water or on moist oil.
		Besides minerals, it also contains hentriacontane, sitosterol, and sitosterol glycoside (Bliss 1973).
		It is a mild laxative and tonic, an antidote for certain types of food poisoning, and is used to treat certain diseases caused by unhealthy water and also intoxication.
		It has been reported that broth from cooking the vine with pork is taken to cure dropsy, general weakness, and leucorrhea. A decoction is a remedy for cough, cachexia, dropsy, and leucorrhea. Externally, it is applied as a dressing to swellings, contusions, and puerperal infections (Perry 1980).
White jute	*Corchorus capsularis*	White jute is high in protein. The dried leaves can be used as a thickener in soups. A tea is made from the dried leaves. Immature fruits are added to salads or used as a potherb.
		The leaves contain a glycoside, quercetin, and capsularin.
		The seeds contain two glycosides, corchorin and corchoritin. A decoction of the leaves is drunk to treat dysentery, consumptive cough, and as a bitter tonic for children. The leaves serve to poultice boils or abscesses and headache (Perry 1980).

English Name	Scientific Name	Nutritional and Therapeutic Values
		It also contains capsularin, cyanidin monoglycoside, β-sitosterol, D-glucoside, corchorol, capsularol, petunidin monoglycosides, corchoraside A, olitoriside, erysimoside, corcherosol, helueticoside, carcharitin, sucrose, raffinose, stachyose, and verbascose (N. Chiu and Chang 1995d). White jute is anti-inflammatory and hemostatic, and relieves summer heat functions. Seeds promotes circulation and are used as a cardiac tonic (K. Lin 1998e).
		Roots, leaves, and seeds are used for prevention of heat stroke and fever caused by heat. It is used to treat dysentery, hemoptysis, and hematemesis (K. Lin 1998e).
		The leaf and flower contain glycosides, capsularin, corchorin, corchoritin, aglycone, strophanthidin, digitoxigenin, coroloside, glucoevatromonoside, erysimoside, olitoriside, linoleic acid, corchoroside, helveticoside, corchotoxin, and oleic, palmitic, and stearic acids (Goda et al. 1998a, 1998b; Yoshikawa et al. 1998).
Winter melon	*Benincasa hispida Lagenaria dasistemon*	The plant contains minerals, thiamine, riboflavin, niacin, and ascorbic acid. It is diuretic and is used to treat diabetes, dropsy, renitis, and splenitis (Perry 1980; Hartwell 1971).
		Winter melon has diuretic and antiswelling functions. Seeds are used as an anti-inflammatory. It is an expectorant, used to treat cough, empyema, and appendicitis (K. Lin 1998f).
		The fruit and seed contain palmitic, stearic, and linoleic acids, thiamine, riboflavin, niacin, and ascorbic acid (Duke and Ayensu 1985).
Yam	*Dioscorea alata D. opposilla D. batatas decaisne*	Yam has steroidal sapogenin, allantoin, arginine, choline, glutamine, leucine, tyrosine, and diosgenin.
		It is anti-inflammatory and used in treatment for arthritis. It also has antitumor activity (Misaki et al. 1972; Y. Xue et al. 1998).
		Yam has dioscorenin, dioscorecin, dioscoretoxin, and diosbulbins A, B, and C (N. Chiu and Chang 1995c).
		It contains diosgenin, choline, dabscisin II, vitamin C, 3,4-dihydroxyphenylethylamine, dopamine, mannan, phytic acid, allantoin, arginine, diosbulbins B and C, and diosgenins A, B, and C (Ye 1999).

English Name	Scientific Name	Nutritional and Therapeutic Values
		Yam can be used as a tonic for spleen, stomach, and lungs and as a stomachic and digestive. It can also be used to alleviate lack of appetite, fatigue, diarrhea, leukorrhea, chronic coughs, nocturnal emissions, spermatorrhea, and frequent or scanty urination (Reid 1993, Gridly et al. 2001).

Note: This information should not be used for the diagnosis, treatment or prevention of diseases in humans. The information contained herein is in no way intended to be a guide to medical practice or a recommendation that herbs be used for medicinal purposes. The information is presented here mainly for educational purpose and should not be used to promote the sale of any product or replace the services of a physician.

2 Vitamins and Minerals of Vegetables

| Scientific Name | Protein (g)[a] | Fat (g)[a] | Sugar (g)[a] | Fiber (g)[a] | A (Re)[b] | Vitamins | | | | Minerals (mg)[a] | | | | | | |
						B$_1$ (mg)[a]	B$_2$ (mg)[a]	B$_6$ (mg)[a]	C (mg)[a]	Na	K	Ca	Mg	P	Fe	Zn
Allium cepa (onion)	1	0	9	0.5	0	0	0	0.02	5	0	50	25	11	30	0.3	0
Allium chinese (scallion)	1	...	4	2	15	...	0	...	35	20	...	2	0	160	...	0
Allium porrum (leek)	0.6	0	12.6	0.3	0	0	0	0	10	1	0	6	0	15	12	0
Allium sativum (garlic)	2.8	0	6.5	1.2	300	0	0.1	0.04	40	6	300	82	15	43	2.2	0
Allium schoenoprasum (chive)	2.7	1	...	...	...	0.1	0.1	...	32	...	...	83	...	41	0.8	...
Allium tuberosum (Chinese leek)	2	1	4.3	0.9	387	0	0.1	0.02	12	4	360	56	20	34	1.3	1
Amaranthus mangosteens (Chinese spinach)	3.7	1	4	3	1,600	0.1	0.24	...	65	80	...	10	...	560	15	...
Amaranthus viridis (slender amaranth)	2.2	1	1.9	0.6	214	0	0.1	0.01	15	25	530	156	37	54	4.9	0
Amorphophallus konjac (konjac)	0.1	0	2.3	0.1	...	...	...	...	...	...	...	17	...	7	0.3	...
Anisogonium esculentum (common bracken)	66.8	18	357	...	2,619	0.5	0.7	...	61.5	...	...	33	...	...	13	...
Anredera cordifolia (Malabar spinach)	25	2	52	8	18.1	...	...	...	19.5	979	38	29	...	...	36	...
Apium graveolens (celery)	0.9	0	3.1	0.7	71.7	0	0.14	0.01	7	71	320	66	11	31	0.9	0
Apium petroselinum (parsley)	2	...	4	2	60	...	...	...	130	35	...	8	...	330	20	...
Arctium lappa (great burdock)	2.5	0	27	5	...	0.25	0.1	...	2	30	180	50	...	58	1.2	6
Armoracia rusticana (horseradish)	1	1	2	...	...	...	...	...	30	0	...	...	...	85	...	...
Asparagus officinalis (asparagus)	2.3	0	4.9	0.7	81.7	0.16	0.1	0.06	16	6	220	11	11	48	0.6	1

Scientific Name	Protein (g)[a]	Fat (g)[a]	Sugar (g)[a]	Fiber (g)[a]	A (Re)[b]	B₁ (mg)[a]	B₂ (mg)[a]	B₆ (mg)[a]	C (mg)[a]	Na	K	Ca	Mg	P	Fe	Zn
Asplenium nidus (bird-nest fern)	...	...	...	...	...	...	...	...	...	...	...	...	...	...	...	...
Benincasa hispida (winter melon)	0.5	0	2.6	0.5	0	0	0	0.01	25	5	120	6	8	25	0.2	0
Beta vulgaris (beet)	30.7	5.8	50	21.7	31.6	0.67	1.58	2.5	...	...	...	3,330	...	368	25	...
Beta vulgaris var. *cicla* (leaf-beet)	1.8	1	4.5	1.3	610	0.1	0.15	0	25	0	0	38	0	28	105	0
Brassica chinensis (Chinese mustard)	1	0	2.1	0.4	236	0	0	0.03	40	40	240	106	15	37	1.4	0
Brassica juncea (leaf mustard)	0.8	1	3.4	0.5	66	0	0.1	0.01	34	35	180	98	12	25	1.4	0
Brassica oleracea (Chinese kale)	2.4	1	3.9	0.8	717	0	0	0	39	55	222	238	33	39	1.9	0
Brassica oleracea var. *botrytis* (broccoli)	2	0	4.2	0.8	1.2	0	0	0.08	73	17	240	28	11	36	0.4	0
Brassica oleracea var. *capitata* (Chinese broccoli)	1.2	0	4.4	0.5	11.7	0	0	0.07	33	17	150	52	11	28	0.3	0
Brassica oleracea var. *italica* (broccoli)	4.3	0	4.6	1.2	103.3	0.1	0.1	0.09	69	21	340	47	22	67	0.8	1
Brassica pekinensis (celery cabbage)	1.1	0	1.8	0.4	5	0	0	0.06	19	15	186	41	10	35	0.4	0
Brassica rapa (turnip)	1	0	2.1	0.4	236	0	0	0.03	40	40	240	106	15	37	1.4	0
Cajanus cajan (pigeon pea)	21.8	1	62.8	4	20	0.59	0.16	...	...	...	...	128	...	287	4.5	0
Canavalia ensiformis (sword bean)	23.2	3	54	65	...	1.13	0	...	...	...	...	190	...	434	12.5	...

| Scientific Name | Protein (g)[a] | Fat (g)[a] | Sugar (g)[a] | Fiber (g)[a] | A (Re)[b] | Vitamins | | | | Minerals (mg)[a] | | | | | | |
						B$_1$ (mg)[a]	B$_2$ (mg)[a]	B$_6$ (mg)[a]	C (mg)[a]	Na	K	Ca	Mg	P	Fe	Zn
Capsella bursa-pastoris (shepherd's purse)	35.6	4	44.1	10	...	2.12	1.44	...	305	...	3,939	1,763	...	729	41	...
Capsicum annuum var. *grossum* (pepper)	0.8	0	5.5	0.9	36.7	0	0	0.08	94	11	130	11	11	26	0.4	0
Capsicum annuum var. *longum* (bell pepper)	2.2	0	13.7	4.5	370	0.17	0.15	0	141	36	330	16	24	55	7.4	0
Chenopodium album (lamb's quarters)	4.2	1	...	...	11,600	0.16	0.44	...	80	...	...	309	...	72	1.2	...
Chrysanthemum coronarium (Japanese honewort)	1.8	1	1.7	0.5	503	0	0	0.08	7	53	390	40	16	25	3.3	1
Citrullus lanatus (watermelon)	7.8	2	85.9	6.3	...	0.5	0.6	...	...	...	1,351	125	...	141	4.7	...
Colocasia antiquorum (taro)	2	...	4	2	70	...	...	...	50	210	380	6	...	...	10	...
Colocasia esculenta (dasheen)	2.5	1	26.4	0.8	6.7	0	0	0.08	8.8	5	500	28	29	64	0.9	2
Corchorus capsularis (white jute)	6.6	5	2.1	0.3	1,950	0.1	...	...	...	...	...	93	...	170	...	2
Coriandrum sativum (coriander)	2.5	0	4.6	0.9	1,033	0	0	0.01	63	29	480	104	23	37	3	0
Cryptotaenia canadensis var. *japonica* (Japanese honewort)	2.8	3	0.4	3.6	6.63	0	0	0.01	176	26	400	222	70	61	7.8	1
Cucumis melo var. *conomon* (oriental pickling melon)	0.9	0	2	0.6	0	0	0	0	18	0	95	25	12	5	0.3	0

Scientific Name	Protein (g)[a]	Fat (g)[a]	Sugar (g)[a]	Fiber (g)[a]	A (Re)[b]	B_1 (mg)[a]	B_2 (mg)[a]	B_6 (mg)[a]	C (mg)[a]	Minerals (mg)[a]						
										Na	K	Ca	Mg	P	Fe	Zn
Cucumis sativus (cucumber)	0.9	0	3.4	0.4	28.3	0	0	0	8	8	90	16	10	13	0.2	0
Cucurbita pepo (pumpkin)	2.4	0	14.2	0.6	874	0.12	0	0.04	3	1	320	9	14	42	0.4	0
Cynara scolymus (globe artichoke)	2	...	17	2	...	...	...	...	6	0	...	...	...	430	20	...
Daucus carota var. sativa (carrot)	1	...	8	2	270	...	...	...	10	40	...	2	...	280	...	0
Dendrocalamus latiflorus (Ma bamboo)	2.4	0	3.6	0.6	0.7	0	0.1	0	3	8	280	9	9	31	0.4	0
Dioscorea alata (Chinese yam)	1.9	2	12.8	0.3	0	0	0	0	4.2	9	370	5	13	32	0.3	0
Dolichos lablab (hyacinth bean)	2.8	0	8.5	2	...	0.13	0.38	1	6	...	...	44	...	51	1.1	0
Eleocharis plantaginea (water chestnut)	2	0	18.8	0.7	4.7	0	0	0	7	25	450	4	12	64	0.7	0
Foeniculum vulgare (fennel)	2.9	1	17	7	1,566	0.12	0.15	...	34	...	338	0.5	...	54	2.9	...
Glycine max (vegetable soybean)	35.1	18	12.5	2.4	6	0.66	0.22	0.07	0	6	620	226	63	226	8.5	2
Gynura formosana (Taiwan velvet plant)	2	0	4.8	3.3	573	0.1	0.85	0.03	24.5	28	380	82	41	42	1.3	0
Helianthus annuus (sunflower)	26.8	39	25.8	4.4	0	0.92	0.22	1.26	1.2	637	536	45	445	726	8.6	7
Hemerocallis fulva (daylily)	2	0	...	...	3,000	0.16	0.21	...	88	24	170	87	...	176	1.2	...
Hibiscus esculentus (okra)	2.4	0	8.3	1	375	0	0.12	0.02	15	16	220	104	54	58	0.9	1

Scientific Name	Protein (g)[a]	Fat (g)[a]	Sugar (g)[a]	Fiber (g)[a]	A (Re)[b]	Vitamins B$_1$ (mg)[a]	B$_2$ (mg)[a]	B$_6$ (mg)[a]	C (mg)[a]	Na	K	Minerals (mg)[a] Ca	Mg	P	Fe	Zn
Hylocereus undatus (night-blooming cereus)	9	3	84.6	9	…	0.26	0.26	…	51.3	…	…	64	…	167	8.3	…
Ipomoea aquatica (water spinach)	1.4	0	4.3	0.8	378	0	0.1	0.03	14	52	440	78	21	37	1.5	1
Ipomoea batatas (leaf of sweet potato vine)	3.3	1	4.1	1	1,269	0	0	0.04	19	21	310	85	20	30	1.5	1
Lactuca indica (Indian lettuce)	1.5	0	1.8	0.7	575	0.1	0.1	0.01	13	0	250	36	18	30	202	0
Lactuca sativa (lettuce)	1.7	0	2.1	0.6	647	0.1	0.1	0.01	14	49	240	34	21	30	2.4	0
Lagenaria siceraria (hairy melon)	0.4	0	4.2	0.4	13.3	0.1	0.1	0.01	69	3	90	18	9	20	0.2	0
Lepidium sativum (cress)	2.6	…	…	…	9,300	0.1	0.26	…	12	…	…	81	…	76	1.3	…
Lilium tigrinum (lily bulbs)	2.4	0.04	6.8	0.4	…	…	…	…	…	…	42	72	…	…	3.2	…
Luffa aculangula (luffa)	1	0	3.4	0.4	…	0	0	0.05	6	…	60	10	9	26	0.2	0
Luffa cylindrica (vegetable sponge)	1	0.2	3.4	0.4	0	0.01	0.02	0.05	6	0	60	10	9	26	0.2	0.2
Lycium chinese (Chinese wolfberry)	12.4	1	72.9	7.8	10.1	0.92	0.39	0.65	9.5	490	1,243	78	69	156	15	1
Lycopersicon esculentum (tomato)	0.9	0	5.5	0.6	84.2	0	0	0.06	21	9	210	10	12	20	0.3	0
Malva verticillata var. *crispa* (Chinese mallow)	4.4	1	…	…	2,190	0.13	0.2	…	35	…	…	249	…	69	13	…
Manihot esculenta (cassava)	0.1	0	88	0.2	…	0	…	…	5.9	…	2.8	37	3	6	…	…
Medicago sativa (alfalfa)	6	0	…	…	3,410	0.13	0.14	…	162	…	…	12	…	51	5.4	…
Mentha arvensis (mint)	3	1	…	…	1,296	0.13	0.16	…	64	2	179	194	…	48	3.8	…

Scientific Name	Protein (g)[a]	Fat (g)[a]	Sugar (g)[a]	Fiber (g)[a]	A (Re)[b]	B$_1$ (mg)[a]	B$_2$ (mg)[a]	B$_6$ (mg)[a]	C (mg)[a]	Minerals (mg)[a]						
										Na	K	Ca	Mg	P	Fe	Zn
Monochoria vaginalis (ducks tongue grass)	5.4	2.5	18.8	4.6	5,290	0.13	0.11	16.2	10	...	...	601	...	30	7.6	...
Momordica charantia (bitter gourd)	0.8	0	3.7	0.6	2.3	0	0	0.06	19	11	160	24	14	41	0.3	0
Morus alba (mulberry)	0.4	30	...	...	0	0.03	0.06	0.7	5	37	152	32	...	3.7	...	...
Nasturtium officinale (watercress)	1	...	1	1	30	...	...	...	25	15	...	4	...	110	...	...
Nelumbo nucifera (lotus)	23.8	1	56.6	3.1	0.4	0.16	0.22	0.18	44	589	437	166	203	667	1.7	2
Ocimum basilicum (sweet basil)	...	...	...	1.2	281.2	...	...	0.48	1.84	...	1	63	13	...	1.3	...
Oenanthe javanica (water celery)	0.8	0.05	1.6	0.7	942	0.02	0.04	0	8	0.5	0.8	34	0	19	1.5	0
Oenanthe stolonifera (water dropwort)	0.2	0.03	1.3	1.28	24	0.64	2.34	10.6	149	192	4,713	1,202	...	585	32	...
Peucedanum sativum (parsnip)	1	...	18	5	...	...	...	...	30	10	...	4	...	380	4	...
Phaseolus angularis (adzuki bean)	19.9	1	64.4	7.8	...	0.1	0.1	...	2	...	...	260	...	9.8	0	...
Phaseolus calcaratus (red bean)	20.8	3	64.9	2.8	...	1	0.1	0.35	1.1	35	1,033	64	161	462	7.8	4
Phaseolus coccineus var. *albanians* (white Dutch runner bean)	1.9	1	63.1	3.8	1.1	0.29	0.12	0.81	1.7	30	930	8.9	161	456	19	29
Phaseolus limensis var. *albanians* (white Dutch runner bean)	8.7	0	18.3	1.6	7.3	0.1	0	0.08	22	8	680	19	71	140	14	1
Phaseolus sureus (mung bean)	19.9	1	64.4	7.8	...	0.1	0.1	...	2	...	...	136	...	260	9.8	...

Scientific Name	Protein (g)ᵃ	Fat (g)ᵃ	Sugar (g)ᵃ	Fiber (g)ᵃ	A (Re)ᵇ	Vitamins B₁ (mg)ᵃ	B₂ (mg)ᵃ	B₆ (mg)ᵃ	C (mg)ᵃ	Na	K	Minerals (mg)ᵃ Ca	Mg	P	Fe	Zn
Phaseolus vulgaris (kidney bean)	1.9	0	7	0.8	0	0.1	0.1	0.03	13	8	20	41	23	45	0.6	1
Phyllostachys makinoi (Makino bamboo)	2.9	0	3	1.4	30	0.16	0.1	...	7	...	...	15	...	71	1.1	...
Phyllostachys pubescens (Moso bamboo)	3.2	0	4.8	1.1	...	0.11	0.13	...	17	...	...	25	...	55	0.4	...
Pisum sativum (pea)	3.2	0	9	0.8	85.8	0.14	0.1	0.04	54	5	160	46	25	68	0.9	1
Portulaca oleracea (purslane)	1.2	0	1.19	1.4	426	0	...	0.08	6.8	94	170	54	62	23	1.3	0
Psophocarpus tetragonolobus (Goa bean)	2.9	0	3.5	2.5	6.5	0.54	0.3	...	13	56	120	330	204	276	1.8	0
Pueraria lobata (kudzu)	2.1	0	...	...	...	0.03	0.91	0.8	...	2	...	15	...	18	0.6	...
Raphanus sativus (leaf of Chinese radish)	5.2	0.1	27.8	0.79	3,000	0.4	0.02	0	22	0	0	290	0	30	1.4	0
Rheum rhaponticum (rhubarb)	1	2	6	...	2	...	...	...	15	0	...	10	...	350	...	...
Rorippa nasturtium-aquaticum (watercress)	1	...	1	1	30	...	...	...	25	15	...	4	...	110	...	...
Saccharum officinarum (sugarcane)	...	...	99.4	...	...	...	0	0.03	5.5	3	61	6	11	1	...	0
Sagittaria sinensis (arrowhead)	4.4	0	24.8	0.4	...	1.6	0.4	...	5	...	729	13	...	165	2.6	...
Solanum melongena (eggplant)	1.3	0	4.7	0.9	3.3	0.1	0	0.02	6	4	200	18	14	28	0.4	0
Solanum nigrum (black nightshade)	0.8	0	3.4	0.7	792	0.1	0.17	0.07	35	32	340	238	60	41	6.7	0

Scientific Name	Protein (g)[a]	Fat (g)[a]	Sugar (g)[a]	Fiber (g)[a]	A (Re)[b]	B$_1$ (mg)[a]	B$_2$ (mg)[a]	B$_6$ (mg)[a]	C (mg)[a]	Minerals (mg)[a]						
										Na	K	Ca	Mg	P	Fe	Zn
Solanum tuberosum (potato)	2.7	0	16.5	0.4	0	0.1	0	0.06	25	5	300	3	25	48	0.5	1
Spinacia oleracea (spinach)	2.1	1	3	0.8	638	0.1	0.1	0.01	9	54	460	77	58	45	2.1	1
Stachys sieboldii (Chinese artichoke)	4	0	13	7	4	...	...	...	25	...	...	6	...	...	10	...
Talinum paniculatum (coral flower)	1.6	2	2.2	2.8	577	0	0	0.01	8.7	17	330	62	84	28	4.2	0
Taraxacum officinale (dandelion)	2.7	1	...	...	14,000	0.19	0.26	...	35	76	397	187	...	66	3.1	...
Toona sinensis (Chinese mahogany)	4.3	2	19.4	2.8	1,222	0.12	0	0.02	255	17	400	514	67	126	2.7	1
Trichosanthes anguina (snake gourd)	1.4	0	3.2	0.6	20	0.1	0	0.04	8.5	22	200	25	15	31	0.9	0
Trigonella foenum-graecum (fenugreek)	2.32	0.08	10	0.98	19	...	...	...	221	...	...	...	...	...	...	...
Vicia faba (broad bean)	31.8	16	45.7	3.3	1.3	0	0.1	0.07	0.1	337	740	58	90	376	3.6	3
Vigna sinensis var. *sesquipedalis* (asparagus bean)	2.2	0	6.1	1	38.3	0.1	0.1	0.04	22	3	160	27	29	42	0.8	1
Wasabia japonica (wasabi)	1.7	0.2	4.3	0.7	1,835	0.06	0.12	0.6	75	...	330	56	87	34	1.0	3
Zanthoxylum ailanthoides (ailanthus)	119	0	23.8	0.9	2,410	0.41	0.1	0.02	116.8	5	640	721	58	77	229	1
Zea mays (sweet corn)	3.5	1	22.1	0.7	400	0.15	0.12	0	12	0	0	3	0	111	0.7	0
Zingiber officinale (ginger)	0	0	4.8	0.5	3.3	0	0	1.03	11	12	270	14	15	22	0.4	0

Scientific Name	Protein (g)[a]	Fat (g)[a]	Sugar (g)[a]	Fiber (g)[a]	A (Re)[b]	B$_1$ (mg)[a]	B$_2$ (mg)[a]	B$_6$ (mg)[a]	C (mg)[a]	Na	K	Ca	Mg	P	Fe	Zn
										Minerals (mg)[a]						
						Vitamins										
Zizania aquatica (water bamboo shoot)	1.5	0	4.3	0.6	0.7	0.1	0	0	6.4	10	180	4	9	43	0.3	0

Sources: Xue, C. X. 2001a. *The encyclopedia of vegetables and fruits in Taiwan.* Vol. 1. Taipei: Taiwan Pu-Lu Publ. Co. (in Chinese); Xue, C. X. 2001b. *The encyclopedia of vegetables and fruits in Taiwan.* Vol. 2. Taipei: Taiwan Pu-Lu Publ. Co. (in Chinese); Duke, J. A., and E. S. Ayensu. 1985. *Medicinal plants of China.* 2 vols. Algonac, MI: Reference Publications.

Note: The information presented here is mainly for educational purposes and should not be used to promote the sale of any product.

3 Flavonoid, Isoflavone, and Carotenoid Contents in Raw Vegetables

Crop	Flavonoid Name & Contents (mg/100 g)		Isoflavone Name & Contents (mg/100 g)		Carotenoid Name & Contents (µg/100 g)	
	Name	Avg.	Name	Avg.	Name	Avg.
Alfalfa sprout (*Medicago sativa*)	⋯	⋯	Isoflavone	0	⋯	⋯
Asparagus (*Asparagus officinalis*)	⋯	⋯	⋯	⋯	a-car	12
					b-car	493
Bean (tao-tou) (*Canavalia gladiata; C. ensiformis*)	Kaempferol	0.42	Isoflavone	0	a-car	68
	Quercetin	3.03			b-car	377
					b-cryp	0
					lut + zea	640
					lye	0
Broad bean (immature) (*Vicia faba*)	(−)-Epicatechin	22.51	Daidzein	0.02	⋯	⋯
	(−)-Epigallocatechin	14.03	Genistein	0.01	⋯	⋯
	(+)-Catechin	12.83	Total isoflavone	0.03	⋯	⋯
Broccoli (Chinese) (*Brassica oleracea* var. *capitata*)	⋯	⋯	⋯	⋯	a-car	1
	⋯	⋯	⋯	⋯	b-car	779
	⋯	⋯	⋯	⋯	b-cryp	0
	⋯	⋯	⋯	⋯	lut + zea	2,445
	⋯	⋯	⋯	⋯	lye	0
Cabbage (Chinese) (*Brassica chinensis*)	Apigenin	0.01	⋯	⋯	⋯	⋯
	Luteolin	0.06	⋯	⋯	⋯	⋯
	Kaempferol	0.37	⋯	⋯	⋯	⋯
	Quercetin	0.01	⋯	⋯	⋯	⋯
Carrot (*Daucus carota* var. *sativa*)	Quercetin	0.07	⋯	⋯	a-car	10,650
	⋯	⋯	⋯	⋯	b-car	18,250

Crop	Flavonoid Name & Contents (mg/100 g)		Isoflavone Name & Contents (mg/100 g)		Carotenoid Name & Contents (μg/100 g)	
	Name	Avg.	Name	Avg.	Name	Avg.
Cauliflower (*Brassica oleracea* var. *botrytis*)	...	...	...	...	b-cryp	0
	...	...	...	...	lut + zea	0
	...	...	...	...	lye	0
	Luteolin	0.08	...	...	...	...
	Kaempferol	0.25	...	...	...	...
	Quercetin	0.03	...	...	...	...
Celery (*Apium graveolens*)	Apigenin	4.61	...	...	a-car	0
	Luteolin	1.31	...	...	b-car	150
	Quercetin	3.5	...	...	b-cryp	0
	...	...	...	...	lut + zea	232
	...	...	...	...	lye	0
Chive (*Allium schoenoprasum*)	Luteolin	0.15	...	...	...	...
	Isorhamnetin	6.75	...	...	...	...
	Kaempferol	10	...	...	...	...
	Quercetin	4.77	...	...	...	...
Corn (*Zea mays*)	Flavonoid	0	...	...	...	...
Cucumber (*Cucumis sativus*)	Kaempferol	0.06	...	...	b-car	138
	Quercetin	0.04	...	...	...	...
Endive (*Cichorium endivia*)	Kaempferol	4.04	...	...	b-car	960
Gourd (bottle gourd) (*Lagenaria siceraria*)	Luteolin	0.01	...	...	...	...
	Myricetin	0.13	...	...	...	...

Crop	Flavonoid Name & Contents (mg/100 g)		Isoflavone Name & Contents (mg/100 g)		Carotenoid Name & Contents (µg/100 g)	
	Name	Avg.	Name	Avg.	Name	Avg.
Kale (Chinese) (*Brassica o leracea*)	Quercetin	0.03	...	...	...	...
	Apigenin	0.01	...	...	a-car	0
	Myricetin	0.01	...	...	b-car	9,226
	Quercetin	0.07	...	...	b-cryp	0
	...	...	...	...	lut + zea	39,550
					lye	0
Leek (*Allium porrum*)	Kaempferol	2.95	...	...	...	...
Lettuce (butterhead) (*Lactuca sativa*)	Kaempferol	0.02	...	...	a-car	0
	Quercetin	1.19	...	...	b-car	1,272
	...	...	...	...	b-cryp	0
	...	...	...	...	lut + zea	2,635
					lye	0
Onion (*Allium cepa*)	Isorhamnetin	1.91	...	...	a-car	6
	Kaempferol	0.18	...	...	b-car	391
	Quercetin	13.27	...	...	...	...
Parsley (*Apium petroselinum*)	Apigenin	302	...	...	...	...
	Luteolin	1.24	...	...	...	...
	Kaempferol	0.44	...	...	...	...
	Myricetin	8.08	...	...	...	...
	Quercetin	0.33	...	...	...	...
Parsnip (*Peucedanum sativum, Pustinaca sativa*)	Quercetin	0.99	...	...	...	...
Pea (edible-podded) (*Pisum sativum*)	Flavonoid	0	...	...	...	...
Pepper (green) (*Capsicum annuum*)	Luteolin	0.69	...	...	...	...

Crop	Flavonoid Name & Contents (mg/100 g)		Isoflavone Name & Contents (mg/100 g)		Carotenoid Name & Contents (µg/100 g)	
	Name	Avg.	Name	Avg.	Name	Avg.
Pepper (hot chili) (*Capsicum annuum* var. *longum*; *C. fructescens*)	Quercetin	0.65	…	…	…	…
	Luteolin	5.11	…	…	…	…
Pepper (red) (*Capsicum annuum*)	Quercetin	16.8	…	…	…	…
	Luteolin	0.63	…	…	…	…
Potato (*Solanum tuberosum*)	Kaempferol	0.05	…	…	…	…
Radish (Chinese) (*Raphanus sativus*)	Kaempferol	0.86	…	…	…	…
Rhubarb (stalks) (*Rheum rhaponticum*)	(−)-Epicatechin	0.51	…	…	…	…
	(−)-Epicatechin 3-gallate	0.6	…	…	…	…
	(+)-catechin	2.17	…	…	…	…
Soybean (*Glycine max*)	Daidzein	46.64	Genistein	73.76	Clycitein	10.88
	Total isoflavone	128.35	…	…	…	…
Soybean (vegetable) (*Glycine max*)	…	…	Daidzein	34.52	…	…
	…	…	Genistein	64.78	…	…
	…	…	Clycitein	13.78	…	…
	…	…	Total isoflavone	118.51	…	…
Spinach (*Spinacia oleracea*)	Luteolin	1.11	…	…	a-car	0
	Kaempferol	0.01	…	…	b-car	5,507
	Myricetin	0.01	…	…	b-cryp	0
	Quercetin	4.86	…	…	lut + zea	11,938
	…	…	…	…	lye	0

Crop	Flavonoid Name & Contents (mg/100 g)		Isoflavone Name & Contents (mg/100 g)		Carotenoid Name & Contents (µg/100 g)	
	Name	Avg.	Name	Avg.	Name	Avg.
Sweet potato (leaves) (*Ipomoea batatas*)	Apigenin	0.12	…	…	a-car	0
	Luteolin	0.2	…	…	b-car	9,180
	Myricetin	9.74	…	…	b-cryp	0
	Quercetin	20.54	…	…	lut + zea	0
	…	…	…	…	lye	0
Tomato (*Lycopersicon esculentum*)	Kaempferol	0.07	…	…	a-car	0
	Quercetin	0.57	…	…	b-car	186
	…	…	…	…	b-cryp	0
	…	…	…	…	lut + zea	40
	…	…	…	…	lye	9,708
Turnip greens (*Brassica rapa* var. *rapa*)	Kaempferol	4.8	…	…	…	…
	Quercetin	0.73	…	…	…	…
Watercress (*Rorippa nasturtium-aquaticum*; *Nasturtium officinale*)	Kaempferol	1	…	…	…	…
	Quercetin	4	…	…	…	…
Water spinach (*Ipomoea aquatica*)	Apigenin	0.01	…	…	…	…
	Luteolin	0.04	…	…	…	…
	Myricetin	0.03	…	…	…	…
	Quercetin	0.18	…	…	…	…

Source: USDA. 2003. Database for the flavonoid content of selected foods. http://www.nal.usda.gov/fnic/foodcomp.

Note: The information presented here is mainly for educational purposes and should not be used to promote the sale of any product.

4 Nutritional and Therapeutic Values of Fruits

English Name	Scientific Name	Nutritional and Therapeutic Values
Abiu	*Pouteria caimito*	The fruit pulp, because of its mucilaginous nature, is eaten to relieve coughs, bronchitis, and other pulmonary complaints. The latex is given as a vermifuge and purge and is applied on abscesses. Triterpenes have been extracted from *Pouteria caimito* (Pellicciari et al. 1972).
		Seed contains saponin, pouterin, a bitter principle (lucumin), and a fixed oil. Leaves contain an amorphous bitter principle and some alkaloid. Latex is used for abscesses, and dried latex is used as an anthelmintic.
		Fruit is used for diabetes. Seeds are used as a tonic for diarrhea and fever. Plant is used in Philippine alternative medicine (www.stuartxchange.org).
Acerola	*Malpighia glabra* var. *florida*	Eaten as a dessert. The fruits may be made into syrup or, with added pectin, into jelly, jam, and other preserves. The acerola fruit is one of the richest natural sources of vitamin C, with about 1.7 g per 100 g of pitted fruit (D. Singh 2006).
		It can be used in the diet of individuals allergic to citrus fruits (www.mercksource.com). Acerola contains anthocyanin and cyanidin-3-glucoside (Einbond et al. 2004).
		Acerola is a folk remedy for breast ailments, diarrhea, dysentery, fever, headache, hepatitis, tenesmus, and sore throat. The juice can be gargled for sore throat. Many of acerola's folk-medicine attributes probably stem from the high vitamin C content (Duke and duCellier 1993).
Apple, paradise apple	*Malus domestica* *M. pumila*	Fruit is used to dispel gas, dissolve mucus, and cure flux; it is also used as a tonic for anemia, bilious disorders, and colic. The seeds contain amygdalin, glucoside, phlorizin, pectin, pectic acid, tannins, essential oils, quercetin, isoquercitrin, and ursolic, oleanolic, pomolic, pomonic, and p-coumaric acids (Duke and Ayensu 1985).
		The bark and root bark are used as an anthelmintic, refrigerant, and soporific. An infusion is used in the treatment of intermittent, remittent, and bilious fevers (Chopra et al. 1986).
		Flavonoids in apple may play an important role in preventing cancer. The flavonoid quercetin can inhibit the growth of colon and prostate cancer cells, and eating quercetin-rich fruits may reduce the risk of lung cancer by 50%. Flavonoids may also reduce the risk of heart disease and stroke.

English Name	Scientific Name	Nutritional and Therapeutic Values
		The bark and roots contain phloretin, an antibioticlike compound that acts on certain bacteria (Rieger 2006). There is insufficient reliable information to rate the effectiveness of apple for other uses (Jellin et al. 2003).
		However, there is some preliminary evidence that increasing apple consumption might decrease the risk of developing lung cancer (Le Marchand et al. 2000).
		There is also some preliminary evidence that apple juice used orally for seven days, with olive oil used on the seventh day before going to bed, might be effective for softening the passage and collection of gallstones in the stool (Dekkers 1999).
		The pectin in apples probably accounts for their effect on diarrhea and constipation. Pectin absorbs water in the gastrointestinal tract and swells to a gummy mass. The mass provides bulk, which tends to normalize bowel function. Apples also contain phloretin, which has antibacterial activity.
		There is some evidence that consuming five or more apples per week can improve lung function as measured by maximum forced expiration in one second (Butland et al. 2000).
		The constituent quercetin is an antioxidant flavonoid found in high concentrations in apples (Butland et al. 2000). Quercetin is thought to be responsible for the potential benefit of apples in preventing lung cancer (Le Marchand et al. 2000).
		It was reported that the fruits of Malus pumila are a tonic for anemia and a remedy for bilious diseases and colic (Perry 1980).
Apricot	Prunus armeniaca Armeniaca vulgaris	Seeds contain toxic compounds, amygdalin, prunasin, and mandelonitrile. Seeds have antitussive, expectorant, and sedative properties for asthma, bronchitis, colds, constipation, cough, and tumors. It is also considered to be anthelmintic, antispasmodic, demulcent, pectoral, and vulnerary (Duke and Ayensu 1985).
		Apricot is rich in beta-carotene, a potent antioxidant. Chemical compounds, cyanogenic glycosides, and laetrile were isolated from seeds, bark, and leaves, a purported alternative treatment for cancer. Apricots are considered to have an aphrodisiac function (http://en.wikipedia.org/wiki/Apricot).
		Apricot seeds are medicinal, with purgative and emetic properties (Gucla et al. 2006). It stimulates the respiratory center reflexively and produces a tranquilizing effect (F. Chen 1997).

English Name	Scientific Name	Nutritional and Therapeutic Values
		Apricot leaves, flowers, seeds, and bark contain toxic compounds that generate cyanide, which is highly toxic. However, in plant tissues, the cyanide concentration is low enough to be considered therapeutic, particularly for cancer treatment (Rieger 2006).
		Apricot oil was used against tumors and ulcers in England. Seeds contain the highest amounts of cyanide-generating compounds and the controversial cancer drug laetrile. Phloretin is an antibioticlike compound found in bark and root extracts. It was reported that phloretin may kill certain types of bacteria (Rieger 2006).
		Seeds contain amygdalin and hydrocyanic acid for use as an astringent, stomachic, and antipyretic (Keys 1976).
		Kernels contain amygdalin, prunasin, fatty acids, and mandelonitrile. The enzyme amygdalase can hydrolyze amygdalin to produce cyanic acid. It is used to stimulate the respiratory center reflexively and to produce a tranquilizing effect (F. Chen 1997).
		In Chinese medicine, very small amounts of toxic kernel constituent (hydrocyanic acid, a source of HCN) is used orally for asthma, cough, and constipation. In folk medicine, apricot is used orally for hemorrhage, infertility, eye inflammation, spasm, and vaginal infections. Historically, laetrile, the semisynthetic derivative of the amygdalin constituent, has been fraudulently acclaimed as a cancer treatment (Jellin et al. 2003).
		In manufacturing, apricot oil is used in cosmetics or as a vehicle for pharmaceutical preparations (Jellin et al. 2003).
		The applicable parts of apricot are the kernel and oil. Apricot contains fruit acids, a variety of sugars, vitamins C and K, β-carotene, thiamine, niacin, and iron. The seed contains the glycoside amygdalin (Jellin et al. 2003).
		Several popular theories that have now been disproved claimed preferential uptake and conversion of amygdalin to hydrogen cyanide in tumor cells. Actually, research shows that amygdalin is slowly hydrolyzed to HCN in the stomach, rapidly absorbed via the gastrointestinal tract, and then diffused throughout the body (Newall et al. 1996).

English Name	Scientific Name	Nutritional and Therapeutic Values
Atemoya	*Annona (atemoya)*	Fruits can be eaten fresh or used for many types of desserts such as milkshakes and ice cream. Atemoya looks very similar in some cases to sugar apple. The bark contains alkaloids, muricine, muricinine, and anonaine. The seeds contain alkaloid, and the leaves have an essential oil, a resin, potassium chloride, and tannin. The crushed leaves are used as a remedy for distention and dyspepsia. The young fruits contain tannin, which is used to treat diarrhea and dysentery (Perry 1980).
		Atemoyacin E, a bis-tetrahydrofuran annonaceous acetogenin, is extracted from *Annona atemoya* seeds (P. Wu et al. 2001). It is used in folk medicine, probably due to the bioactive compounds found in the roots, leaves, bark, fruits, and seeds. Flavonoids present in the seeds, roots, bark, stem, and fruits are potential chemopreventive agents, given evidence that they decrease tumor incidence (Pinto et al. 2005).
Avocado	*Persea americana*	The avocado fruit is an important food in South America and is nutritious, with high levels of mainly unsaturated oils, minerals, vitamins (A, B, C, D, and E), and protein.
		Avocado is used for labial tumors. It is also reported to be abortifacient, antibiotic, antifertility, aperient, aphrodisiac, diuretic, emmenagogue, and vermifuge. A leaf decoction is taken for diarrhea, sore throat, and hemorrhage (Duke and duCellier 1993). The fruit skin is antibiotic and is employed as a vermifuge and remedy for dysentery. The leaves are chewed as a remedy for pyorrhea. Heated leaves are applied on the forehead to relieve neuralgia. Seeds contain tannin as well as myristic, palmitic, stearic, oleic, linoleic, and linolenic acids. Unripe avocados are said to be toxic (Morton 1987c).
		Unripe avocado fruit has activity against six human tumor cell lines in culture and shows selectivity for human prostate adenocarcinoma cells, being nearly as potent as adriamycin (Oberlies et al. 1998).
		It has been reported that avocado can help reduce cholesterol (Duke 1997). The avocado fruit is used to reduce serum cholesterol levels. Avocado oil is applied topically to soothe and heal skin and to treat sclerosis of the skin, pyorrhea, and arthritis. The fruit pulp is used topically to promote hair growth and hasten wound healing.

English Name	Scientific Name	Nutritional and Therapeutic Values
		In folk medicine, avocado fruit has been used as an aphrodisiac and to stimulate menstrual flow. The seeds, leaves, and bark have been used to treat dysentery and diarrhea and to relieve toothache (Jellin 2003). The applicable parts of avocado are the fruit, leaves, and seeds. The cholesterol-lowering and skin-soothing effects may be due to the high content of unsaturated fatty acids and other compounds in avocado (Jellin 2003).
Banana	*Musa sapientum* *M. paradisiaca*	The common banana is eaten raw as a dessert fruit. It is also dried and made into flour. The shoots and leaves contain protein, fat, carbohydrate, fiber, minerals, and vitamins. Banana pulp contains serotonin, norepinephrine, and dopamine. Its high potassium content makes the banana useful in treatment of high blood pressure (Duke and duCellier 1993). All parts of the banana plant have medicinal applications. The flower is used in treatment of bronchitis and dysentery and on ulcers. The unripe peel and the leaves are taken in treatment of dysentery and diarrhea and are used to treat malignant ulcers. Antifungal and antibiotic principles are found in the peel and pulp of fully ripe bananas (Morton 1987b).
		It was reported that banana lipids did not affect the concentration of serum cholesterol. Feeding of dopamine, n-epinephrine, and serotonin tended to raise the concentration of serum cholesterol (Horigone et al. 1992).
		Freeze-dried banana pulp showed a marked cholesterol-lowering effect when incorporated into a diet at the level of 300 or 500 g/kg, while the banana pulp dried in a hot-air current (65°C) did not (Horigone et al. 1992). Banana contains vitamin A, B, C, and E. It also has serotonin, noradrenaline, dopamine, and muscarin (Y. Chang 2000).
		Banana contains potassium, physiologically active compounds, serotonin, norepinephrine, and dopamine. Some extracts have shown hypoglycemic activity in lab studies. It can be used to treat ailments of the skin, back, and blood; headaches, fever, and flu; and diarrhea and constipation (Rieger 2006).
		The root, trunk juice, and flower contain serotonin and norepinephrine, which are used to treat carbuncles, tumors, swelling, measles, headache with fever, and sunburn. It is also used to stimulate the smooth muscle of the infecting, and to treat certain forms of heat collapse (Perry and Metzger 1980).

English Name	Scientific Name	Nutritional and Therapeutic Values
Barbados cherry	*Malpighia glabra* var. *florida* *M. emarginata*	The fruit of acerola is one of the richest natural sources of vitamin C (about 1.7 g per 100 g of pitted fruit) (D. Singh 2006). It can be used in the diet of individuals allergic to citrus fruits (see www. mercksource.com). It contains anthocyanin and cyanidin-3-glucoside (Einbond et al. 2004). A crude acerola polyphenol (C-AP) fraction appeared to have an inhibitory effect on alpha-glucosidase and, particularly, on maltase activities.
		The results of an experiment to elucidate the antihyperglycemic effect of crude acerola polyphenol indicated that C-AP significantly suppressed the plasma glucose level after administering both glucose and maltose. Results also suggested that C-AP had a preventive effect on hyperglycemia in the postprandial state. The mechanism for this effect is considered to have been both the suppression of intestinal glucose transport and the inhibition of alpha-glucosidase (Hanamura et al. 2006).
		It is a folk remedy for breast ailments, diarrhea, dysentery, fever, headache, hepatitis, tenesmus, and sore throat. The juice may be gargled for sore throat. Many of acerola's folk medicine attributes probably stem from the high vitamin C content (Duke and duCellier 1993).
Betel nut	*Areca catechu*	It is known commonly as betel palm or betel nut tree.
		The nut and leaves contain arecoline, arecaine, areca red, catechin, homoarecoline, arecolidine, guvacoline, and guvacine. Seeds contain arecoline, arecaidine, guvacine, guvacoline, and leucocyanidin. Betel nut is used to treat taeniasis and is also used as an insecticide, antifungal, and virus.
		The leaves have anticarcinogenic agents; the nut has cholinomimetic and acetylcholine sterase inhibitory constituents (T. Li 2006). It was reported that waist size was strongly related to betel usage, independent of other factors such as age. Betel use interacted with sex, relating to increasing glycemia only in females, since waist size and age were the major markers of increasing glycemia. It is suggested that betel chewing, a habit common to about 10% of the world population, may contribute to the risk of developing type 2 diabetes mellitus (Mannan et al. 2000).
		The fruit contains arecoline, arecaine, guvacine, guvacoline, arecoline, homoarecoline, areca red, and catching (N. Chiu and Chang 1995b). It contains arecoline, arecolidine, guvacoline, and guvacine. Betel nut is used to treat throat taeniasis (Huang 1999).

English Name	Scientific Name	Nutritional and Therapeutic Values
Bilimbe	*Averrhoa carambola*	Betel nut also contains lauric, myristic, palmitic, stearic, oleic, linoleic, capric, dodecanoic, and tetradecanoic acids. Amino acids include proline, tyrosine, phenylalanine, and arginine. Juice from the fruit contains catechin and leucoanthocyanidin (Huang 1999).
		The star fruit is a uniquely flavorful fruit. The fruit's flavor ranges from very sour to mildly sweetish and tastes something like a mix of apple, pineapple, and kiwifruit. Medicinally, bilimbe has numerous functions, including vermifuge, laxative, refrigerant, antiscorbutic, febrifuge, sialogogue, antiphlogistic, stimulant, emmenagogue, anodyne, and emetic properties.
		This edible fruit is a source of iron and vitamins B1, B2, and C, oxalate and potassium (N. Chiu and Chang 1995a).
		In folkloric medicine, a tea of boiled leaves is used for aphthous stomatitis.
		Crushed shoots or leaves are used externally for headaches and ringworm. Seed is used for asthma and colic (www.stuartxchange.org).
Biriba	*Rollinia mucosa*	The fruit is regarded as refrigerant, analeptic, and antiscorbutic. The powdered seeds are said to be a remedy for enterocolitis. It contains vitamins, methionine, threonine, tryptophan, and lysine (Morton 1987b).
		Biriba produces furofuranic lignans (magnolin, epiyangambin, yangambin) that are antagonists of platelet-activating factor (Figueiredo et al. 1999).
Bitter orange	*Citrus aurantium*	In China, bitter orange juice and peel have been used as a digestive tonic. It soothes gas and bloating in the stomach.
		In Chinese medicine, it is an expectorant with laxative properties. The juice can be used as medicine for cough. The roots and leaves are taken as an astringent drink to treat dysentery (Perry 1980).
		Bitter orange extract is a noncentrally acting sympathicomimetic agent, which when combined with caffeine and St. John's wort — as well as caloric restriction and exercise — can induce weight loss to a greater extent than diet and exercise alone (Colker et al. 1999).

English Name	Scientific Name	Nutritional and Therapeutic Values
Black nightshade	*Solanum nigram*	Leaf, root, and stalk are used for cancerous sores, leucoderma, and wounds. Young shoots eaten as potherb are considered a tonic for virility in men and for dysmenorrhea in females. They are also used for dysentery, sore throat, and whitlow. Extracts depress the central nervous system, decrease cardiac activity, reduce blood pressure, and function as a vasodilator, analgesic, and antispasmodic (Duke and Ayensu 1985).
		It has been used as an analgesic, antispasmodic, and sedative. However, it is very dangerous, and internal use is not advised.
		A decoction of leaves can be used against skin diseases, ulcer, arthritis, and bruises (www.botanical online.com). Black nightshade contains solanine, solasonine, solamargine, solanumariculare, solasodine, diosgenin, tigogenin, and vitamin C.
Blueberry	*Vaccinium corymbosum*	In a USDA Human Nutrition Research Center lab, neuroscientists discovered that feeding blueberry to laboratory rats slowed age-related loss in their mental capacity, a finding that has important implications for humans (Kowalchuk 1976).
		Blueberry contains compounds known as anthocyanosides. In studies with experimental animals, these compounds have been shown to offer significant protection against ulcers. They help stimulate the production of mucus that protects the stomach lining from digestive acids (Duke 1997).
		In folklore medicine, decoctions of fruit and root bark are used to treat dysentery. The leaves contain arbutin, a chemical that acts as a diuretic and produces an antiseptic effect in the urinary mucus membrane, reducing the incidence of urinary tract infections.
		It was reported that blueberry is supposedly useful for everything from controlling bed-wetting to kidney stones, and even in the treatment of gonorrhea. In females, a tea made from blueberry can be used as a bath or douche after childbirth to aid healing and prevent infections. Indians used a tea derived from the fruits or leaves to control weight.
		Anthocyanin from blueberry functions as an antioxidant and anti-inflammatory in mammals. The antioxidant properties are known to reduce the incidence of heart disease and cancer in humans (Rieger 2006).

English Name	Scientific Name	Nutritional and Therapeutic Values
		Blueberry is used to prevent cataracts and glaucoma, ulcers, urinary tract infection, multiple sclerosis, fever, varicose veins, and hemorrhoids and to improve blood circulation. The dried fruit and leaves are used as a treatment for diarrhea. Tea made from the dried leaves is used to treat sore throat and other inflammations of the mouth or mucus membranes of the throat. Blueberry juice is also used as a contrast agent in magnetic resonance imaging (Jellin 2003).
		In traditional medicine, blueberry is used as a "blood purifier" for colic and labor pains and as a tonic after miscarriage. By inhalation, fumes of burning dried blueberry flowers have been used for treatment of insanity (Jellin 2003). The applicable parts of the blueberry are the fruit and leaves (Robbers and Tyler 1999). Blueberry fruit is high in fiber and vitamin C (Jellin 2003). It also contains anthocyanins and proanthocyanidins, which appear to have antioxidant activity (Youdim et al. 2000).
		Preliminary research from animal models suggests that the antioxidant effects of blueberry extracts might have anticancer activity and potentially reduce normal oxidative cellular damage that occurs with aging (Bomser et al. 1996). Blueberry, like its relative, the cranberry, also appears to prevent bacterial adhesion to the bladder and bacterial colonization (Howell et al. 1998), although clinical studies have not yet been performed.
		According to research originally conducted in Japan, blueberry juice is effective as a contrast agent to improve, or delineate, the structures of the stomach, duodenum, small and large bowel, pancreas, and bile ducts. That is because blueberry juice is rich in manganese, a metal found in nature and an essential element in our diet.
Breadfruit	*Artocarpus altilis* A. *lakoocha*	Breadfruit is a staple food in many tropical regions. It can be eaten once cooked, or it can be further processed into a variety of other foods. It is used as a cataplasm for tumors in Brazil. Powder of roasted leaves is applied for enlarged spleen, and ashes of the leaves are applied in treatment of herpes (Duke and duCellier 1993).
		The juice and seeds are purgative, and the bark is astringent. The root is tonic and deobstruent. The leaves are used to treat dropsy. It contains two triterpenes, amyrin acetate and lupeol acetate (Perry and Metzger 1980).

English Name	Scientific Name	Nutritional and Therapeutic Values
		The latex and bark are part of the native pharmacopoeia. Latex is massaged into the skin to treat broken bones and sprains and is bandaged on the spine to relieve sciatica. The root is astringent and is used as a purgative. The bark is used to treat headaches. The tea made from this plant is thought to control diabetes. The leaves are used to treat liver disease and fever in Taiwan (Ragone 1997).
		Breadfruit seeds contain protein, carbohydrate, fat, calcium, potassium, phosphorus, iron, and magnesium. They also contain niacin, sodium, thiamine, riboflavin, amino acids, and vitamin C (Dalessandrik and Boor 1994).
		Medicinally, the latex and bark of breadfruit are part of the native pharmacopoeia. The yellowing leaf is brewed into tea and is taken to reduce high blood pressure. The tea is also thought to control diabetes; gamma-aminobutyric acid is the active ingredient (Dalessandrik and Boor 1994).
		Fruit contains sugar, starch, protein, calcium, cerotic acid, ceryl cerotate, α-amyrin, and acetate. It is used to relieve pain, kidney disorders, and diabetes (N. Chiu and Chang 1995d).
Bullock's heart	*Annona reticulata*	The compounds (squancone and isoannon areticin) isolated from this plant showed potential cytotoxicities against CCM2 and four cancer cell lines (Yu et al. 1997).
		It has been reported that a compound (acetogenin) extracted from the seeds of Annona reticulata showed anticancer properties (F. Chang et al. 1998a).
Cacao tree	*Theobroma cacao*	The seeds are used in the manufacture of cocoa, cocoa butter, and chocolate. A decoction of the root is considered to be emmenagogic, ecbolic, and abortive. It contains theobromine, cacao-red, tannin, fixed oil, starch, protein, caffeine, and phenylethylamine. It has been reported that fresh fruits and vegetables are the best sources for antioxidants and vitamins (R. Lee and Balick 2001).
		The oil contains glycerides of arachic, oleic, palmitic, and stearic acids; aliphatic hydrocarbons; stigmasterol; and a mixture of sitosterols. It has antiseptic, diuretic, emmenagogic, parasiticidal, and vulnerary properties (Perry and Metzger 1980; N. Chiu and Chang 1995f; Rieger 2006).
		It is used principally for its diuretic effect due to stimulation of the renal epithelium. It is especially useful when there is an accumulation of fluid in the body resulting from cardiac failure, when it is often given with digitalis to relieve dilatation. It is also employed in high blood pressure, as it dilates the blood vessels (Grieve 1971).

English Name	Scientific Name	Nutritional and Therapeutic Values
		Cocoa butter is applied to soothe minor skin irritation, including burns, chapped lips, sores, wrinkles, and wounds. It is also used to treat cough, fever, malaria, rheumatism, and snakebite, and is considered to be an aphrodisiac (Rieger 2006).
		Cacao is antiseptic, diuretic, ecbolic, emmenagogic, and parasiticidal. It is a folk remedy for alopecia, burns, cough, dry lips, eyes, fever, listlessness, malaria, nephrosis, parturition, pregnancy, rheumatism, snakebite, and wounds (Duke and duCellier 1993).
Caimito	*Pouteria caimito*	The fruit pulp, because of its mucilaginous nature, is eaten to relieve coughs, bronchitis, and other pulmonary complaints.The latex is given as a vermifuge and purge and is applied on abscesses.
		Triterpenes have been extracted from *Pouteria caimito* (Pellicciari et al. 1972).
		Seeds contain saponin, pouterin, a bitter principle (lucumin), and a fixed oil. Leaves contain an amorphous bitter principle and some alkaloid. Latex is used for abscesses; dried latex is used as an anthelmintic.
		Fruit is used for diabetes. Seeds are used as a tonic for diarrhea and fever. The plant is used in Philippine alternative medicine (www.stuartxchange.org).
Calamondin orange	*Citrus microcarpa*	In China, the leaves and root have the same uses as the peel of the fruit for treatment of anorexia, cold, cough, malignant breast sores, and phlegm. A decoction of the root may be taken as a bechic-expectorant and to care for lumbago (Perry 1980).
		It has been reported that rubbing calamondin juice on insect bites can alleviate itching and irritation. The juice also bleaches freckles and helps to clear up acne vulgaris and pruritus vulvae. It is taken orally as a cough remedy and an antiphlogistic (www.geocities.com).
		It has been reported that mixing honey with *Citrus microcarpa* juice relieves colds and fever and serves as a general health tonic (Lacuna-Richman 2002).

English Name	Scientific Name	Nutritional and Therapeutic Values
Cantaloupe	*Cucumis melo* *C. sativus*	Seeds contain citrulline, cystine, galactane, histidine, lysine, myristic acid, and tryptophan. Fruit contains peptidase, protease, and vitamins A, B, and C. Root contains melonemetine. Elaterin, melotoxin, and the antitumor cucurbitacin B occur in the plant (Duke and Ayensu 1985). *Cucumis melo* is used for treatment of heat and thirst, sore throat, sore eyes, high blood pressure, burns, and scalds (K. Lin 1998e). It is used as a food and to sustain the nutritional quality of diets in Moshaweng Tlokwa, Botswana (Grivetti 1978). The pedicel is used with compounds, including melotoxin, cucurbitacins B and E, and sterol. Cantaloupe can be used to induce vomiting for drug intoxication. It is also used to treat toxic and chronic hepatitis and cirrhosis (Akihisa et al. 1987). Cantaloupe contains elaterin; unripe cantaloupe contains elaterin, melotoxin, and cucurbitacins and has anticancer properties (Ye 1999). The flower buds contain a bitter principle that causes nausea and vomiting. The roasted young buds can be made into a powder that is used as an emetic and to clean the stomach, either from illness or poisoning. The powder is also used as a remedy for jaundice and for an ulcerated nose. The seeds are used as a digestive and a bechic, and the fruit as a stomachic. The peduncle of the fruit is used as an antiemetic. The seeds contain myristic acid, phosphates, galactane, lysine, citrulline, histidine, tryptophan, and cystine (Perry 1980). Cantaloupe is a folk remedy for anasarca, bruise, cancer, cold, coryza, cough, diabetes, dyspepsia, dysuria, eczema, extravasation, gonorrhea, jaundice, menorrhagia, oliguria, polypus, stomatitis, and tumors (Duke and duCellier 1993)
Carambola	*Averrhoa carambola*	Fruit can be pounded and applied to treat wounds; it is also used to quench thirst, increase salivation, and allay fever (Duke and Ayensu 1985). Fruit is astringent to bowels. It is digestible, tonic, and strengthening. It causes biliousness in the body. The juice can be used as an eye drop to improve vision. The leaves are antipruritic, antipyretic, and anthelmintic (Dr. Chiranjit Parmar, horticultural consultant on lesser known Indian plants; www.ibiblio.org). The fruit is regarded as thirst quenching, increasing saliva secretion, and as a diuretic. It acts as a styptic when pounded and applied to wounds. The flowers are said to be vermifuge. Fruits or leaves may be rubbed on as an embrocation to combat skin afflictions (Perry 1980). Crushed leaves are used to treat chicken pox, fever, headache, and ringworm. Leaf decoctions are given to stop emesis (Duke and duCellier 1993).

English Name	Scientific Name	Nutritional and Therapeutic Values
Carissa	*Carissa grandiflora* *C. carandas*	The green fruits are astringent, and the ripe fruits are used to treat bilious afflictions, as a remedy for septicemia, and for cooling. The root is bitter, stomachic, and antiscorbutic. The acrid juice of the root is used to treat itch, but the latex is considered to be an irritant. An extract of the bark is cardiotonic and cardiac (Perry 1980). Aqueous extracts from the roots of Carissa have exhibited anti-HSV (Herpes simplex virus) activity in vitro and in vivo for both wild-type and resistant strains of HSV (Tolo et al. 2006).
Cashew nut	*Anacardium occidentale*	Oil from the fruit is used against leprosy and worms. Experimental results suggest that the oil is hypoglycemic. The oil contains anacardic acid, which is bactericidal and nematicidal, and anacardol, both of which have been suggested as antitumor compounds (Duke and Ayensu 1985). Compounds, tannins, anacardic acid, and cardol from the ethanol extraction of cashew nut have antimicrobial and cytotoxic activities with minimum inhibitory concentration and lethal concentration values (Mackeen et al. 1997). Many medicinal uses of cashew nut bark and leaves have been reported in the native region of Brazil. Bark teas have been used for treatment of diarrhea, and the caustic shell oil has been used to treat skin infections, warts, worms and botfly larvae beneath the skin. It is antimicrobial, anti-inflammatory, astringent, diuretic, and hypoglycemic, among other medicinal properties. Clinical studies have documented the anti-inflammatory properties of tannins and the antimicrobial properties of anacardic acid against several species, including Escherichia coli and Helicobacter pylori. Leaf extracts produce hypoglycemic activity in rodents and a reduction in artificially induced diabetes (Rieger 2006).
Ceylon olive	*Elaeocarpus serratus* *E. grandiflorus*	The unripe fruit is first boiled, then squashed flat so the flesh cracks open around the seed. The ripe fruit is softer and somewhat sweeter and is eaten with jaggery. The plant is a home remedy for flatulence, colic, and diarrhea. The plant contains a poisonous bitter principle, elaeocarpid, the leaves have a small content of saponin. A decoction of the fruits is mildly diuretic. It treats bilious attacks. The leaves show some antibiotic activity against staphylococcus (Perry 1980).

English Name	Scientific Name	Nutritional and Therapeutic Values
Chestnut	*Castanea crenata* *C. mollissima*	The flower is used for treatment of scrofula; stem bark is used for poisoned wounds; and sap is used for lacquer poisoning. Husk is astringent and is used to treat dysentery, nausea, and thirst (Duke and Ayensu 1985).
		The flower is also used as a remedy for tuberculosis and scrofula. A decoction of the fresh leaves contains hyperin and can allay irritation of the skin caused by lacquer (Perry 1980).
		The green or dried leaves, inner bark, and fruit are used for medicinal purposes such as relief of whooping cough or nagging distressing coughs and controlling paroxysmal or infrequent hiccoughs and other irritable and excitable conditions for the respiratory organs. It is tonic and mildly sedative (Hutchens 1991). It is an astringent herb that is used to treat diarrhea, varicose veins, leg ulcers, hemorrhoids, neuralgia, and sunburn (Lust 1979).
		The bark contains tannin; vitamins A, B, and C; and β-carotene. Seeds contain protein, fat, starch, and sugar (N. Chiu and Chang 1995b).
		Flower and stem bark contain quercetin, urea, protein, β-carotene, riboflavin, thiamine, and ascorbic acid. It is used to treat diarrhea, poisoned wounds, and lacquer poisoning (Zhu 1989).
		Chestnut contains tannins, plastoquinones, and mucilage. It is used to treat whooping cough, bronchitis, and sore throats (Chevallier 1996).
		A decoction of the shells is an astringent used to treat nausea, thirst, and dysentery (Perry 1980).
Chicle	*Manilkara zapota* *M. kauki*	The plant yields fruit twice a year. The fruit has a high latex content and does not ripen until picked. It is also known as chikoo. It tastes like sweet candy or caramel.
		Flower and seeds are used medicinally. Immature sapodillas are rich in tannin (proanthocyanidins). Because of the tannin content, young fruits are boiled and the decoction taken to stop diarrhea. An infusion of the young fruits and the flowers is drunk to relieve pulmonary complaints. A decoction of old, yellowed leaves is drunk as a remedy for coughs, colds, and diarrhea. A "tea" of the bark is regarded as a febrifuge and is said to halt diarrhea and dysentery. The crushed seeds have a diuretic action and are claimed to expel bladder and kidney stones. The latex is used in the tropics as a crude filling for tooth cavities (www.hort.purdue.edu/newcrop/nexus/Manilkara_zapota).

English Name	Scientific Name	Nutritional and Therapeutic Values
		A decoction of young fruits is used to relieve diarrhea. The crushed seeds have a diuretic action and are claimed to expel bladder and kidney stones (Morton 1987).
		Anthocyanin and cyanidin-3-glucoside have been identified in chicle (Einbond et al. 2004).
		Chicle has been selected and used to treat gastrointestinal illnesses (Heinrich 2000).
Chinese cherry	*Cerasus avium* *runus avium*	The fruit contains amygdalin and prunasin, substances that break down in water to form hydrocyanic acid. In small amounts, this exceedingly poisonous compound stimulates respiration and aids digestion (Bown 1995).
		It also has antimutagenic activity (Miyazawa et al. 2003).
Chinese gooseberry	*Actinidia deliciosa*	Chinese gooseberry contains metastable acid, iridomyrmecin, allomatatabiol, dihydronepetalactol, isoneomatatabiol, and neomatatabiol (T. Li 2006).
		A decoction of branches and leaves has been used to cure mange in dogs, and a compound has been isolated from the fruit that is irresistible to cats, both wild and domesticated. Juice from the stalk is used to treat gravel. The astringent, antiscorbutic fruit is used for quenching thirst and to treat gravel. Chinese use the insecticidal plant to treat esophageal, liver, mammary, and stomach cancers as well as rheumatoid arthritis, urinary stones, fever, and tension. It is also used as an antidote for cinnabar (Duke and duCellier 1993).
Chinese jujube	*Zizyphus vulgaris* var. *inermis*	The seeds contain no alkaloid; the oil contains oleic, linoleic, and palmitic acids and phytosterol.
		The fruits are considered to be pectoral. The bark is a remedy for diarrhea, the root for fever, and the leaves for scorpion stings. The fruits or kernels of the seeds are probably the most important part of the plant in medicine. They are administered as having nervine, tonic, roborant, stomachic, sedative, laxative, bechic, antipyretic, and diuretic properties (Perry 1980).
		Chinese jujube can help in maintaining a healthy appetite and effective digestion. It is used to treat weak spleens and stomachs (J. Chen 2005).
		The fruit is recommended for antirheumatoid arthritis, insomnia, neurasthenia, pain and weakness of rheumatism, and splenetics.

English Name	Scientific Name	Nutritional and Therapeutic Values
		The seeds are hypnotic, narcotic, sedative, stomachic, tonic, and used for insomnia, night sweats, neurasthenia, palpitations, apprehension, amnesia, clamminess, epihydrosis, and vertigo. Root is for dyspepsia. In folk medicine, it is used as a remedy for anemia, hypertonia, nephritis, and nervous disease. The extracts are said to demonstrate tranquilizing, hypotensive, and uterotonic activities. They contain betulic acid, betuline, ebelin, lactone, jujuboside, jujubogenin, jujuboside, flavone C-glycoside, and spinosin. The shoots contain fiber, protein, carbohydrate, fat, minerals, thiamine, and ascorbic acid (Duke and Ayensu 1985).
Chinese olive	*Canarium album*	Fruit raw or cooked is used like olives. It also provides fibers for making cloth, rope, paper, etc.
		The fruit contains beta-carotene and vitamins. The juice from leaves is used to treat lacquer poisoning. Fruit is antiphlogistic, astringent, sialogogic, and stomachic. It is an antidote after eating poisonous fish, and it is also used as a remedy for sore and swollen throat, toothache, tonsillitis, dysentery, alcoholic intoxication, and diarrhea (Duke and Ayensu 1985; K. Lin 1998d).
		In traditional Chinese medicine, Chinese olive fruit is used to relieve anxiety. The roots are used to treat diabetes and gonorrhea (Newman 2000).
		Fruits are used as a remedy for pharyngitis, tonsillitis, cough, summer fever and thirst, enteritis, dysentery, epilepsy, and sore throat (K. Lin 1998e).
		Chinese olive contains tannin, chebulinic acid, chebulagic acid, terchebin, gallic acid, ellagic acid, shikimic acid, dehydroshikimic acid, quinic acid, amino acid, glucogallin, sennoside A, chebulin, corilagin, 1,3,6-trigalloyl glucose, 1,2,3,4,6-pentagalloyl-β-glucose, arabinose, rhamnose, glucose, polyphenol oxidase, tannase, catechol, and β-sitosterol (N. Chiu and Chang 1995f).
		It also contains hepatoprotective compounds (integrisglobal.com).
		Seeds from Chinese olive contain β-carotene, thiamine, riboflavin, niacin, and ascorbic acid. It has antiphlogistic, astringent, and pharyngitic properties (Duke and Ayensu 1985).

English Name	Scientific Name	Nutritional and Therapeutic Values
Citron	*Citrus medica*	The leaves and root have the same uses as the peel of the fruit. A decoction of the root may be taken as a bechic-expectorant and as a remedy for lumbago. The seeds are anthelmintic and febrifuge. A cyanogenetic substance is found in the seeds (Perry 1980). Citron contains essential oils, citral, and limonene (Y. Chang 2000). It is used as a remedy for seasickness, pulmonary troubles, and intestinal ailments. The flowers are used medicinally by the Chinese. Seeds are used as a vermifuge. The essential oil of the peel is regarded as an antibiotic (Morton 1987d).
		It has been reported that the remedies of the Citrus species range from oral hygiene and toothache relief to use as a contraceptive, laxative, purgative, and sedative, to use as a treatment for a wide variety of common ailments such as diarrhea and vomiting. Hesperidin, a bioflavonoid from Citrus peels, is a strong vasopressor agent that may lower the blood pressure. Pectin from the Citrus species is reported to reduce cholesterol.
		The limonene oils in Citrus peels may cause contact dermatitis. Furocoumarin may enhance sunburn on skin exposed to ultraviolet light. Citromellar, another volatile oil, has mutagenic properties. Limonene and petitgrain oils from peels or leaves are used as essential oils and also have an insecticidal property (Rieger 2006).
		The juice, bark, and rind are used in folk remedies for cancers and tumors. They are astringent, expectorant, refrigerant, stimulant, stomachic, and tonic. Citron is a folk remedy for asthma, colic, cough, diarrhea, dysentery, fever, jaundice, nausea, sclerosis, stomachache, stomach ailments, syphilis, thirst, and tumors of the abdomen (Duke and duCellier 1993).
Coconut	*Cocos nucifera*	The coconut palm is a large palm, growing to 30 m tall. The term "coconut" refers to the nut of the coconut palm, which is commonly referred to as a fruit.
		The green fruit juice is used as a remedy for poisoning and cholera and is used as a diuretic. Root bark is astringent and styptic and is used as a remedy for fluxes and hemorrhages. Fresh coconut juice with rice flour is poulticed onto carbuncles, gangrenous sores, and indolent ulcers (Duke and Ayensu 1985).
		Coconut is used for many medicinal uses, from treating skin conditions to regulating bodily functions, to eliminating fungal infections such as athlete's foot, jock itch, diaper rash, and toenail fungus (Fife 2005).

English Name	Scientific Name	Nutritional and Therapeutic Values
		Coconut has the ability to scavenge free radicals, inhibit lipid peroxidation, and protect hemoglobin from nitrite-induced excitation. The scavenging ability and protection of hemoglobin from oxidation may be partly attributed to the ascorbic acid in coconut (Kumar et al. 2003, Mantena et al. 2003).
		Coconut milk (liquid from endosperm) is used as an anthelmintic (eliminates intestinal worms). It contains sugars and is sterile. It is used to treat abscesses and tumors, dysentery, cold and flu, constipation, scurvy, and venereal diseases.
		Lauric and capric acids found in coconut may be converted to monolaurin and monocaprin in the body; these compounds have shown antibacterial, antiviral, and antiprotozoal activities and have proved to be useful in defending against various bacteria, including HIV and herpes viruses and the protozoan Giardia.
		Coconut oil may protect the liver from the damaging effects of alcohol and improve the anti-inflammatory response of the immune system. Coconut oil does not form harmful trans-fatty acids when used in cooking.
		Major fatty acids from coconut include lauric, myristic, palmitic, caprylic, and oleic acids (Rieger 2006).
Coffee	*Coffea arabica*	Coffee is said to be an antidote to poisoning from alkaloids, which accounts for its antisoporific property. The raw berries are prescribed to treat hemicrania and intermittent fevers. Application of the powdered seeds is an effective treatment for burns and scalds. A decoction of the unroasted beans is used to treat colic of the bladder and kidneys (Perry 1980).
		Coffee is rich in antioxidants. It reduces the risk of a number of diseases and ailments, including type 2 diabetes, Parkinson's, colon cancer, cirrhosis, gallstones, and depression (www.coffeescience.org).
		It has been reported that green coffee bean extract can be used as a mineral absorption enhancer to relieve mineral deficiency (European patent EP 1424076; www.freepatentsonline.com). Seeds contain 1,2-cyclopentandione, 1,2-propandione, acetylacrolein, furfuryl alcohol, and caffeine. These are used to improve digestion, appetite, stomach function, and urination (N. Chiu and Chang 1995f).

English Name	Scientific Name	Nutritional and Therapeutic Values
		Caffeine (1,3,7-trimethylxanthine) is an alkaloid that may have allelopathic properties. Caffeine acts as a diuretic, vasodilator, laxative, and appetite suppressant. Caffeine is sold commercially as a component in pain medication, diet pills, over-the-counter stimulants, and medicines administered to hyperactive children, for whom it has a calming effect.
		Moderate coffee consumption has been reported to reduce the risk of colon cancer, cirrhosis, gallstones, Parkinson's disease, asthma, and suicide (Reiger 2006). It has been reported that coffee may help in type 2 diabetes prevention (Van Dam et al. 2006). Several large studies have reported an inverse association between coffee consumption and the risk of type 2 diabetes mellitus (Pereira et al. 2007).
		Caffeine extracted from coffee beans of Coffea arabica is used in combination with analgesics and ergotamine to treat migraine headaches. It is used orally with analgesics for simple headaches and for preventing and treating postoperative and postdural puncture headaches.
		It is also used orally to treat asthma, increase blood pressure in hypotension, increase mental alertness, enhance athletic performance, and treat neonatal apnea. Caffeine is used in combination with ephedrine or other stimulants and diuretics for weight loss. Very high doses are used as euphoriants, often in combination with ephedrine as an alternative to illicit stimulants (Jellin 2003).
		Topical caffeine cream preparations have been used to reduce erythema and itching in dermatitis. Recently, caffeine has been used in combination with ergotamine to relieve migraine headaches.
		Caffeine is also used for postoperative and postdural puncture headache, neonatal apnea, acute respiratory depression, and as a diuretic. It is also used to extend the length of seizure with electroconvulsive therapy (Jellin 2003).
		Caffeine is a methyl xanthine compound, structurally related to theophylline, theobromine, and uric acid (Suleman and Siddiqui 2000). It is 100% bioavailable after oral administration and is metabolized principally in the liver to paraxanthine, theophylline, and theobromine (Sinclair and Geiger 2000).
		Caffeine stimulates the central nervous system, heart, muscles (15), and possibly the pressor centers that control blood pressure (Schulz et al. 1998).

English Name	Scientific Name	Nutritional and Therapeutic Values
Common fig	*Ficus carica* *F. pyriformis*	The common fig can be eaten fresh or dried and is used in jam-making. Most commercial production generates dried or otherwise processed forms, as the ripe fruit does not transport well and, once picked, does not keep well. Leaves contain bergapten, cerotinic acid, ficusin, glutamine, papain, pepsin, quercetin, rhamnose, rutin, sitosterol, tyrosine, and urease. Leaves are slightly poisonous, but they are utilized in treating hemorrhoids. A decoction of the leaves is helpful in treating stomachache (Perry 1980; Duke and Ayensu 1985). The common fig is used as an anti-inflammatory, diuretic, and analgesic as a remedy for nephritis, cystitis, urethritis, nephrotic edema, cardiac edema, and epigastric pain (K. Lin 1998f). The fruits are used as a remedy for pharyngitis, hoarseness, asthma, constipation, and hemorrhoids. Roots and leaves are used to treat tuberculous cervical lymphadenopathy, hemorrhoid infection, enteritis, and diarrhea. The fruits contain quinic acid, shikimic acid, and auxin are used externally as a remedy for pyodermas (K. Lin 1998c; 1998d). Animal studies of fig and fig leaf have shown both short-term and long-term hypoglycemic effects (Mossman 2005). Stems are used as an anti-inflammatory, diuretic, and analgesic to treat nephritis, cystitis, urethritis, nephrotic edema, cardiac edema, and epigastric pain (K. Lin 1998g). Root and root bark contain psoralen, bergapten, guaiazulene, β-amyrin, lupeol, valeric acid, guaiacol, octacosane, quinic acid, shikimic acid, and auxin (N. Chiu and Chang 1995b). Leaf and fruit contain bergapten, carotinin, ficusin, glutamine, papain, pepsin, psoralen, guaiaxulene, amyrin, lupeol, retin, octacosane, guaiacol, quercetin, rhamnose, sitosterol, tyrosin, and urease acid. It is used internally to treat stomachache and externally as a remedy for swollen piles, corns, and warts. Fruit has laxative, digestive, anthelmintic, hypolipidemic, and hypotriglyceridemic activities (C. Perez et al. 1999).
Cucumber tree	*Magnolia acuminata*	A decoction of the leaves is used as a postpartum protective medicine. Crushed leaves are used to treat rheumatism and diabetes.

English Name	Scientific Name	Nutritional and Therapeutic Values
		A paste of the leaves is applied to patients short of breath. Fruit is pounded and applied to wounds and used to quench thirst, increase salivation, and allay fever (Perry 1980; Duke and Ayensu 1985).
		It is antiperiodic, aromatic, diaphoretic, laxative, stimulant, and tonic.
		Tea made from the bark is antipyretic, mildly diaphoretic, and laxative (Foster and Duke 1999).
		Stem contains oxoushinsunine, salicifoline, magnoflorine, stephanine, anolobine, and magnococline (N. Chiu and Chang 1995b).
Custard apple	*Annona reticulata*	The fruit is reported to contain calories, protein, fat, carbohydrate, fiber, ash, riboflavin, and ascorbic acid. Bark contains tannin and anonaine. Custard apple is considered to be astringent, diuretic, insecticidal, pectoral, poisonous, stomachic, tonic, and vermifuge. The resin from the seed can be hazardous to humans (Duke and duCellier 1993).
		The compounds squancone and isoannon areticin, isolated from this plant, showed potential cytotoxicities against CCM2 and four cancer cell lines (Yu et al. 1997). Acetogenins extracted from seeds of *Annona reticulata* showed anticancer properties (F. Chang et al. 1998).
Durian	*Durio zibethinus* *D. oxleyanus*	The fruit can grow up to 30 cm long and 15 cm in diameter. Its shape ranges from oblong to round, the color of its husk green to brown, and its flesh pale-yellow to red. The taste of the flesh has been described as nutty and sweet.
		The leaves are used in poultices, and a decoction is used as a bath for people with jaundice. The milky juice of the fruit is used as an aphrodisiac. Juice from pounding the inner bark is taken as a medicine for malaria. The grated seeds are applied to ulcers and wounds. A decoction of the leaves and roots is used as an antipyretic. It is also a remedy to treat fevers (Perry 1980).
		Durian polysaccharide gel is able to entrap lipids, and it seems to have potential use as a medicinal dietary food for patients requiring lipid control (Tippayakul et al. 2005).
		The fruit contains butyric acid (N. Chiu and Chang 1995b).
Dwarf flowering cherry	*Prunus japonica*	Broth of leafy shoot is used to stop hemorrhage. The kernels are demulcent, deobstruent, diuretic, and lenitive. They are used as a remedy for cardialgia, constipation, dropsy, dyspepsia, fever, ophthalmia, and rheumatism (Perry 1980; Duke and Ayensu 1985).

English Name	Scientific Name	Nutritional and Therapeutic Values
		Fruit of *Prunus japonica*, a Chinese member of subquenus *Lithocerasus* sect. *Microcerasus*, showed a complex anthocyanins profile distinct from *P. besseyi* and *P. pumila* (Werner et al. 1989).
		Leaf and fruit contain amygdaline, citric acid, and fatty acids. It is diuretic and laxative (F. Chen 1997).
Egg fruit (canistel)	*Lucuma nervosa* *Pouteria campechiana*	The edible canistel fruit is oval in shape, 5–10 cm long, and orange-yellow in color.
		Pulp is eaten fresh or used in beverages, jams, and desserts. Flavor is very sweet. Pulp is high in niacin and vitamins A and C. In Mexico, the astringent decoction of the bark is used as a febrifuge, while in Cuba it is applied for skin problems. A preparation of the seeds is used to treat ulcers (Morton 1987e).
		Total dietary fiber in egg fruit reaches 8.6 g (50%). It contains uranic acid, polysaccharides, lignin, and dietary fiber (S. Chang et al. 1998).
Egg tree	*Garcinia xanthocymus* *G. morella*	Garcinia xanthocymus is a tropical evergreen tree. The pericarp of the edible fruit is deep reddish-purple when ripe.
		The fragrant flesh is sweet and creamy, citrous with some peach flavor.
		This plant contains two antibiotic compounds, morellin and guttiferin. It is considered bactericidal, cathartic, and ecbolic and is used as a vermifuge. It is also used as a remedy for dropsy, sores, and worms. A preparation of the fruit of the egg tree is given to treat bilious conditions, diarrhea, and dysentery. Resin from the stem is used to treat cancerous sores and indolent ulcers (Perry 1980). It contains gum, resin, starch, and gambogic acid. The Chinese regard it as very poisonous. The main symptoms of poisoning are abdominal pain, diarrhea, and lowering of blood pressure (Perry 1980).
		Two new benzophenones, guttiferone and gambogenone, that were extracted from fruits displayed cytotoxicity in the SW-480 colon cancer cell line (Baggett et al. 2005).
		The serum from leaves contains α-guttiferin, β-guttiferin, morellic acid, isomorellic acid, morellin, isomorellin, dihydroisomorellin, ethoxydihydroisomorellin, neomorellin, and morelloflavone. It is used to treat cancer and inflammation caused by cancer (Rieger 2006).

English Name	Scientific Name	Nutritional and Therapeutic Values
Elephant apple	*Dillenia indica*	The astringent bark and fruit and leaves are used to treat fever and diarrhea. The fruit pulp cleanses the hair or the cooling juice may be used. The fresh inner bark rubbed to a paste with the sap squeezed out of fresh leaves is a remedy suggested to treat flabby gums, thrush, and scurvy (Perry 1980).
		Substances from the stem bark contain anthocyanins, anthraquinones, and flavonoids (Tiwari and Srivastava 1979). According to Ayurvedic medicine, its bark and leaves are astringent. The bruised bark is applied as cataplasm in treatment of arthritis. The pulp of the fruit is used as a hair wash. The juice of unripe fruits allays cough, assists expectoration, and cures angina and aphthae (Oudhia 2007).
European blackberry	*Rubus fruticosus* *R. japonica* *R. reflexus*	The blackberry can be reasonably deduced to have been consumed by humans for thousands of years. The blossoms are good nectar producers. It is known to contain polyphenol antioxidants, naturally occurring chemicals that can upregulate certain beneficial metabolic processes in mammals.
		Roots and leaves are used as an antirheumatic to strengthen bones and muscles and to treat rheumatic pains, traumatic injury, and fractures.
		Leaves are mashed or pulverized and applied to bleeding wounds or lesions (K. Lin 1998d).
		It has been reported that the polyphenols in European blackberry have the ability to act as antioxidants and free-radical scavengers (K. Lin 1998a).
		The roots are used to treat contusion and hematoma, hepatosplenomegaly, urinary tract infection or stones, nephritis, common colds, pharyngitis, hemoptysis, hematemesis, rheumatic pain, traumatic injury, and fractures (K. Lin 1998a.c).
		Leaves are used externally for bleeding wounds. Mashed or pulverized roots are applied to lesions. It is an anticarcinogen/antimutagen that inhibits HIV binding to cells inhibits blood clotting, and scavenges free radicals (K. Lin 1998a.c).
		European blackberry contains ellagic acid, tannins, organic acid, and vitamin C. It is mildly astringent, antiseptic, antifungal, diuretic, and has tonic properties (Bunney 1992).

English Name	Scientific Name	Nutritional and Therapeutic Values
		European blackberry juice is used to treat infections of the mouth and eyes. The powdered bark is used for toothache relief. A tea made from leaves is said to aid digestion. Stems are peeled and boiled to produce a liquid to arrest vomiting. Root decoctions are used as a remedy for dysentery.
Fiji longan	*Pometia pinnata*	Fiji longan contains saponin and polycyclic compounds. It is used only externally. A decoction of the bark or leaves is used to bathe patients with fever. The bark is used in a dressing for festering sores or wounds (Perry 1980).
		In Papua, New Guinea, the masticated bark is applied to burns. In Fiji, bark extracts are used to treat ailments, including stomach complaints, diarrhea, dysentery, pain relief, cold, flu, diabetes, and mouth ulcers (Thomson and Thaman 2006).
Fingered citron	*Citrus medica* var. *sacrodactylis*	In China, the leaves and root of this species have the same uses as the peel of the fruit. A decoction of the root may be taken as a bechic-expectorant and as a remedy for lumbago. The seeds are anthelmintic and febrifuge (Perry 1980).
		Fruits are used. Flowers, leaves, and roots are also useful. The fruit cut and macerated in alcohol has antiasthmatic properties. An infusion of the fresh shoots is appetitive and vermifuge and is a remedy for stomachache. A decoction of the rind may be used to treat coughs, colds, dyspepsia, and as an antidote for fish poison. The rind may also be used in ointments or used fresh on acne and eczema. The essential oil is reported as having some value as an antibiotic to treat typhus, meningococcus, and other bacilli (Perry 1980).
		It is used to induce productive cough and as a remedy for abdominal distention, gastric pain, anorexia, vomiting, chronic gastritis, and gastric neuralgia (K. Lin 1998d).
		It contains arsenic, calcium, citral, copper, dipentene, geranyl acetate, hesperidin, iron, d-limonene, linalyl acetate, magnesium, manganese, nordentatin, phellandrene, potassium, sodium, 3,5,6-trihydroxyl-7,3,4-trimethoxyflavone, xanthyletin, and zinc (Duke 2001).
		Fruit contains pinene, α-limonene, citropten, limettin, diosmin, and hesperidin (N. Chiu and Chang 1995c).

English Name	Scientific Name	Nutritional and Therapeutic Values
Flowering quince	*Chaenomeles speciosa*	The fruits are considered to be tonic and sedative, administered against sunstroke, nausea, indigestion, colic, cholera, and other bowel troubles, rheumatism, and muscle cramps of beri-beri, which is caused by vitamin B1 deficiency. The fruits also have soothing, stomachic, and astringent functions (Perry 1980).
		The fruits are analgesic, anti-inflammatory, antispasmodic, astringent, and digestive. A decoction is used internally in the treatment of nausea, joint pains, cholera, and associated cramps (Duke and Ayensu 1985). Fruit contains triterpenoids and oleanolic acid, which are used in Chinese medicine. It also contains vitamin C, and lalic, tartaric, citric, and hydrocyanic acids. It is used to treat arthralgia, diarrhea, cholera, gout, and arthritis (Keys 1976). Flowering quince contain malic, tartaric, citric, ascorbic, fumaric, and oleanolic acids as well as catalase, peroxidase, phenol oxidase, and vitamin C.
Ginkgo	*Ginkgo biloba*	Ginkgo contains ginkgocides A, B, C, J, and M. flavonoids, bilobalide, sciadopitysin, ginkgetin, isoginkgetin, bilobetin, and carotenoids. It is used to treat dementia and cerebral insufficiency and disorders. It also can relieve asthma (T. Li 2000).
		It reduces the clotting tendency of platelets, dilates blood vessels, and reduces inflammation.
		Ginkgo is used to improve blood flow to the brain and in the lower legs. It may be useful in treating dizziness, headache, noise in the ears, and memory loss. It may also prevent damage to the kidneys caused by immunosuppressants (Beers 2004).
		It has been reported that the sesquiterpene bilobalide reduces increased water and electrolyte levels in damaged brain tissue. The diterpene ginkgolides are potent platelet activating factor (PAF) inhibitors. PAF can contribute to brain damage not only by inducing thrombosis, but also by increasing the permeability of blood vessels, allowing liquid to seep through them into brain tissue. This is likely to result in nerve damage (Tyler 1999).
		Ginkgo leaves contain shikimic acid and flavonoids. Leaves also contain phenolic components, sesquiterpene, bilobalide, and beta-sterol. Ginkgolides and diterpenes have also been extracted from leaves and root bark. Phenolic toxic substances can be extracted from fruit pulps and sensitizers from seeds. Ginnol identical with celidoniol has also been found. Fruit extracts contain anacardic acids; seeds contain alkaloids-ginkgotoxin and amino acids (Chauhan 1999).

English Name	Scientific Name	Nutritional and Therapeutic Values
		Ginkgo has antitussive, antiasthmatic, and anodyne properties. It treats coronary artery disease, angina pectoris, hypercholesterolemia, and Parkinson's disease, and inhibits the growth of human cancer cell lines (J. Lee et al. 1998).
		Ginkgo contains kaempferol, kaempferol-3-rhamnoglucoside, heptaacetyl kaempferol glucoside, kaempferol-3-6-p-coumaroyl-glucosyl-β-1,4-rhamnoside, quercetin, isorhamnetin, octaacetyl quercetin 3-qlucoside, heptaacetyl luteoline quteolin 3-glucoside, octaacetyl delphidenon glucoside, (+)-catechin-pentaacetate, (-) epicatechin-pentaacetate, (+)-gallocatechin-hexacetate, (-)-epigallo catechin-hexacetate, bilobetin, ginkgetin, ginkgol, sciadopitysin, 1-5-methoxy-bilobetin, and ginkgolic, hydroginkgolic, ginkgolinic, anacardic, quinic, linoleic, shikimic, ascorbic, formic, propionic, butyric, and caprylic acids. It also contains α-hexenol, sequoyitol, pinite, hexacosanol-1, octacosanol, β-sitosterol, nonacosyl alcohol-10, ginnol, d-sesamin, cyanophoric glucoside, gibberellin, carotene, riboflavin, and asparagine (J. Lee et al. 1998).
Grape	*Vitis vinifera* *V. labrusca*	Fruits contain malic, tartaric, and racemic acids. It is considered to be antiemetic, antilithic, diuretic, and galactagogue. It is used to treat scrofula. Decoction of leaves is used for abortion, cholera, dropsy, and nausea. The fruit is considered constructive, cooling, and strengthening and is used to treat kidney afflictions (Perry 1980; Duke and Ayensu 1985).
		Grape seed is used for treating and preventing vascular or circulatory disorders, including venous insufficiency, varicose veins, atherosclerosis, and peripheral vascular disease (Jellin 2003).
		Grape leaves are used to stop bleeding and as a remedy for inflammation and pain, such as the kind brought on by hemorrhoids. Unripe grapes are used to treat sore throat, and dried grapes are used to treat consumption, constipation, and thirst. Extracts of grape seed are used to treat a range of health problems related to free-radical damage, including heart disease and cancer (Anderson et al. 2002).
		Historically, grape has been used to treat cancer. A compound, resveratrol, extracted from grape shows anticarcinogenic activity. It can inhibit tumor formation in three ways: by stopping DNA damage, by slowing/halting cell transformation from normal to cancerous, and by slowing tumor growth.

English Name	Scientific Name	Nutritional and Therapeutic Values
		Resveratrol may be important in reducing heart disease; it has anti-inflammatory properties and may be useful for prevention of colon cancer and a wide variety of other tumors. The ellagic acid that occurs in grapes may have a number of health effects on humans. It has anticancer properties and may act as a free-radical scavenger (Rieger 2006).
		The potential cancer-chemopreventive activity of trans-astringin, a plant stilbenoid recently found in wine, may function as a potential cancer-chemopreventive agent (Waffo-Teguo et al. 2001).
		Grapes, including grape skin and grape juice, are used to prevent coronary heart disease. They are also used as a dietary source of antioxidants. Grapes have also been used as a remedy for varicose veins, hemorrhoids, capillary fragility, and as a mild laxative for constipation.
		Grape fasts have been used for detoxification. Dried grapes, raisins or sultanas, have been used as an expectorant for cough. In beverages and drink mixes, including wine, grape skin extract is used as a coloring agent (Jellin 2003). Grapes provide a variety of constituents that are thought to be pharmacologically active. Various types of phenolic compounds, including anthocyanins, cinnamates, and flavan-3-ols, are thought to provide benefit in the prevention of heart disease. These phenolic compounds are thought to have antioxidant properties and play a role in prevention of low-density lipoprotein (LDL) oxidation.
		Red grape varieties tended to produce more oxidation protection than other varieties. A similar trend has been seen with red versus white wines. There was a significant correlation between total phenol content and anthocyanin content and antioxidant activity. Phenol content in red grapes is primarily from anthocyanins, which are responsible for producing the color in red grapes (Meyer et al. 1997).
		Grapes are also reported to have laxative and expectorant properties (Chevallier 1996). Some evidence suggests that anthocyanins might strengthen capillaries and have antifungal and antibacterial activity (Leung and Foster 1996).
Grapefruit	*Citrus paradis*	Grapefruit juice contains less quercetin than grape juice; it primarily contains the flavonoids naringin, luteolin, and apigenin glucoside (Osman et al. 1988).
		Seven flavanones (didymin, eriocitrin, hesperidin, naringin, narirutia, neohesperidin, and poncirin) are present in grapefruit. It had a total flavanones content of 27 mg/100 g as aglycones and a distinct flavanone profile, dominated by naringin (Peterson et al. 2006).

English Name	Scientific Name	Nutritional and Therapeutic Values
		Grapefruit is used for reducing cholesterol and reversing atherosclerosis; as a supplemental source of potassium, vitamin C, and fiber; for reducing hematocrit; as an anticancer agent; for psoriasis; and as an aid in weight reduction (Jellin 2003). For food uses, grapefruit is consumed as fruit and juice. There is insufficient reliable information available about the effectiveness of grapefruit. However, there is some evidence that consumption of vitamin C-rich citrus fruits, including grapefruit and others, might improve lung function in people with asthma. Intake of citrus fruit one or two times per week has produced this benefit in some studies. However, other studies have not found this benefit (Butland et al. 2000).
		The applicable parts of grapefruit are the fruit and juice. The potential benefits of grapefruit in asthma might be due to the antioxidant properties of vitamin C or other fruit constituents (Forastiere et al. 2000).
		Grapefruit juice contains furanocoumarins, including bergamottin and dihydroxybergamottin, which inhibit cytochrome P450 3A4 (CYP3A4) (Fukuda et al. 1997). Juice also contains naringin, naringenin, limonin, quercetin, kaempferol, and obacunone, which are known to inhibit human hepatic microsomes (Chan et al. 1998).
		Drug interactions with grapefruit juice are well-documented. The chemistry of the grapefruit varies by the species, the growing conditions, and the process used to extract the juice. Because grapefruit juice is not standardized, use as an adjunct to drug therapy is not recommended (Ameer and Weintraub 1997).
		Whole grapefruit is high in water and fiber. It is a good dietary source of potassium, vitamin C, pectin, and other nutrients. Grapefruit pectin, which is found in whole fruit but not the juice, can reduce cholesterol and promote regression of atherosclerosis. Studies suggest grapefruit can affect blood components. Some evidence suggests that the constituent naringin might induce red cell aggregation.
		Consuming one half to one grapefruit per day can reduce an individual's hematocrit level (Jellin 2003).

English Name	Scientific Name	Nutritional and Therapeutic Values
Grapefruit seed	*Citrus paradis*	The effect of grapefruit juice on drugs is difficult to predict because the bioavailability of compounds such as naringenin varies greatly among individuals, and the chemical constituents of grapefruit vary (Ameer and Weintraub 1997; Ho et al. 2000). Grapefruit seed extract is used for preventing and treating infections due to bacteria, viruses, fungi, and parasites. It is particularly promoted for yeast infection and intestinal parasites, including intestinal infections associated with travel. Topically, grapefruit seed extract is used as a facial cleanser, first-aid treatment, and treatment for mild skin irritations. It is also used as an ear or nasal rinse for prevention and treatment of infections, a throat gargle for sore throat, a dental rinse to prevent gingivitis and promote healthy gums and fresh breath, and a vaginal douche for candidiasis. It has also been nebulized for the treatment of lung infections (Jellin 2003). Grapefruit seeds contain numerous constituents including naringin, nomilin, deacetyl-nomilin, and nomilinic-acid-17-O-beta-D-glucoside (Duke 2001), and naringin has been reported to induce red blood cell aggregation in vitro.
Guajilote tree	*Parmentiera edulis*	Hypoglycemic activity-guided fractionation together with chemical analysis led to the isolation of one guaianolide (lactucin-8-O-methylacrylate) from the chloroform extract of the dried fruits of Parmentiera edulis. Identification was based on spectroscopic methods. The compound lowered blood sugar levels after administration to alloxan-diabetic mice (Perez, 2000). Guajilote tree fruits are used in Guatemala for the treatment of gonorrhea (Caceres et al. 1995).
Guava	*Psidium guajava*	The fruits contain numerous seeds that can produce a mature fruit-bearing plant within four years. The tree is easily identified by its distinctive thin, smooth, copper-colored bark when it flakes off, and showing a greenish layer beneath. A decoction of the leaves is antidiarrhetic and is used internally as a remedy for stomachache or externally as a lotion for skin disease, ringworms, wounds, and ulcers. Fresh leaves have shown a certain effectiveness in treating mild and moderately chronic cases, reducing blood glucose and urine glucose, and the frequency of urination (Perry 1980; Duke and Ayensu 1985).

English Name	Scientific Name	Nutritional and Therapeutic Values
		Leaves are used for medicinal purpose, as a remedy for acute gastroenteritis, dysentery, acute and chronic enteritis, and infantile indigestion. Fresh leaves are useful in treating traumatic injury, bleeding wounds, and pretibial ulcer (K. Lin 1998b).
		The Tikuna Indians use guava to treat diarrhea and dysentery, sore throat, vomiting, and stomach upsets by infusion or decoction of leaves and bark. Guava is rich in tannins, phenols, triterpenes, flavonoids, essential oils, saponins, carotenoids, lectins, vitamins, fiber, and fatty acid. It has an antioxidant function (Qian and Venant 2004).
		It also has antioxidant activities from peel, pulp, and seed fractions (Guo et al. 2003)
		Guava contains essential oils, quercetin, avicularin, guaijaverin, eugenol, crataegolic acid, and arjunolic acid (Y. Chang 2000).
		Fruit contains avicularin, guaijaverin, arabinose ester, amritoside, and crataegolic, luteioic, and argamolic acids. It is used to treat dysentery and acute gastrointestinal inflammation (Huang 1999).
Highbush blueberry	*Vaccinium corymbosum*	The fruits contain compounds known as anthocyanosides, which have been shown to offer significant protection against ulcers. It helps stimulate the production of mucus that protects the stomach lining from digestive acids. Dried fruits are rich in both tannins and pectin, which help relieve diarrhea (Duke 1997).
		Resveratrol, pterostilbene, and piceatannol were isolated from highbush blueberry. These naturally occurring stilbenes, known to be strong antioxidants and to have cancer chemopreventive activities, will add to the purported health benefits derived from the consumption of these small fruits (Rimando et al. 2004).
		Extracted from highbush blueberries, ursolic acid and 19-alpha-hydroxyursolic acid have been isolated and identified. All compounds have been shown to inhibit the growth of human tumor cells (Schmandke 2004).
Honey tangerine "Murcott"	*Citrus tangelo*	The fruit contains umbelliferone, which is antifungal. Fruit is antiemetic, antitussive, diaphoretic, digestive, and carminative. It is also used as a remedy for abdominal pain, diarrhea, and chest congestion. The peel is bitter, aromatic, stomachic, and antivinous, and it is used as a remedy for dyspepsia, vomiting, cholera, and colds (Perry 1980).

English Name	Scientific Name	Nutritional and Therapeutic Values
		Flavonoid glycosides have been identified in honey tangerine (Robards et al. 1999).
		Honey tangerine contains d-limonene, citrial, nobiletin, hesperidin, and vitamin B1 (Y. Chang 2000).
Indian dillenia	*Dillenia indica*	Bark is used to treat fever and diarrhea. The fruit pulp cleanses the hair (Perry 1980).
		Substances from the stem bark include anthocyanins, anthraquinones, and flavonoids (Tiwari and Srivastava 1979).
		According to Ayurvedic medicine, its bark and leaves are astringent. The bruised bark is applied as a cataplasm for arthritis. The pulp of the fruit is used as a hair wash. The juice of the unripe fruit allays cough, assists expectoration, and is used as a remedy for angina and aphthae (Oudhia 2007).
Indian jujube	*Zizyphus mauritiana*	The flowers are yellowish and borne in clusters. The edible fruits are round and 3–4 cm in diameter, and each fruit has one rounded knobby seed.
		A bark decoction is used as a gargle and mouthwash to treat angina and gingivitis. It is astringent and used to treat dysentery. The leaves are an antifebrile (Perry 1980).
		The fruits are applied on cuts and ulcers. The dried ripe fruit is a mild laxative. The seeds are sedative to halt nausea, vomiting, and abdominal pains in pregnancy. The leaves are applied as poultices and are helpful in relieving liver troubles, asthma, and fever (Morton 1987f). Indian jujube is rich in sugars, vitamins C and A, and carotene. It is also rich in calcium and magnesium (Leakey 1998).
Jaboticaba	*Myrciaria cauliflora*	The nuts are used to treat diarrhea and are used as an aphrodisiac. The red sap from the bark is taken against retention of water. Oil from the seeds or pulp of the bark is applied to treat skin affictions (Perry 1980).
		A new depside, jaboticabin, together with 17 known compounds were isolated from the fruit of jaboticaba. Two anthocyanins, cyanidin 3-glucoside and delphinidin 3-glucoside, also showed good activity in these assays (Reynertson 2006).
		The astringent decoction of the sun-dried skins is prescribed in Brazil as a treatment for hemoptysis, asthma, diarrhea, and dysentery.
		It is also used as a gargle for chronic inflammation of the tonsils (Morton 1987g).

English Name	Scientific Name	Nutritional and Therapeutic Values
		Jaboticaba has high antioxidant capacity. It contains cyanidin-3-O-β-glucopyranoside, and anthocyanin (Einbond et al. 2004).
Jackfruit	*Artocarpus heterophyllus* *A. odoratissimus*	Jackfruit is the largest tree-borne fruit in the world. The exterior of the compound fruit is green or yellow when ripe.
		The interior consists of large edible bulbs of yellow, banana-flavored flesh. Leaves are used as a remedy for diarrhea; the latex from the stem contains cerotic acid and is used to treat abscesses and ulcers.
		The bark is used as a gargle. The root is taken after childbirth for diarrhea and worms (Duke and Ayensu 1985). The Chinese consider jackfruit pulp and seeds to be tonic, cooling, and nutritious, and to be useful in overcoming the influence of alcohol on the system. The root is used as a remedy for skin diseases and asthma. An extract of the root is used for fever and diarrhea (Morton 1987h).
		The biological conversion of provitamin A in the jackfruit kernel appears to be satisfactory. It could be advocated as part of a strategy to prevent and control vitamin A deficiency (Chandrika et al. 2004).
		Fruit contains cycloheterophyllin, morin, cyanomaclurin, and acetylcholine. It is used to lower the blood pressure and improve sexual activity (N. Chiu and Chang 1995c).
Japanese apricot	*Prunus mume*	Dried petals are decocted for treatment of fever and sore throat. White flower buds are used to treat glandular tuberculosis, phlegm in chest, poor vision, and summer cold. Dried green fruits are used for abdominal pain, achlorhydria, cough, diarrhea, dysentery, fever, inappetence, and intestinal worms (Duke and Ayensu 1985).
		An active compound named B-1 (2-hydroxy-1-(7-hydroxy-2-oxo-2H-chromen-6-yl)), isolated from the fruit of Prunus mume, showed an ability to inhibit cancer cells (Jeong et al. 2006).
		Fruits are primarily used, although flowers and roots are also useful. Japanese apricot can be used for prolonged coughs, dryness in mouth and thirst, biliary ascariasis, cholecystitis, bacillary dysentery, and chronic diarrhea. It is externally used to treat granulomas, nasal polyps, and corns. Carbonized fruit is ground into a powder and applied as a poultice (K. Lin 1998e).
		It is used to treat cough, diarrhea, vomiting, and digestion problems (N. Chiu and Chang 1995a).

English Name	Scientific Name	Nutritional and Therapeutic Values
		Fruit contains prudomenin, amygdalin, and malic, succinic, citric, and tartaric acids. It is used to treat biliary ascariasis and hookworm (F. Chen 1997). Japanese apricot contains lactrile, cyanide, β-carotene, thiamine, oligopeptides, polysaccharide, and ascorbic, malic, citric acids. It is used internally as a remedy for chronic coughs and externally to treat fungal skin infections and warts and to improve blood fluidity. It has immunochemical properties (Fang and Huang 1999).
		Japanese apricot contains n-hexanal, trans-z-hexanal, n-hexanol, trans-2-hexen-1-ol, cis-3-hexen-1-ol, linalool, α-terpineol, geraniol, trimethyltetrahydronaphthalene, tetradecanoic acid, benzaldehyde, terpinen-4-ol, benzylalcohol, hexadecanoic acid, neutral lipids, glycolipids, phospholipids, free sterols, sterol esters, ceryl alcohol, fumaric acid (lup-20(29)-ene, 7β-15α-3-β-palmitate, stearate, arachidate, behenate, lignocerate, rhamnocitrin-3-O-rhamnoides, kaempferol-3-O-rhamnoside, rhamnetion-3-O-rhamnoside, quercetin-3-O-rhamnoside (Rieger 2006).
Java apple	*Syzygium aqueum*	The fruits and seeds are used when making a cooling beverage to be taken for eruptive fevers. The leaves macerated in water are a part of baths and lotions. The dried powdered leaves may be applied to a cracked tongue.
		The astringent bark has been used to make a mouthwash to treat thrush (Perry 1980). Four flavonoids isolated from the hexane extract were tested for a possible spasmolytic activity. All flavonoids showed dose-dependent spasmolytic activity (Ghayur et al. 2006).
		These results indicated that the presence of compounds with spasmolytic acid calcium antagonist activity may be responsible for the medicinal use of the plant in diarrhea (Ghayur et al. 2006).
Jujuba	*Zizyphus jujuba*	Fruit is eaten fresh or candied, which is used in desserts. The fruit, which is native to China, has a long history of medicinal uses. Jujuba contains polyphenolic compounds with antioxidative activity (Jong-Chan et al. 2006).
		A new cyclopeptide alkaloid, jubanine, together with known alkaloids, scutianine and zizyphine, have been isolated from the stem bark of *Zizyphus jujuba* and identified by spectral analysis (Tripathi et al. 2001).

English Name	Scientific Name	Nutritional and Therapeutic Values
		The fruits are considered to be pectoral; the bark is a remedy for diarrhea; the roots are used for fever; and the leaves are used for scorpion stings. The stone seeds are used as hypnotics and narcotics. The fruits or kernels of the seeds are probably the most important part of the plant in medicine, although the leaves, bark, wood, and root also are indicated as useful (Perry 1980).
		The plant has been used in China since ancient times and, apart from its virtues as a medicine, it acts as an adjuvant with other drugs that are combined in medicines. It is mentioned as antagonistic to Aconitum as well as to Gentiana species.
		It is administered as having nervine, tonic, roborant, stomachic, sedative, laxative, bechic, antipyretic, and diuretic properties. The leaves, root, and bark are used to treat fevers, to promote hair growth, and as a collyrium. A decoction of the root is taken to relieve a sensation of fullness in the stomach and to aid digestion. The seed oil contains oleic, linoleic, and palmitic acids and phytosterol (Perry 1980).
Kiwifruit	*Actinidia deliciosa* A. *chinensis* A. *latifolia*	The fruit is astringent and antiscorbutic and is used for quenching thirst and treating gravel. The plant is used to treat esophageal and liver cancers, rheumatoid arthritis, urinary stones, and fever.
		The vitamin C properties are beneficial for the treatment of scurvy, allergic purpura, the common cold, and coronary heart disease and the prevention of certain cancers (Duke and Ayensu 1985). A decoction of roots is used to treat rheumatoid arthritis, sore throat, diarrhea, boils, and pyodermas. Kiwifruit is a good source of vitamin C, potassium, and folate. Crushed fresh leaves are used for topical application to treat snakebites, burns, and scalds (K. Lin 1998e).
		Kiwifruit is a good source of vitamin C, potassium, and folate. It has been reported that kiwifruit may also be a source of vitamins E and K. It has laxative properties that are particularly beneficial for elderly consumers (Ferguson and Ferguson 2003).
		The whole herb, including the root, is used as an anti-inflammatory and an antiswelling analgesic to treat sore throat, diarrhea, rheumatoid arthritis, boils, and pyodermas (K. Lin 1998e). Kiwifruit contains actinidine, quercetin, kaempferol, caffeine, pocumaric acid, leucodelphinidin, leucocyanidin, matatabic acid, iridomyrmecin, allomatatabiol, neonepetalactone, dihydronepetalactol, matatabiether, isoneomatabiol, matatabistic acid, neomatabiol, and vitamins B and C.

English Name	Scientific Name	Nutritional and Therapeutic Values
		It is used to treat esophageal and liver cancer, rheumatoid arthritis, urinary stones, and fever (Zhu 1989). It also has antioxidant activities from peel, pulp, and seed fractions (Guo et al. 2003).
Lansat	*Lansium domesticum*	The bark and fruit peel contain lansium acid. The seeds contain a bitter principle and traces of alkaloid. A decoction of the astringent bark or leaves is used to treat dysentery. The seeds are antipyretic and anthelmintic.
		A tincture of the resin and tannin extracted from the rind has been found to relieve abdominal pain, diarrhea, and gastrointestinal disorders (Perry 1980).
		Cyclocaratanoid triterpenes isolated from the leaves have novel inhibitors for skin tumors (Nishizawa et al. 1989). It was reported that five tetranortriterpenoids, domesticulides A–E (1–5), were isolated from seeds of *Lansium domesticum Corr.* together with 11 known triterpenoids (6–16). Their structures were elucidated by analysis of their spectroscopic data. Compounds 2, 3, 4, 7, 8, 10, 11, and 15 showed antimalarial activity against Plasmodium falciparum with IC50s of 2.4–9.7 (g/ml (Saewan et al. 2006). Three new natural onoceranoid triterpenes — lansionic acid (1), 3-beta-hydroxyonocera-8 (26), 14-dien-21-one (2), and 21-alpha-hydroxyonocera-8 (26), 14-dien-3-one (3) — were isolated from the fruit peel of *Lansium domesticum* together with two known triterpenoids (4 and 5), and their structures were elucidated from spectral data. These triterpenoids exhibited mild toxicity against brine shrimp (Artemia salina) (Tanaka et al. 2002).
Lemon	*Citrus limon*	Plant provides essential oils that are antibiotic to Bacillus, Meningococcus, and Typhus bacteria. The juice is recommended as an antidote for poisoning by euphorbiaceous plants. The bark is bitter, tonic, and stomachic (Duke and Ayensu 1985; Perry 1980).
		Fruits are used to treat anorexia, vitamin C deficiency, bronchiolitis, and heat stroke. Root is used for epigastric pain, hernial pain, orchitis, coughs, and bronchial asthma. Leaves treat asthma, bloatedness, and diarrhea. Fresh lemon juice with rock sugar diluted with water has appetizing and thirst-quenching effects (K. Lin 1998f).
		There are five flavonoids (naringin, hesperidin, neohesperidin, sinensetin, and nobiletin) in the peel of lemon. It is used as a traditional Chinese medicine (Y. Lu et al. 2006).

English Name	Scientific Name	Nutritional and Therapeutic Values
		Fruit, roots, and leaves are used to promote salivary secretion and are stomachic, expectorant, and antitussive. Roots are used to promote circulation and are analgesic, antitussive, and antiasthmatic. Leaves are antitussive and expectorant and are used to stimulate appetite (K. Lin 1998g).
		Lemon contains coumarins, bioflavonoids, vitamins A, B, and C, mucilage, volatile oils, limonene, l-linalool, d-limonene, linalyl acetate, flavonoids, benzoic acid, cinnamic acid, coumarins, and carotenoids. It is antiseptic, antirheumatic, antibacterial, antioxidant, carminative, laxative, liniment, and vermifuge. Juice is used to treat tumors and warts (Mansell and McIntosh 1991).
Litchi	*Litchi chinensis*	The fruit is a drupe, 3–4 cm long and 3 cm in diameter. The outside is covered by a red, roughly textured rind that is inedible. The inside consists of a layer of sweet, translucent white flesh that is rich in vitamin C.
		It contains amino acids (lysine, leucine, valine, and alanine), glutamic acid, serine, and traces of proline. A total of 42 volatile constituents has been identified; β-phenethyl alcohol and its derivatives and terpenoids comprised the major portion of the volatiles. Fruit is antidiarrhetic, antitussive, tonic, and recommended for enlarged glands and tumors. The rind is used to treat smallpox eruptions and bowel fluxes. The seeds are analgesic and astringent and are used to treat colic, gastralgia, orchitis, pains of hernia, and anemic pain (Duke and Ayensu 1985).
		It was reported that aqueous extract of litchi seeds may lower feeding and improve the metabolic status in diabetic conditions. This is probably due to its hypoglycemic and hypocholesterolemic effects (Babu and Srinivasan 1997).
		It also contains polyphenoloxidase, vitamins A, B, and C, α-(methylene-cyclo-propyl)-glycine, saponin, and leucocyanidin (N. Chiu and Chang 1995e).
		Leaf, fruit, and seeds contain vitamins A, B, and C, sugar, lysine, leucine, valine, alanine, serine, proline, threonine, arginine, lysine, β-phenethyl alcohol, and amino, asparagic, citric, and glutamic acids. It is used as a remedy for gland enlargement and tumors and to treat bites of poisonous animals. It is an astringent and analgesic and is used in treatment of gastralgia, colic, and orchitis (Johnston et al. 1980).

English Name	Scientific Name	Nutritional and Therapeutic Values
Lobi-lobi	*Flacourtia inermis* *F. rukam*	The astringent juice is used to treat diarrhea and dysentery. The sap of the leaves is applied to inflamed eyelids. The dried and pounded leaves are dusted on wounds. The fruit is used as a remedy for dysmenorrhea (Perry 1980). In the Philippines, the roots are considered to be medicinal, and their decoction is given internally to women after childbirth.
Longan	*Dimocarpus longan*	The fruit is edible, which is often used in East Asian soups, snacks, desserts, and sweet and sour foods. They are round with a thin brown-colored inedible shell. The flesh of the fruit, which surrounds a big, black seed, is translucent, white, soft, and juicy. Seeds contain saponin and are used to wash the hair. Bark contains tannin, and the leaves contain quercetin and quercitron. The fruit is antidotal and anthelmintic and acts on the spleen. Seeds are a nutrient tonic and are used as a remedy for insomnia, neurasthenia, and excessive sweating. It is an antifatigue tonic in anemic, convalescent, debilitated, or postpartum individuals. Plant is used to treat anemia, hyperactive mental activity, forgetfulness, and uterine cancer (Duke and Ayensu 1985). Longan is very nutritious, with high values for energy, protein, and potassium (Hoe and Siong 1999).
Loquat	*Eriobotrya japonica*	The loquat fruit grows in clusters. It is oval rounded with a smooth or downy yellow or orange skin. Each fruit contains five ovules, of which three to five mature into large brown seeds. It has high sugar, acid, and pectin contents. Fruits are consumed throughout Asia. It is an important crop in Thailand. The fruit contains gallic acid, corilagin, and ellagic acid. Seed and pulp contain phenolics (Rangkadilok et al. 2005). The leaves contain d-sorbitol and ascorbic acid oxidase and are rich in vitamin B. The seeds contain saponins, amygdalin, emulsin, and hydrocyanic acid. The fruits contain citric and succinic acids, oxidase, amylase, invertase, and vitamin C. Leaves contain large amounts of saponin and are used to treat chronic bronchitis and coughs. It is bitterish and used to treat lungs and stomach. It is prescribed for phlegm, high fever, and nausea (Perry 1980). Logistic regression was used to develop a multivariate model, which indicated that alternative medicine such as loquat is positively associated with age- and diabetes-related problems (Noel et al. 1997). Leaves are used to treat bronchitis, cough, gastritis, and vomiting (K. Lin 1998e).

English Name	Scientific Name	Nutritional and Therapeutic Values
Manggis	*Garcinia mangostana*	Leaf, flower, and fruit contain levulose, sucrose, amygdalin, cryptoxanthin, carotenes, phenyl ethyl alcohol pentosans, essential oils, and malic, citric, tartaric, and succinic acids. Loquat is antitussive and expectorant and is used to treat bronchitis, cough, fever, and nausea. It is externally applied to treat epistaxis, small pox, and ulcers (Duke and Ayensu 1985).
		The parts, pericarp, bark, dried leaves, and powdered rind of the fruit are astringent. The bark and pericarp are used in treating diarrhea and dysentery. A decoction of the root may be given to treat irregular menstruation (Perry 1980).
		It is used as a remedy for dysentery, diarrhea, urinary tract infections, gonorrhea, thrush, tuber calluses, menstrual disorders, cancer, and osteoarthritis. It is also used to stimulate the immune system and improve mental health (Jellin et al. 2003).
		Fruit skin contains mangostin. It is used as a remedy for diarrhea, cough, and intestinal infection and to improve blood circulation (N. Chiu and Chang 1995b).
Mango	*Mangifera indica*	The plant is bactericidal and fungicidal. It contains arabinan, carotenoids, galacturonan, glucan, isoquercitrin, mangiferin, quercetin, violaxanthin, and m-digallic, ellagic, embolic, mangiferonic, ambonic, and isomangiferolic acids.
		Leaf ashes are used to treat burns, scalds, and skin ailments. Smoke from a burning leaf is inhaled as a remedy for hiccups, asthma, cough, and other throat ailments. Seeds are used as a remedy for stubborn colds, coughs, and diarrhea (Duke and Ayensu 1985).
		Vimany and mangiferin were isolated from mango recently, and these may be useful in the treatment of diseases of pathogenesis or allergic diseases (Garcia et al. 2003).
		The nutshell and juice are used in folk remedies for warts in Brazil.
		It is anodyne, antiseptic, antitussive, aperitif, ascaricide, and vermifuge. It is also used as a remedy for anasarca, anemia, asthma, bladder ailments, bronchitis, burn, catarrh, chest ailments, cholera, circulation, cough, cracked feet, diarrhea, diphtheria, and dropsy (Duke and duCellier 1993).
		The mango seeds are powdered and mixed with "Mishri" and dried "bras" (*Rhododendron arboreum*) flowers as a treatment for dysentery. The kernel is the principal part used for medicinal purposes (Chauhan 1999).

English Name	Scientific Name	Nutritional and Therapeutic Values
		Mango sap is toxic and can cause a rash similar to poison ivy on the skin. The active principles in sap are mangiferin, mangiferic acid, and mangiferol.
		Mango is an astringent and is used in variety of folk remedies for various ailments. Remedies for bronchitis, internal hemorrhage, bladder ailments, diarrhea, syphilis, ringworm, and warts are made from twigs and leaves (Rieger 2006).
Marang	*Artocarpus odoratissimus* *A. heterophyllus*	Leaves are used to treat diarrhea. Stem latex is used to treat abscesses and ulcers. The pulp and seeds of the fruit are regarded as cooling, tonic, and pectoral.
		The sap is antisyphilitic and is used as a vermifuge; the wood contains a yellow pigment, morin and cyanomaclurin; the bark has tannin; and the latex contains cerotic acid (Perry 1980; Duke and Ayensu 1985).
		The biological conversion of provitamin A in the kernel of marang appears satisfactory. It could be advocated as part of a strategy to prevent and control vitamin A deficiency (Chandrika et al. 2004).
		It is a tonic to treat discomfort from alcohol influence. Marang contains caoutchoue, resin, cerotic acid, protein, and minerals (Duke and Ayensu 1985).
Mazzard cherry	*Cerasus avium* *Prunus avium*	The fruit is used as a folk remedy for aches and pain. The fruit stalks are astringent, diuretic, and tonic.
		A decoction is used in the treatment of cystitis, edema, bronchial complaints, looseness of the bowels, and anemia. An aromatic resin can be obtained by making small incisions in the trunk (Perry 1980).
		This has been used as an inhalant in the treatment of persistent coughs. Although no specific mention has been seen for this species, all members of the genus contain amygdalin and prunasin, substances that break down in water to form hydrocyanic acid. In small amounts, this exceedingly poisonous compound stimulates respiration, improves digestion, and gives a sense of well-being (Chiej 1984; Bown 1995).
		It has been reported that stalk extract of cherry has anti-inflammatory effects (Blazso and Gabor 1994).
Miracle fruit	*Synsepalum dulcificum*	The single-seeded berry is bland and insipid, but contains a glycoprotein, miraculin.

English Name	Scientific Name	Nutritional and Therapeutic Values
		The fruit is given to reduce fevers and as a treatment for diabetes, malaria, piles, and acute coughs (Theerasilp and Kurihara 1988).
		It has been reported that miracle fruit may be used as an adjuvant for treating diabetic patients with insulin resistance because this fruit has the ability to improve insulin sensitivity (C. Chen et al. 2006).
		The lipid fraction of crushed seeds from miracle fruit contains neutral lipids, including glycolipids, phospholipids, triglycerides, diglycerides, monoglycerides, fatty acids, and unsaponifiable matter. The unsaponifiable material contained hydrocarbons, steryl esters, triterpene alcohols, free sterols, and an unknown substance (Guney and Nawar 1977).
		The red pigments of miracle fruit were cyanidin-3-monogalactoside, cyanidin-3-monoglucoside, and cyanidin-3-monoarabinoside. The major flavonol pigments were quercetin-3-monogalactoside, kaempferol-3-monoglucoside, myricetin-3-monogalactoside, and traces of similar flavonoids (Buckmire and Francis 1976).
Monkey jack	*Artocarpus lakoocha*	The fruit contains β-amyrin acetate and lupeol acetate. The juice and seeds from this plant are purgative. The bark is astringent. The root is tonic and deobstruent, and the leaves are used in treating dropsy (Perry 1980).
		Monkey jack's major active ingredient, oxyresveratrol, was dissolved in propylene glycol and applied daily. This preliminary study suggested that the heartwood extract may have a promising potential for use as an effective and economical skin-whitening agent (Tengamnuay et al. 2006).
		Fruit and bark are used for medicinal purposes (Chauhan 1999).
Moraceae	*Ficus pumila* var. *awkeotsang*	A gelatinous dessert is made from the seeds of this fig-like fruit. The stem and leaves are bitter and cooling and are used to bandage wounds and to treat boils, sore throat, and rheumatism. A decoction of a whole young plant is prescribed to treat piles. A fermented infusion of the leaves is used to relieve painful and protruding piles (Perry 1980).
		Fruits are used as a remedy for oligogalactia, amenorrhea, nocturnal ejaculation, impotence, and chyluria. The branch of the plant is used as a remedy for rheumatism, arthritis, and traumatic injury. Boiled in equal amounts of water and wine, the branch of the plant can be used to treat oral disorders (K. Lin 1998a).

English Name	Scientific Name	Nutritional and Therapeutic Values
		Moraceae has been used in Chinese medicine for its powerful scavenging activity. It is used to treat inflammation, diseases of blood circulation, and for tumors (W. Lu et al. 2001).
		Root and stem contain meso-inositol, β-sitosterol, taraxeryl acetate, and β-amyrin acetate. Fruit buds contain meso-inositol, β-sitosterol, taraxeryl acetate, and β-amyrin acetate (N. Chiu and Chang 1995b)
		Latex from Moraceae can be used to treat carbuncle, dysentery, hematuria, piles, hernia, and bladder inflammation (Duke and Ayensu 1985). It is used to treat carbuncle, dysentery, hematuria, hemorrhoids, hernia, oligogalactia, amenorrhea, nocturnal ejaculation, impotence, chyluria, and bladder inflammation (K. Lin 1998a).
Mulberry	*Morus alba*	The fruit is insipid. It varies from white to pink, but the natural fruit color of the species in the wild is deep purple. It is used for ethnomedical uses in traditional Chinese medicine.
		Mulberry is native to China. It is restorative, tonic, pectoral, and diuretic. It is prescribed to treat cough, asthma, phthisis and other chest complaints, dropsy, and rheumatism. The leaves contain carotene, succinic acid, adenine, choline, and amylase. They are depurative, cooling, and resolvent.
		The fruits are thirst relieving and promote vigor. The root bark, young branchlets, leaves, and fruit are all medicinal, containing β-amyrin, sitosterol, resinotannol, and some volatile oils. The plant is used especially to treat high blood pressure and numbness in hands and feet. The root bark is antivinous and is used to treat rheumatism (Perry 1980; Duke and Ayensu 1985).
		Roots are used as a remedy for cough and edema; branches are used to treat rheumatic arthritis and lumbago; leaves are used to treat influenza, cough, and sore eye; and fruits are used to treat chronic hepatitis, anemia, and neurasthenia (K. Lin 1998a).
		It has been reported that mulberroside F, isolated from mulberry leaves, might be used as a skin-whitening agent (Lee et al. 2002). Mulberry contains vitamin B1, adenine, choline, isoquercitrin, and trigonelline. It is used to treat high blood pressure and diabetes and to lower the blood sugar level (Y. Chang 2000).
		Mulberry has antioxidant activities from peel, pulp, and seed fractions (Guo et al. 2003).

English Name	Scientific Name	Nutritional and Therapeutic Values
		Leaves, branches, fruit, bark, and roots of mulberry are used for their therapeutic properties. Root is antitussive, antiasthmatic, diuretic, and antiswelling. Branches are antipyretic and analgesic.
		Leaves are antipyretic, and fruits are nourishing to the blood. Leaves contain inokosterone, ecdysterone, moracetin, quercetin-3-triglucoside, astragalin, α-β-hexenal, pipecolic acid, glutathione, and myoinositol (K. Lin 1998a).
		Young twig from mulberry contains morin, dihydromorin, maclurin, dihydrokaempferol, mulberrin, 2,4,4-tetrahydroxybenzophenone, mulberrochromene, cyclomulberrochromene. It is antirheumatic, antihypertensive, and diuretic, and it is used to remove obstructions of the intestinal tract (Huang 1999).
		It contains two antibiotic compounds, morellin and guttiferin, which are active against gram-positive and gram-negative bacteria.
		The pounded seed of this plant is applied externally to resolve glandular swellings. Resin from stem is used for cancerous sores, indolent ulcers, and tooth extraction (Duke and Ayensu 1985).
Mundo	*Garcinia dulcis*	Two major phenolic compounds, dulcisxanthones and dulcinone, were isolated from the flowers of *Garcinia dulcis*. These compounds act as radical scavengers and antibacterial agents (Deachathai et al. 2006).
		Five xanthones, including symphoxanthone, were isolated from the bark of *G. dulcis*. All five inhibited the growth of Plasmodium falciparum (Likhitwitayawuid et al. 1998). *Garcinia dulcis* is used in traditional medicine to treat lymphatitis, parotitis, and struma.
		A new xanthone, dulciol A, and two known xanthones were isolated from the bark. Four novel xanthones and eight known xanthones were isolated from the roots (Iinuma et al. 1996).
		A preparation of the fruit is used to treat bilious conditions, diarrhea, and dysentery. The gum resin is used in China for external medicinal use only, either alone as a powder or as an ingredient in treatment of wounds of all kinds, cancerous sores, and indolent ulcers, and to cause decayed teeth to drop out.
		The plant contains gum, resin, starch, and gambogic acid (Perry 1980).

English Name	Scientific Name	Nutritional and Therapeutic Values
Myrobalan	*Phyllanthus emblica*	Fresh fruits (emblics) are baked in tarts or added to other foods and seasoned during cooking. The juice is used to flavor vinegar. Both ripe and half-ripe fruits are candied whole and also made into jam and other preserves, sweetmeats, pickles, and relishes.
		The fruit contains the piscicidal compound phyllanthin. Root is used as a stimulant for kidneys. Whole plant is decocted as a remedy for conjunctivitis, diarrhea, edema, enteritis, hepatitis, jaundice, marasmus, nephritis, ophthalmus, urogenital ailments, and worms (Duke and Ayensu 1985).
		Fruits are used as a remedy for colds, fever, cough, sore throat, toothache, diabetes, and vitamin C deficiency. Roots are used to treat hypertension, epigastric pain, enteritis, and tuberculous lymphadenopathy. Leaves used externally for edema and eczema (K. Lin 1998b). Leaves of myrobalan have antineutrophil and antiplatelet properties in vitro. This agrees with the anti-inflammatory and antipyretic usage of this tree in traditional medicine by rural populations in Asia (Summanen 1999).
		Fruits, leaves, bark, and roots are used. Fruits are cool, antipyretic, anti-inflammatory, throat soothing, nourishing to the lungs, and antitussive. Leaves are acrid tasting, neutral, and diuretic, and these are used to treat edema and eczema. Root is bland tasting, neutral, and astringent. It is used to treat hypotension, epigastric pain, enteritis, tuberculous lymphadenopathy, headache, and liver and stomach disorders (Y. Chang 2000).
		Myrobalan contains chebulinic acid, mucic acid, α-leucodelphinidin, and vitamin C. It is used as a remedy for conjunctivitis, diarrhea, abdominal tumors, nephritis, and urogenital ailments (Shishoo et al. 1997). It also contain emblicanins A and B and pedunculagin (Chevallier 1996).
Papaya	*Carica papaya*	Papaya contains antitumor agents, including benzyl isothiocyanate, β-carotene, carpaine, carposide, cryptoxanthin, cryptoxanthin monepoxide, lycopene, papain, rennin, and violaxanthin. Dried pulp is used as a remedy for inflamed and swollen feet. The latex is used for burns and pains and as a vermifuge (Duke and Ayensu 1985).
		Papaya is one of the main fruits that has been recommended for prevention of vitamin A deficiency. The major carotenoids of yellow- and red-fleshed papaya were the provitamin A, carotenoids, β-carotene, and β-cryptoxanthin (Chandrika et al. 2003).

English Name	Scientific Name	Nutritional and Therapeutic Values
		It contains carpaine, φ-carpaine, pseudocarzyl isothiocyanate, nicotine, choline, carposide, saponin, cotinine, myosmine, papain, rennin, cryptoxanthin, violaxanthin, β-carotene, monoepoxide, lycopene, 5,6-monopoxy-β-carotene, and vitamins A, B1, B2, C, and G (N. Chiu and Chang 1995f).
		Fruit pulp is the basic component of facial creams, salves, and shampoos. Papaya culls are ground into a puree that can be used for cosmetic purposes. The puree has two proteolytic enzymes, papain and chymorpapain, and it retains proteolytic activity over a wide pH range.
		Papain can be used during surgical procedures to dissolve ruptured spinal discs. Folk-medicine uses of the fruits, leaves, and latex may be related to papain content. Fresh latex can be smeared on boils, warts, corns, or freckles to remove them from the skin. It is also used for treating psoriasis and ringworm. Both the latex and plant part are considered antiseptic, antibacterial, anthelmintic, and amebicidal. Papain is used in remedies for ulcers, diphtheria, swelling, toothache, fever, relief of gas, and sour stomach (Rieger 2006).
Passion fruit	*Passiflora edulis* *P. foetida*	Passion fruit pulp is often eaten fresh, and the seeds are edible. The fresh root is considered to be a powerful narcotic and poisonous. The leaves produce hydrocyanic acid and hence are poisonous (Perry 1980).
		The fruit is used as a flavoring in drinks, desserts, sauces, and many other foods. This plant contains fixed oil, lethicin, choline, phytin, globulin, and sesamin. It has therapeutic values as an anodyne, nerve sedative, diuretic, and antispasmodic. It is also useful in controlling convulsions (particularly in the young, as indicated by muscular twitching and asthenic insomnia in childhood, and the elderly), irritative and neuralgic pains with debility, nervous headache, and hysteria (Hutchens 1991).
		The fruit is edible, but the fresh root is considered to be a powerful narcotic and poisonous. The leaves are applied as a dressing to wounds. In small doses, the root is vermifuge. However, it is poisonous in larger doses (Perry 1980).
		The fruits are used as a remedy for cervical lymphadenitis, pyodermas, scabies, and ulcer of the leg. Fruits are boiled in water for washing or mashed and applied topically (K. Lin 1998b).
		Passion fruit has been used for the treatment of insomnia, anxiety, and various other disorders of the central nervous system since antiquity (Dhawan et al. 2003).

English Name	Scientific Name	Nutritional and Therapeutic Values
		The whole herb and fruits are used as a remedy for cough, cervical lymphadenitis, and pyodermas. Externally, fruits are boiled in water for washing, or the fresh herb is macerated for topical use (K. Lin 1998b). The fruit is used in folk remedies to treat cancer of the stomach. It is reported to be cyanogenic, narcotic, and sedative. Passion fruit is a folk remedy for epilepsy, insomnia, morphinism, neuralgia, and spasm (Duke and duCellier 1993).
Peach	*Prunus persica* *Amygdalus persica*	The kernel contains emulsin, prussic acid, choline, allantoinase, vitamin B1, acetylcholine, naringenin, catechin, and lycopene.
		The kernels are laxative, depurative, and antispasmodic against cough, rheumatism, dysmenorrhea, amenorrhea, contusion, hematoma, constipation, and hemorrhages. The bark contains a heteroside persicoside, and the leaves and branches are smygdonitrile. The inner white bark of the root is used as a prophylactic in epidemics and as a remedy for dropsy and jaundice (Perry 1980; Y. Chang 2000).
		Leaves of peach are used for their antipyretic, antitoxic, insecticidal, and antipruritic properties. They are used as a remedy for malaria, furunculosis, hemorrhoids, eczema, and vaginal trichomoniasis. Flowers are used as a laxative and diuretic (K. Lin 1998a).
		Total and soluble dietary fibers are low in peach (7.0%) compared with fruits such as fig, mango, orange, papaya, and sweet lime (Ramulu and Rao 2003).
		Kernel, leaves, and flowers are used. Kernel is used for dysmenorrhea, amenorrhea, contusion, hematoma, and constipation. Leaves are used for malaria, furunculosis, hemorrhoids, eczema, and vaginal trichomoniasis. Flowers are used for edema, ascites, and constipation (K. Lin 1998b).
		Amygdalus persica has a high contents of oxalic acid in the leaves (P. Singh 1973). It is used for headache, eye sore, flu, and inflammation (Y. Chang 2000).
		Peach leaves, flowers, and especially seeds and bark contain cyanogenic glycosides, such as amygdalin and prunasin. These compounds yield cyanide. However, in plant tissues, cyanide is low enough in concentration to be considered therapeutic, particularly for cancer treatment (Rieger 2006).
		Peach bark has been used as an herbal remedy for a wide variety of ailments. It has use in encouraging menstruation in females with delayed menses.

English Name	Scientific Name	Nutritional and Therapeutic Values
		It also relieves bladder inflammation and urinary tract problems; functions as a mild laxative; has expectorant activity for the lungs, nose, and throat; and relieves chest pain and spasms.
		Bark and root extracts contain phloretin, which has antibiotic activity on gram-positive and gram-negative bacteria (Rieger 2006).
		Leaf, flower, and fruit contain malic acid, citric acid, octalactone, leucoanthocyanins, tannins, hexalactone, hectalactone, benzyl alcohol, nonalactone, decalactone, ethanol, hexanol, acetaldehyde, benzaldehyde, acetic acid, pentanoic acid, and hexanoic acid. They have astringent, febrifuge, parasiticide, diuretic, sedative, and vermifuge properties (Duke and Ayensu 1985).
Pepino	*Solanum verbascifolium* *S. melongena* *S. muricatum* *S. xanthocarpum*	A pepino melon or melon pear is a fruit with variable shapes and sizes, rounded or oblong. When ripe, pepino has a yellow cream skin with purple stripes. The flesh is juicy and moderately sweet, with the same texture as a melon.
		In Taiwan, it is administered to treat dysentery, intestinal pain, and fever. A poultice of the leaves is a headache remedy; a decoction is drunk as a remedy against vertigo and is also used to bathe the body after childbirth. The leaves are considered to be a potent medicine for expelling all impurities through the urine, and in particular to treat leucorrhea. Decoction of roots is used as a remedy for dyspepsia and violent pain. Decoction taken with ginger and onion is used to treat hematuria (Perry 1980; Duke and Ayensu 1985).
		The root of this plant is used to treat acute dysentery, mental depression, and disorders of the spine. Leaves are used as a remedy for rectal prolapse in infants. The ripe fruit is effective in treatment of swelling and abscesses (K. Lin 1998e). Primary constituents (starches, proteins, sugars, fatty acids, minerals, vitamins, and glucosides) and secondary metabolites (saponins, alkaloids, tannins, oxalates, carotenes, anthocyanins, and betalains) have been identified in pepino (Jacobsen et al. 2003).
		Roots and leaves are used. Roots are used to treat stomachache, fractures, traumatic injury, and chronic granulocytic leukemia. Leaves are used as a topical in treatment of pyodermas ulcer, cuts, and abrasions (K. Lin 1998g).

English Name	Scientific Name	Nutritional and Therapeutic Values
		Pepino contains solasonine, solanine, solanidine, solasodine, carpesterol, and diosgenin (N. Chiu and Chang 1995a). Root contains solasonine and is used to treat dysentery, intestinal pain, and fever (N. Chiu and Chang 1995a).
Persimmon	*Diospyros kaki*	It is a native of China. Juice squeezed from the unripe fruit reduces high blood pressure, stops hemorrhage, helps to reduce congestion of hemorrhoids, acts as a laxative, and is a remedy for typhus and typhoid. The calyx and the exudation on the dried fruit are medicinal. The fruit contains 3681–7598 g β-carotene equivalent. It is stomachic, astringent, and pectoral. Persimmon contains the antitumor compounds betulinic acid, acetylcholine, choline, and shibuol (Perry 1980; Duke and Ayensu 1985).
		Persimmon fruits are used to treat dry coughs, sore throat, gastrointestinal bleeding, hemorrhoidal bleeding, and hypertension. Fruit stalks are used to treat hiccups and night frequency. Roots are used to treat hemoptysis, hemorrhoids, and uterine bleeding, and leaves are used for thrombocytopenic purpura, functional uterine bleeding, and bleeding peptic ulcer. Young and tender leaves are used as a tea in treatment of coronary artery insufficiency, especially in seniors (K. Lin 1998f).
		Persimmon has been used traditionally in Korea to promote maternal health. The extract of persimmon fruit was found to be the most potent, with an IC50 value of 0.11 mg/ml (Han et al. 2002).
		Whole herb is used. Fruits are used to treat dry coughs, sore throat, gastrointestinal bleeding, hemorrhoidal bleeding, and hypertension. Fruit stalk is a remedy for hiccups and night frequency. Roots are used to treat hemoptysis, bleeding hemorrhoids, and uterine bleeding. Leaves are used for thrombocytopenic purpura, functional uterine bleeding, bleeding peptic ulcer, hemoptysis, bleeding hemorrhoids, and hypertension (K. Lin 1998f).
		Fruit and crushed leaves are used for medicinal purposes (Chauhan 1999). It contains oleanolic acid, ursolic acid, astragali, myricitron, vitamin C, L-citrulline, mannitol, shibuol, choline, acetylcholine, hydroxytriterpenic acid, oleanolic acid, and betulinic acid. Persimmon can be used to treat toothache by cooking the powdered bark and adhering it onto the tooth (Y. Chang 2000).

English Name	Scientific Name	Nutritional and Therapeutic Values
		In modern medicine, the juice squeezed from the unripe persimmon fruit, the calyx, and part of the stalk below it as well as the exudation of the dried fruit are used as a medicine. The fruit is stomachic, astringent, and pectoral. It is used to treat hiccups, and the juice from unripe fruit reduces high blood pressure, stops hemorrhage, helps to reduce congestion of hemorrhoids, acts as a laxative, and is a remedy for typhus and typhoid. A decoction of the calyx and peduncle is a remedy for obstinate cough, difficult breathing, and retching from a cough. The stalk is stomachic, antiemetic, and bechic (Perry 1980).
Phoenix eye	*Sterculia nobilis*	Ping-pong or phoenix eye has been identified as one of the important medicinal plants in Japan (Fuju et al. 2003).
Pineapple	*Ananas comosus*	The ripe fruits are considered to be depurative and diuretic. The roots are used to treat gonorrhea. The juice of the unripe fruit acts as a violent purgative, an abortifacient, and, in small quantities, an anthelmintic. The fruit or its juice promotes digestion and is also useful in treating throat troubles. The young leaves are used to treat fever. The ripe pineapple contains sugars, free organic acid, a trace of vanillin, and the enzyme bromelin (Perry 1980). Flowers are used to regulate menstruation, especially menorrhagia. Leaves are used as a treatment for abundant menses. The fruit is used to treat uterine fibroids and menorrhagia (Arias 1989; Estevez and Baez 1998). It is used to treat various women's health conditions in the Dominican Republic (Andreana et al. 2002). Bromolain is a mixture of protein-digesting enzymes found in pineapples. It aids digestion and helps reduce inflammation, bruising healing time, and pain following surgery and physical injuries (Taussig and Batkin 1988). It also has properties of interference with growth of malignant cells, inhibition of platelet aggregation, fibrinolytic activity, anti-inflammatory action, and skin debridement properties (Taussig and Batkin 1988). Pineapple fruit contains vitamins A, B, C, and G and bromelin. Leaves contain ergosterol peroxide, 5-stigmautena-3β-3α-diol, 3,4-dihydroxycinnamic acid, and ananasic acid (Y. Chang 2000). Pineapple contains vitamins A, B, C, and G. It also contains ergosterol peroxide, 5-stigmantena-3β, 7α-diol, 3,4-dihydroxycinnamic acid, 4-hydroxycinnamic acid, ananasic acid, and bromelin (Y. Chang 2000).

English Name	Scientific Name	Nutritional and Therapeutic Values
		It has papaia and pepsis functions. Pineapple is used to improve digestion and as a remedy for diarrhea (Y. Chang 2000).
		Bromelain is a proteolytic enzyme from pineapple juice that has uses as an anti-inflammatory, for muscle relaxation, and in the treatment of warts, abscesses, bruises, and ulcers. Juice from unripe fruits is said to be purgative and also anthelmintic (Rieger 2006).
		Pineapple leaf contains ergosterol peroxide, ananasic acid, 5-stigmantena-3β, 7d-diol, 3,4-dihydroxycinnamic acid, and vitamins. It has antioxidant activity and is used to aid digestion, lower blood pressure, and as an anticancer agent (N. Chiu and Chang 1995d).
		Unripe fruit improves digestion, increases appetite, and relieves dyspepsia. It is used as a uterine tonic. Ripe fruit reduces excessive gastric acid, and the juice is used as a digestive tonic and diuretic (Rieger 2006).
Pineapple guava	*Feijoa sellowiana*	The composition and amount of liposoluble substances in the flesh and peel of feijoa fruit were isolated. The identified substances included triacylglycerols, sterols, cerebrosides, digalactosyldiacylglycerols, ceramide oligosides, and phosphatidyl glycerols (Kolesnik et al. 1992).
Ping-pong	*Sterculia nobilis*	The fruits of the noble bottle tree are as big as dove eggs. The seeds are wrapped in red legumes that crack when the fruit is ripened. Ping-pong or Phoenix's eye produces chemicals that kill off surrounding plants as a defense mechanism (Fuju et al. 2003).
Pitanga	*Eugenia uniflora* *E. urceolata* *E. jambos*	A poultice made with roots is applied to eruptions on the skin. The root is also utilized in a decoction after childbirth.
		The bark, leaves, and root are used in poultices to treat itch. An infusion of the leaves and bark is said to be efficacious in treating diarrhea. Pitanga contains trace elements of vital importance for human metabolism and prevention and healing of diseases (Obiajunwa et al. 2002).
		Dichloromethane and ethanol extracts of 12 plants were tested for antiviral activity. It was found that the most potent inhibition was shown by extracts of Eugenia jambos (Adab et al. 1998).

English Name	Scientific Name	Nutritional and Therapeutic Values
		Flower bud and bark are used. Pitanga contains rhamnetin, eugenitin, kaempferol, oleanolic acid, isoeugenitin, ellagic acid, β-sitosterol, and mairin. Essential oils include eugenol, humulene, acetyl eugenol, chavicol, α-caryophylline, β-caryophylline, and ylangene. It is used to stimulate gastric secretions, increase digestion, dispel gases, and as an antibacterial and antifungal (Huang 1999).
Plum	*Prunus salicina*	This plant is recommended to treat liver troubles. The white bark of the root is considered to be cooling, thirst relieving, and antifebrile. It is used to treat nausea and fever in children (Perry 1980).
		Plum contains amino acids, including threonine, isoleucine, leucine, lysine, methionine, cystine, tyrosine, valine, aspartic acid, glutamic acid, glycine, proline, and serine. It also has gallic acid, tannin, volatile oils, olein, linolein, stearin, phytosterin, myricyl alcohol, and hentriacontane. The fruit and bark are used as a disinfectant, antimellin. It also treats diarrhea and gingivitis (chinesemedicalpsychiatry.com).
		The plant contains amygdalin, prunasin, hydrocyanic acid, and prussic acid.
		The fruit is stomachic. It is said to be good for allaying thirst and is given in the treatment of arthritis (Chopra et al. 1986).
		Plum leaves, flowers, seeds, and bark contain toxic compounds that generate cyanide. However, in plant tissues, cyanide is low enough in concentration to be considered therapeutic, particularly for cancer treatment.
		Plum juice is used as a natural laxative. Phloretin extracted from bark and root is able to kill certain bacteria (Rieger 2006).
Pomarrosa	*Eugenia jambos*	A decoction of the leaves is used to treat sore eyes. The bark is supposed to be a good astringent.
		All parts of the plant are stimulant and remedial for toothache.
		The astringent seeds and bark are administered to treat diarrhea, dysentery, and catarrhal fever. The fruit and leaves are rich in tannin. Powdered leaves are rubbed on the body to cool the fever of smallpox and also made into a poultice for itch. The astringent seeds and bark are administered to treat diarrhea, dysentery, and catarrhal fever. The fruit and leaves are rich in tannin and jambosin also has been isolated (Perry 1980).

English Name	Scientific Name	Nutritional and Therapeutic Values
		Rose apple is an antipyretic and anti-inflammatory herb of Asian folk medicine. A 70% acetone extract yielded castalagin and casuarina, which exerted the strongest cytotoxic effects on human leukemia cell HL-60 (L. Yang et al. 2000).
Pomegranate	*Punica granatum*	The pomegranate is native from Iran to the Himalayas in northern India. The fruit is between an orange and a grapefruit. The edible parts are the seeds and the red seed pulp surrounding them.
		The flowers are used for stomachache, and the juice for cough and as an astringent in treatment of diarrhea. Stem bark is used for dysentery. The dried pericarp from the fruit is decocted for treatment of colic, colitis, diarrhea, dysentery, leucorrhea, menorrhagia, oxyuriasis, paralysis, and rectocele.
		The seeds contains lignin hydrochloride and lignocarbohydrate complexes (Dalimov et al. 2004). It has been reported that the fermented juice and pericarp extract of pomegranate have cancer-preventive and -suppressive potential (Kawaii and Lansky 2004).
		The rind contains about 28% of gallotannic acid together with a yellow coloring matter. Flowers yield sitosterol and ursolic, maslinic, ellagic, and gallic acids. Edible portion of the fruit contains glucose, fructose, maltose, starch, carotene, thiamine, riboflavin, nicotinic acid, vitamin C, pectin, amino acid, etc. (Chauhan 1999).
		It contains isopelletierine, pseudopelletierine, methyl isopelletierine, friedelin, ursolic acid, and isoquercitrin (N. Chiu and Chang 1995a). It has antioxidant activities from peel, pulp, and seed fractions (Guo et al. 2003).
		It is anthelmintic, astringent, cardiac, cooling, and expectorant. It is useful in treating brain afflictions, coughs and colds, diarrhea, and dysentery. It is also used as a heart tonic, to increase seminal flow, and to stop bleeding from the nose. Seed, fruit, and root bark are used (Chauhan 1999).
		Pericarp and root back from pomegranate contain pelletierine, isopelletierine, methyl isopelletierine, methyl pelletierine, pseudopelletierine, sitosterol, and gallotannic, ursolic, maslinic, ellagic, and gallic acids. It can be used to purge intestinal parasites (Chauhan 1999).
		It has been regarded as a food medicine from all parts of the tree.

English Name	Scientific Name	Nutritional and Therapeutic Values
		It is a tonic for the heart and is used to treat inflammation of the stomach. Juice from the fresh fruit is a cooling beverage for fever and sickness. It also acts on the liver, heart, and kidneys. It can treat digestive disorders, diarrhea, and dysentery, and it has anthelmintic properties to destroy parasitic worms (Perry 1980; Duke and Ayensu 1985).
Pomelo	*Citrus grandis*	The peel is antitussive and is used as a remedy for cough and asthma. It is also stomachic and aids digestion and liquefies sputum. Leaves are anti-inflammatory and antiswelling (K. Lin 1998d).
Pond apple	*Annona glabra*	The fruits of *Annona glabra* have two new kaurane diterpenoids, annoglabasins A and B, along with 11 known kaurane derivatives. The bark contains two alkaloids, muricine and muricinine. The seeds contain alkaloid, and the leaves have an essential oil, a resin, potassium chloride, and tannin (Perry 1980).
		It was found to show significant inhibition of HIV replication in H9 lymphocytic cells (F. Chang et al. 1998b).
		It is used to treat infantile diarrhea, abdominal illnesses, pulmonary diseases, burn baths, jaundice, and coughing associated with TB. It has vermifuge, antiparasitic, and rheumatism properties. The flower is used for kidney ailments.
		It was reported that three acetogenins (squamocin, asimicin, and desacetyluvaricin) extracted from seeds have activity against insects and mites (Ohsawa et al. 1991).
		Ferric chelate reductase activity was found in the root and leaf of Annona glabra (Ojeda et al. 2004).
Ponkan orange	*Citrus reticulata*	Citrus species contain a wide range of active ingredients, and research is still underway to discover their uses.
		Ponkan oranges are rich in vitamin C, flavonoids, acids, and volatile oils. They also contain coumarins such as bergapten, which sensitizes the skin to sunlight. Bergapten is sometimes added to tanning preparations, as it promotes pigmentation in the skin. It is used to treat dyspepsia, gastrointestinal distension, cough with phlegm, hiccup, and vomiting (Bown 1995).
		Citrus fruits have been known to reduce the proliferation of many cancer cells.

English Name	Scientific Name	Nutritional and Therapeutic Values
		The antiproliferative effects of *Citrus reticulata* extract, the immature tangerine peel, on human gastric cancer cell line SNU-668 were evaluated. Results suggest that *Citrus reticulata* extract may induce apoptosis through the caspase-3 pathway in human gastric cancer cells (Kim et al. 2005).
		Ponkan orange is an expectorant and has antitussive and antiemetic properties. The external layer of pericarp is used is used to treat indigestion.
		It contains citral, geraniol, linalool, methyl anthranilate, stachydrine, putrescine, apyrocatechol, naringin, poncirin, hesperidin, neohesperidin, and nobiletin (Huang 1999).
Prickly pear cactus	*Opuntia dillenii*	One disclosed U.S. patent is a treatment of existing scars and prevention of new scars in humans and animals using a topical application containing alcoholic extracts cortex phellodendri and *Opuntia ficus indica* in a specific combination (Niazi 2002).
		The fleshy stem of prickly pear cactus can be macerated in a little water or baked and applied to deep-seated abscesses on the soles of the feet and to congested or inflamed parts of the body. The plant, pounded and boiled, is used to fatten livestock.
		The fresh plant is cut longitudinally, and the outer part and some of the inner flesh are used to dress abscesses. The broth or a decoction of the plant cooked with pork or eggs is used as a tonic; the preparation is said to cure numbness (Perry 1980).
		It may be used as an insecticide (Perry 1980).
Rambutan	*Nephelium lappaceum*	Rambutan is an evergreen tree growing to a height of 10–20 m. The fruit is a round-to-oval drupe 3–6 cm long and 3–4 cm wide, borne in a loose pendant cluster of 10–20 together. The fruit flesh is translucent, whitish, or very pale pink, with a sweet, mildly acidic flavor.
		The seed is glossy brown, 2–3 cm long, with a white basal scar. It is poisonous and should not be eaten with the fruit flesh.
		The fruit of Nephelium lappaceum is recommended as an antidysenteric and a worming carminative. It is used as an astringent and antifebrile. A decoction is given to treat diarrhea and fever. The seeds contain fat, ash, protein, fiber, starch, oleic acid, arachidic acid, and traces of stearic acid (Perry 1980).

English Name	Scientific Name	Nutritional and Therapeutic Values
		Seeds yield 40–48% rambutan tallow. The insoluble fatty acids of the tallow contain 45% oleic acid. The tallow contains rachis, stearin, and olein acids. The seed is toxic due to the presence of nephelium saponin and tannin.
		A root decoction is used for fevers; the leaves are used as a poultice; bark is used as an astringent for tongue malachis. Fruit is used to treat dysentery and as a warm carminative in treatment of dyspepsia. Fruit decoction is used as a remedy for diarrhea (www.stuartxchange.org).
		Aerial part of the plant and the kernel are used. It has glucose, sucrose, tartaric acid, vitamins A and B, saponin, and tannins. It is styptic and also a nutrient tonic in treatment of neurasthenia and insomnia (Keys 1976).
Rose apple	*Eugenia jambos*	A decoction of the leaves is used to treat sore eyes. The bark is supposed to be a good astringent. All parts of the plant are stimulant and remedial for toothache.
		The astringent seeds and bark are administered to treat diarrhea, dysentery, and catarrhal fever. The fruit and leaves are rich in tannin (Perry 1980).
		Rose apple is an antipyretic and anti-inflammatory herb of Asian folk medicine. A 70% acetone extract yielded castalagin and casuarina, which exerted the strongest cytotoxic effects on human leukemia cells HL-60 (L. Yang et al. 2000).
Roselle	*Hibiscus sabdariffa* *H. tiliaceus* *H. schizopetalus*	The seeds are used to treat debility; the leaves are emollient. In Taiwan, the seeds are regarded as gently laxative, diuretic, and tonic. Roselle contains saponin, saponaretin, and vitexin (Perry 1980; Duke and Ayensu 1985).
		It can be used to treat bronchitis coughs. The tender leaves and stem can be eaten as a vegetable for its anti-inflammatory properties, to promote digestion, and as a remedy for boils in axilla. Mashed fresh leaves are used as a poultice (K. Lin 1998e). The root has emetic action (K. Lin 1998f).
		It is valued for its mild laxative effect and for its ability to increase urination, attributed to two diuretic ingredients, ascorbic and glycolic acids. It is used as a cooling herb, providing relief during hot weather by increasing the flow of blood to the skin's surface and dilating the pores to cool the skin (Ya et al. 2005).

English Name	Scientific Name	Nutritional and Therapeutic Values
		Roots and leaves are used as a neutral anti-inflammatory, to promote digestion, and as a remedy for boils in axilla.
		The seed contains rich protein, fat, and dietary fiber and is a good source of minerals. It also contains lysine and tryptophan (Udayasekhara 1996).
		Leaf, flower, and stem bark contain saponin, saponaretin, and vitexin. It has stomachic, diuretic, and expectorant properties and is used as a remedy for hematochezia, gas, and vertigo (Duke and Ayensu 1985).
		It contains mucilage, hibiscus, thiamine, gossypetin, anthecyanin, and citric, malic, tartaric, myristic, and palmitic acids. It has a soothing effect on the mucous membranes that line the respiratory and digestive tracts. Seeds are used for cramps, and flowers as an astringent (Small and Catling 1999).
		Bark, leaves, and flowers are used for bronchitis and cough, fever, and cassava poisoning. Externally used to treat boils and abscesses by applying mashed fresh leaves or bark to affected parts (K. Lin 1998g).
Round kumquat	*Fortunella japonica* *F. margarita* (*Note: Fortunella japonica are mostly cultivated as kumquat*)	This plant is used as an antiphlogistic, an antivinous, a carminative, a stimulant, and for deodorizing (Duke and Ayensu 1985).
		It contains the aromatic oil fortunellin, and 80% of the vitamin C is in the rind. It is used for chest oppression, alcoholism, thirst, indigestion, and excessive sputum. Root is used to promote blood circulation, aid digestion, stimulate the appetite, relieve gastric pain and indigestion, remove excessive sputum, and treat hernia. Seeds are used to treat eye infection, sore throat, furuncles, and carbuncles (K. Lin 1998f).
		Kumquats are known as a tonic and have diuretic and laxative properties. They contain vitamin C, zinc, potassium, phosphorus, manganese, copper, calcium, bioflavonoids, and pectin. They may help with coughs, colds, dyspepsia, liver disorders, and cholesterol (Cousin and Hartvig 2006).
		It contains fortunellin, essential oil, and vitamins A and C. Fruits, roots, and seeds are used for chest oppression, alcoholism, thirst, indigestion, and excessive sputum (K. Lin 1998g).
		Kumquats contain glucosides, galactose, essential oils, pentosane, and vitamin C. They have antiphlogistic, antivinous, carminative, deodorizing, and astimulant properties (Perry and Metzger 1980).

English Name	Scientific Name	Nutritional and Therapeutic Values
Sand pear	*Pyrus serotina* *P. sinensis* *P. betulaefolia*	The fruit is used to treat dysentery, and the cooked fruit used to treat mucous diarrhea. The fruit peel is also a remedy for colds, dry cough, vomiting, inflammation, and pulmonary troubles. The bark of the root is an astringent applied to wounds and itches (Perry 1980). Leaves are used for cholera, colic, and cramps. The fruit contains lysine, phenylalanine, leucine, tryptophan, biotin, and pantothenic, folic, α-ketoglutaric, ursolic, malonic, succinic, lactic, glycolic, shikimic, glyceric, mucic, and citramalic acids (Duke and Ayensu 1985). Sand pear has antiseptic, astringent, febrifuge, nervine, and pectoral properties (Stuart 2004). Sand pear has antidiarrhetic properties. It was considered as a medicinal plant in folk medicine (Pieroni 2000). With respect to medicinal properties, pears are similar to apples. Seed has cyanogenic glucosides, which are poisonous. The bark and roots contain phloretin, an antibiotic-like substance that acts on gram-positive and gram-negative bacteria. Pear juice has been implicated in the cause of chronic, nonspecific diarrhea in infants and children. Pear peel is listed as an ingredient in a Chinese tea for "winter colds without sore throat." The decoction is prepared with ginger, cinnamon, green onion, and black pepper. Tangerine peel is added if there is a cough, and pear peel is added if there is severe cough (Rieger 2006).
Santol	*Sandoricum koetjape*	Santol is a cultivated crop in Thailand; the root is an aromatic, a carminative, an antispasmodic, an astringent, and a stomachic. It contains gallic acid, tannin, volatile oil, fat, antimellin, jambulol, olein, linolein, palmitin, stearin acids, phytosterin, myricyl alcohol, and hentriacontane (Perry 1980). The root is employed to treat dysentery. It is used as a tonic and in postpartum protective medicine. The leaves are made into a poultice for itches. A decoction of the leaves is used to treat diarrhea. A decoction of the bark is suggested to correct irregularities in menstruation, and a decoction mixed with the fruit juice is taken to treat dysentery (Perry 1980).

English Name	Scientific Name	Nutritional and Therapeutic Values
		Decoction or infusion of leaves is used for baths to reduce fever. It is also used for diarrhea and as a tonic after childbirth. A bark poultice is used for ringworm. Bitter roots, bruised with vinegar and water, are carminative and used for diarrhea and dysentery (www.stuartxchang.org/santol.html).
		Extract from Sandoricum koetjape exhibited toxicity to killifish (Oryzias latipes). Of the triterpenoids active in vitro, koetjapic acid appears to be a promising cancer chemopreventive agent (Ismail et al. 2003).
Shaddock	Citrus grandis	Shaddock contains deacetylnomilin, geraniol, limonene, linalool, methyl anthranilate, naringinin-4(-glucoside-7-neohesperidoside, naringin, neohesperidin, obaculactone, obacunone, and poncirin.
		The leaves of pomelo are boiled and placed on painful places and swelling as well as ulcers. It is depurative. Gargling with the juice is said to help throat cancer. It is reported to be alterative, antiseptic, aperitive, carminative, digestive, refrigerant, stomachic, and tonic. It is a folk remedy for chorea and convulsion (Duke and duCellier 1993).
		The fruit is antivinous, aromatic, bitter, and stomachic. It is used as a remedy for boils, cholera, cold, dyspepsia, itch, and nausea. The seeds are cooked and used to treat bladder pain, hernia, and swollen genitals (Duke and Ayensu 1985).
		The peel is stomachic and antitussive and is used to relieve cough and asthma, to aid digestion, and to liquefy sputum. Leaves are anti-inflammatory and antiswelling (K. Lin 1998d).
		Flavonoids-enriched tissues of Citrus grandis peel, immature fruit, and flowers are consumed as culinary seasonings and, in China, as tea ingredients for contraries. It contains citrus flavonoids, naringin, hesperidin, neohesperidin, sinensetin, and nobiletin (Y. Lu et al. 2006).
		Fruit peel and leaves are used. Fruit peel is stomachic and antitussive. It is used to aid digestion, liquefy sputum, relieve gastric and hernial pain, reduce abdominal distention, relieve indigestion, induce productive cough, and alleviate asthma. Leaves are anti-inflammatory and antiswelling and are used as a remedy for mastitis and tonsillitis (K. Lin 1998e).
Soursop	Annona muricata	The crushed leaves may be applied for boils or abscesses. It is used as a remedy for distention, dyspepsia, scabies, and skin diseases of children. A lotion containing crushed leaves is used to treat rheumatism, coughs, and colds. The semimature fruit and the bark are strongly astringent and are indicated for use in treating diarrhea and dysentery (Perry 1980).

English Name	Scientific Name	Nutritional and Therapeutic Values
		All parts of the tree are used in natural medicine in the tropics. The fruit and juice are taken for worms and parasites and to cool fevers. They are also used as an astringent for diarrhea and dysentery. The crushed seeds are used against internal parasites, head lice, and worms (Raintree Nutrition: tropical plant database). Seeds from soursop contain annonaceous acetogenins, annocherines A and B, cherianoine, romucosine H, artabonatine B, and acetogenins. They are antiparasitic and are used to treat acute dysentery, mental depression, spine disorders, rectal prolapse, and swelling (Kooiman 1972).
		Soursop is antibilious, astringent, cicatrizant, cyanogenetic, depurative, emetic, hypotensive, insecticidal, pectoral, pediculicide, piscicide, sedative, soporific, stomachic, and tranquilizer (Duke and duCellier 1993).
		Leaves are used in Ecuador as an analgesic and antispasmodic. The leaf tea is often used in Latin America as a sedative and tranquilizer, but also for asthma, cholecystosis, lithiasis, and nephrosis (Duke and duCellier 1993).
Strawberry	*Fragaria ananassa* *F. vesca*	Strawberry is reported to be alterative, astringent, depurative, discutient, diuretic, laxative, and refrigerant. It is used to treat bladder ailments, blennorrhagia, blood ailments, calculus, cancer, and diabetes. It contains pentosans, pectins, and citric and malic acids. A chromoglucoside, fragarianin, has been extracted from the roots (Duke and duCellier 1993).
		Leaves are mildly astringent and diuretic. The plant is rarely used medicinally today, but it can be taken to treat diarrhea and dysentery. The leaves were also used as a gargle for sore throats, and in a lotion for minor burns and scrapes (www.herbs2000.com).
		Strawberry is a significant source of natural antioxidants due to its rich phenolic composition (Kahkonen et al. 1999). It can be dried for future use. The leaves are high in vitamin C and are also said to increase one's appetite. The leaves make a pleasant tea (Willard 1992).
		The amounts of flavonols (quercetin, myricetin, and kaempferol) and phenolic acids (ellagic, p-coumaric, caffeic, and ferulic acids) were analyzed in strawberry cultivars (Hakkinen and Torronen 2000).
		Strawberry contains myricetin to treat gastric pain, diarrhea, and dysentery (Huang 1999). It also has tannins, vitamin C, pectin, and malic acids. It stimulates the appetite. It has antidyspeptic properties (Rogers 1997).

English Name	Scientific Name	Nutritional and Therapeutic Values
		It has antioxidant activities from peel, pulp, and seed fractions (Guo et al. 2003).
		Roots and leaves are made into lotions and gargles in England and used for fastening loose teeth. Fruit juice is used for mouth ulcers. A tea from leaves and used it against diarrhea.
		Fruits are considered folk remedies for diarrhea, gonorrhea, gout, stomachache, and kidney stones. Strawberry is an astringent used as a diuretic or a mild laxative.
		Medicinally, strawberries have been shown to kill certain viruses, polio and herpes, in vitro, and they may block the formation of nitrosamines, which can cause cancer. Strawberry contains high quantities of ellagic acid, which has a wide range of biological activities.
		It was reported that ellagic acid inhibits cancer or mutation induced by benzopyrene aflatoxin in rats. This may be through inhibition of metabolic activation of carcinogens.
		Ellagic acid may inhibit absorption of HIV onto cells and HIV enzyme activity on DNA. Blood clotting is promoted and hemorrhage inhibited by ellagic acid, perhaps through aggregating and metal-chelating activity (Rieger 2006).
		A cut strawberry, rubbed over the skin immediately after washing will whiten it and help remove slight sunburn. For a badly sunburnt face, it is recommended to rub the juice well into the skin and to leave it on for about 1 h before washing it off with warm water (Willard 1992).
Strawberry guava	*Psidium cattleianum*	A decoction of the pods with leaves of *Psidium cattleianum* is indicated as efficacious in some cases of profuse uterine bleeding.
		All parts of the plant, including the young fruits, are astringent. In China, a decoction of the leaves is antidiarrhetic.
		It is taken to treat stomachache or used externally as a lotion for skin complaints, ringworms, wounds, and ulcers. The boiled leaves can be applied as a poultice to take heat away from wounds (Willard 1992).
		In Taiwan, dried ripe fruits are recommended as a remedy for dysentery. They are pectoral, tonic, and slightly laxative. This plant is a good source of vitamin B. It also contains triterpinoid, essential oils, tannin, fixed oils, and eugenol (Perry 1980).

English Name	Scientific Name	Nutritional and Therapeutic Values
		Strawberry guava has a high level of total phenolics and vitamin C. It is a significant source of phenolic antioxidant, which may have potential beneficial effects on human health (Luximon-Ramma et al. 2003).
		Strawberry guava is high in pectin. The fruits are good for mixing with high-acid, low-pectin fruits for making jellies. The leaves are used for medicinal purposes as a remedy for diarrhea and for their supposed antimicrobial properties. In Asia, a tea is made from guava fruits and leaves.
Strawberry tree	*Myrica rubra*	Besides fresh consumption, the fruits are commonly dried, canned, and fermented into an alcoholic beverage.
		The plant is also used as ornamental trees for parks and streets. Root and bark are used for hematemesis, massive uterine bleeding, hemorrhoidal bleeding, traumatic injury, fractures, gastric and duodenal ulcer, enteritis, dysentery, and toothache. Fruits are used for mouth dryness and anorexia (K. Lin 1998c).
		The bark of this plant contains diarylheptanoids (Inoue et al. 1984). It also has antiviral properties (Cheng et al. 2003).
		The strawberry tree possesses chemopreventive properties that, in some cases, can be used therapeutically.
		It has significant antiproliferative activity against various cancer cells. This activity is supposed to be associated with the modulation of cell-cycle progression and induction of apoptosis (Kuo et al. 2005).
Sugar apple	*Annona squamosa*	An infusion of the leaves is quieting. The crushed leaves may be applied for boils or abscesses. They can also be used as a remedy for distention and dyspepsia, on scabies and skin diseases of children, in a lotion to treat rheumatism, and as a remedy for coughs and colds. The young fruits contain tannin, and the bark is strongly astringent and is indicated for use in treating diarrhea and dysentery (Perry 1980).
		Chemical compounds from sugar apple showed significant activity against HIV replication in H9 lymphocyte cells, with an EC50 value of 0.8 g/ml (Y. Wu et al. 1996).

English Name	Scientific Name	Nutritional and Therapeutic Values
		Crushed leaves make a good maturative poultice for abscesses and can also be inhaled as a remedy for syncope. A decoction of leaves and powdered seeds is used to destroy vermin and relieve itch (Duke and duCellier 1993).
		The fruit pulp of sugar apple has nutritional value in normal as well as in diabetic rabbits. It increased the absorption and digestibility of dietary proteins and the net utilization of protein and decreased the urinary excretion of protein and sugar (R. K. Gupta et al. 2005).
		Roots, leaves, and fruits are used. Root is anti-inflammatory and antidepressive. It is used to treat acute dysentery, mental depression, and disorders of the spine. Leaves are anti-inflammatory and astringent and are used to treat rectal prolapse in infants, swelling, and abscesses. The ripe fruit is also effective for swelling and abscesses. The unripe fruits and seeds are antiparasitic (K. Lin 1998f).
		Root contains hydrocyanic acid, vitamin C, protein, and starch (N. Chiu and Chang 1995b).
		Sugar apple has many alkaloids, such as aporphine, roemerine, norcorydine, corydine, norisocorydine, glaucine, and anonaine in different parts of the plant (Kowalska and Puett 1990).
		The roots are used to treat dysentery, depression, and spinal marrow diseases, while leaves have been used in cases of prolapse of anus, sores, and swelling (Chao-Ming et al. 1997).
Sugarcane	*Saccharum officinarum* *S. sinense*	In China, the juice of sugarcane is considered to be cooling, stomachic, and expectorant. It is often applied to wounds, ulcers, and boils.
		A decoction of the crushed stem, with rhizomes of thatch grass (*Imperata cylindrica*), is taken internally to soothe the bronchial tubes and is also considered useful for clearing the blood (Perry 1980).
		Refined sugar is used for dry cough, fever, lack of secretion, and splenitis (Duke and Ayensu 1985).
		Policosanol and octacosanol isolated from sugarcane has been shown to lower cholesterol in animal models (Ioanna and Berthold 2002).
		It contains calcium, iron, vitamins C, B1, and B6, 24-methylene-lophenol, and 24-ethylidene-lophenol (N. Chiu and Chang 1995e).

English Name	Scientific Name	Nutritional and Therapeutic Values
Sweet cherry	*Prunus avium* *Cerasus avium*	Sweet cherry is used as a folk remedy for aches and pain. The fruit stalks are astringent, diuretic, and tonic. A decoction is used in the treatment of cystitis, edema, bronchial complaints, looseness of the bowels, and anemia. An aromatic resin can be obtained by making small incisions in the trunk. This has been used as an inhalant in the treatment of persistent coughs. Although no specific mention has been seen for this species, all members of the genus contain amygdalin and prunasin, substances that break down in water to form hydrocyanic acid. In small amounts, this exceedingly poisonous compound stimulates respiration, improves digestion, and gives a sense of well-being (Chiej 1984; Bown 1995).
		It has been reported that stalk extract of cherry has anti-inflammatory effects (Blazso and Gabor 1994).
		Leaves, flowers, and especially the seeds and bark contain toxic compounds that generate cyanide. However, in plant tissues, cyanide is low enough in concentration to be considered therapeutic, particularly for cancer treatment.
		Cherry stalk tea is a diuretic and is thought to cure kidney diseases. Cherry stalk extract (Novicardin) is used to reduce inflammation (Rieger 2006).
Sweet orange	*Citrus sinensis*	The rinds of the fruits and the juice are fragrant, stomachic, carminative, antiscorbutic, antiemetic, antivinous, diuretic, and expectorant. A decoction of the rind may be used to treat coughs, colds, dyspepsia, and as an antidote for fish poison (Perry 1980).
		Flavonoid glycosides in the sweet orange peel have hypotensive effects (Kumamoto et al. 1996).
		A beverage including *Citrus sinensis* is claimed to have hypotensive, stomachic, depurative, and diuretic properties (Volpato and Godinez 2004).
		Orally, the peel of sweet orange is used as an appetite stimulant. Sweet orange peel is also used to reduce phlegm, and to treat coughs, colds, anorexia, and malignant breast sores. It is also used as a tonic, antiflatulent, and for dyspepsia. In conjunction with other fruits and vegetables, sweet orange juice is used for prevention of hypertension and stroke, and for the improvement of blood lipid profiles (Leung and Foster 1996; Ishiwa et al. 2000; Jellin 2003).

English Name	Scientific Name	Nutritional and Therapeutic Values
		The fruit and juice are used dietarily as a cancer treatment. They are reported to be antiseptic, aperitif, astringent, carminative, expectorant, nervine, hypnotic, sedative, stimulant, stomachic, sudorific, tonic, and vermifuge (Duke and duCellier 1993).
Tahitian quince	*Spondias dulcis*	The bark is astringent and, with the bark of terminalis, is used to make a decoction taken as an antidiarrhetic. The bark and leaves are macerated and the liquid drunk as a medicine (Perry 1980).
		There were strong correlations between antioxidant activity, total phenolics, and proanthocyanidins. It is high in total phenolics, which may have potential beneficial effects on human health (Luximon-Ramma et al. 2003).
		Polysaccharide isolated from the gum of Tahitian quince contains galactose, arabinose, mannose, rhamnose, glucuronic acid, and its 4-O-methyl derivative (Martinez et al. 2003).
Tamarillo	*Cyphomandra betacea*	Tamarillo is a fruit crop with agronomic, organoleptic, physicochemical, and nutritive properties. It contains vitamins A, B6, C, and E, iron, and citric, malic, and quinic acids. It is used to alleviate respiratory diseases and combat anemia (Bermejo et al. 1994; Prohens and Nuez 2000).
		The broad-spectrum antimicrobial activity of an invertase inhibitory protein (IIP) isolated from *Cyphomandra betacea* ripe fruits is documented. This IIP inhibited the growth of xylophagous and phytopathogenic fungi and phytopathogenic bacteria. The results indicate the possible participation of IIP in the plant defense mechanism and its potential application as a biological control agent against phytopathogenic fungi and bacteria (Ordonez et al. 2006).
		As a folk medicine, Wayapi Indians use decoctions of the shoots in baths for their children to protect them from progressive debility (Duke and duCellier 1993).
Tamarind	*Tamarindus indica*	Stem is used as a diuretic and purgative and is used to treat liver disorders, inappetence, and anuria with constipation. The plant has a folk reputation as a remedy for amenorrhea, anasarca, anthrax, anuria, apoplexy, asthma, bilious problems, boils, carbuncles, chills, colds, colitis, conjunctivitis, cough, diarrhea, dropsy, dysentery, fever, hangover, headache, hemorrhage, hepatosis, hypertension, inflammation, jaundice, myalgia, piles, rheumatism, scurvy, snakebite, sore throat, sores, sprue, sunstroke, swelling, syphilis, tumors, and worms (Duke and Ayensu 1985).
		The seeds are a good source of zinc. Seed is used to make dawwa (porridge), commonly consumed during pregnancy (Lockett et al. 2002).

English Name	Scientific Name	Nutritional and Therapeutic Values
		Stem and fruit contain tannins, β-sitosterol, campesterol, pectins, mucilage, vitamin B, arabinose, xylose, galactose, glucose, and palmitic, oleic, linoleic, eicosanoic, and uronic acids. It has diuretic, purgative, hypoglycemic, and hypocholesterolemic properties. It is used as a remedy for liver disorders and inappetence and to improve digestion (Ibrahim et al. 1995).
		The pulp of the tamarind has been used as an antiscorbutic, laxative, and carminative. It is also used as a digestive and to treat bile disorders. It is used in a gargle for sore throat, as a liniment for rheumatism when mixed with salt, applied on inflammations, administered to alleviate sunstroke and alcoholic intoxication, to aid the restoration of sensation in cases of paralysis, and as part of a vermifuge ointment (Duke and duCellier 1993).
Tankan	*Citrus tankan*	In China, the peel, immature fruit, and flower are consumed as culinary seasonings and tea ingredients. There are five citrus flavonoids: naringin, hesperidin, neohesperidin, sinensetin, and nobiletin were extracted. A major ingredient of citrus-related TCM is also a suitable source of naringin and neohesperidin, and a good juice source for flavanone glycosides (Y. Lu et al. 2006). The Chinese have used preparations of tankan for medicinal purposes.
Tava	*Pometia pinnata*	This plant contains saponin and polycyclic compounds. It is used only externally. A decoction of the bark or leaves is used to bathe patients with fever. The bark is contained in a dressing for festering sores or wounds (Perry 1980).
		In Papua New Guinea, the masticated bark is applied to burns. In Fiji, bark extracts are used for pain relief and to treat such ailments as stomach complaints, diarrhea, dysentery, cold, flu, diabetes, and mouth ulcers (Thomson and Thaman 2006).
Tobacco nightshade	*Solanum verbascifolium* *S. melongena* *S. muricatum* *S. xanthocarpum*	In Taiwan, tobacco nightshade is administered to treat dysentery, intestinal pain, and fever.
		A poultice of the leaves is a headache remedy. A decoction is drunk against vertigo and is also used to bathe the body after childbirth.
		The leaves are considered a potent medicine for expelling all impurities through the urine, and in particular to treat leucorrhea. Decoction of roots is used for dyspepsia and violent pain, and it is taken with ginger and onion as a remedy for hematuria (Perry 1980; Duke and Ayensu 1985).

English Name	Scientific Name	Nutritional and Therapeutic Values
		The root of this plant is used as a remedy for acute dysentery, mental depression, and disorders of the spine. Leaves are used as a treatment for rectal prolapse in infants. The ripe fruit is effective for treating swelling and abscesses (K. Lin 1998e).
		Primary constituents (starches, proteins, sugars, fatty acids, minerals, vitamins, and glucosides) and secondary metabolites (saponins, alkaloids, tannins, oxalates, carotenes, anthocyannins, and betalains) have been identified in pepino (*S. muricatum*) (Jacobsen et al. 2003).
		Root, leaf, flower, and fruit contain trigonelline, stachydrine, choline, solanine, nasunin, shisonin, delphinidin-3-monoglucoside, adenine, solasodine, arginine, and glucoside. It is used to treat arthritis, respiratory disorders, swelling, cough, diarrhea, and blood in the urine (Zhu 1989).
Tree tomato	*Cyphomandra betacea*	Tamarillo is a fruit crop with agronomic, organoleptic, physico chemical and nutritive properties. It contains vitamin A, B6, C and E and iron, citric, malic, and quinic acids. It is used for alleviating respiratory diseases and combating anaemia (Bermejo and Leon, 1994; Prohens and Nuez, 2000).
		The broad-spectrum antimicrobial activity of an invertase inhibitory protein (IIP) isolated from Cyphomandra betacea ripe fruits is docomented. This IIP inhibited the growth of xylophagous and phytopatogenic fungi and phytopathogenic bacteria. The results indicate the possible participation of IIP in the plant defence mechanism and its potential application as a biological control agent against phytopathogenic fungi and bacteria (Ordonez et al., 2006).
		As a folk medicine, Wayapi Indians use decoctions of the shoots in baths for their children, to protect them from progressive debility (Duke and duCellier, 1993).
Triangular cactus	*Hylocereus undatus*	Triangular cactus is used both as an ornamental vine and as a fruit crop. The fruit is oblong to ovoid (6–12 cm long, 4–9 cm thick), red with large bracteals, and the pulp is white and edible.
		This plant is used as a remedy for cervical lymphadenitis. The flowers are used for bronchitis, tuberculous lymphadenopathy, pulmonary diseases, and tuberculosis (K. Lin 1998c).
		It was reported that a potential COX-2 inhibitor has been extracted from triangular cactus (Obukowicz and Hummert 2004).
		The whole herb is used. It contains hentriacontane and β-sitosterol. It is used to lower blood pressure and to treat lung, kidney, and liver infections, and sore throat (N. Chiu and Chang 1995d).

English Name	Scientific Name	Nutritional and Therapeutic Values
Wampi	*Clausena lansium*	In China, wampi is considered to be stomachic, cooling, and anthelmintic.
		The rind of the fruit is a resolvent for rheumatic swellings and cures enlarged spleen that causes fever. Warmed in gin, it is taken to help urination.
		The seed is a treatment for hernia. The leaves are employed in the care of the hair, as they are reputed to be useful against dandruff (Perry 1980).
		The hepatoprotective actions of compounds isolated from the leaves of wampi significantly depressed the elevated serum transaminase in mice intoxicated with CCl4. Compounds have hepatoprotective activity in mice. Secoclausenamide and clausenamide demonstrated that both compounds decreased the hepatotoxicity of thioacetamide and acetanin openin mice (Geng et al. 1996).
		Roots, leaves, fruits, and seeds are used. Leaves are used for prevention of influenza, colds and fever, epidemic encephalitis, and malaria. Roots and seeds are used for stomachache, epigastric pain, hernial pain, dysmenorrhea, and rheumatic bone pain. Fruits are used for indigestion and to induce productive cough (K. Lin 1998b).
		Wampi leaves contain flavonoids and amino acids. They are used as a diuretic and to alleviate pain, inflammation, stomachache, flu, and windpipe infection (N. Chiu and Chang 1995e).
Watermelon	*Citrullus vulgaris* *C. lanatus*	Watermelon contains one or more of the antitumor compounds called cucurbitacins. It also contains caprylic, capric, lauric, myristic, palmitic, stearic, oleic, and linoleic acids. The fruit is rich in pectin, and the juice contains citrulline. The rind is prescribed for alcoholic poisoning, diabetes, and nephritis. The pulp is used to treat alcoholism, sore throat, and stomatitis. The seed is demulcent and pectoral (Duke and Ayensu 1985).
		Watermelon contains high concentrations of free citrulline and arginine. It developed markedly elevated plasma citrulline and moderately elevated plasma arginine in six healthy adult volunteers (Mandel et al. 2005).
		Watermelon can also induce citrullinemia (Mandel et al. 2005).
Water wax apple	*Syzygium aqueum* *S. samarangense* *S. malaccense*	The fruits and seeds are used to make a cooling beverage to be taken for eruptive fevers. The leaves macerated in water are used in baths and lotions. The dried powdered leaves may be applied to a cracked tongue. The astringent bark has been used to make a mouthwash to treat thrush (Perry 1980).

English Name	Scientific Name	Nutritional and Therapeutic Values
		It is a tropical tree growing to 12 m tall with evergreen leaves. The fruit is a bell-shaped edible berry of green, red, or purple color.
		Four flavonoids isolated from the hexane extract were tested for a possible spasmolytic activity. All flavonoids showed dose-dependent spasmolytic activity (Ghayur et al. 2006).
		These results indicated that the presence of compounds with spasmolytic acid calcium antagonist activity may be responsible for the medicinal use of the plant in diarrhea (Ghayur et al. 2006).
Wax jumbo	*Syzygium aqueum*	The fruits and seeds are used when making a cooling beverage to be taken for eruptive fevers. The leaves macerated in water are used in baths and lotions. The dried powdered leaves may be applied to a cracked tongue. The astringent bark has been used to make a mouthwash to treat thrush (Perry 1980).
		Four flavonoids isolated from the hexane extract were tested for a possible spasmolytic activity. All flavonoids showed dose-dependent spasmolytic activity (Ghayur et al. 2006).
White sapote	*Casimiroa edulis*	White sapote is an evergreen tree, it contains sugars, phenolic aglycones, and tannins (Saleh et al. 2005). It contains phellopterin, isopimpinellin, psoralen, casimiroin, gamma-fagarine, flavonoids, zapotin, and 5,6,2(-trimethoxyflavone (Ito et al. 1998). Aqueous extract of the leaves has anticonvulsant activity (Ruiz et al. 1995).
		It contains antimutagenic constituents with potential cancer chemopreventive activity. An ethyl acetate extract derived from the seeds inhibited mutagenicity induced by 7,12-dimethylbenz[a]anthr acetate with Salmonella typhimurium strain TM677 (Ito et al. 1998).

Note: This information should not be used for the diagnosis, treatment, or prevention of diseases in humans. The information contained herein is in no way intended to be a guide to medical practice or a recommendation that herbs be used for medicinal purposes. The information presented here is mainly for educational purposes and should not be used to promote the sale of any product or replace the services of a physician.

5 Vitamins and Minerals of Fruits

Scientific Name	Protein	Fat	Sugar	Fiber	Vitamins (mg)					Minerals (mg/100 g)						
					$A_{(RE)}$	B_1	B_2	B_6	C	Na	K	Ca	Mg	P	Fe	Zn
Actinidia deliciosa, A. chinensis (kiwifruit)	0.79	0.07	17.5	1.1	175	0.02	0.05	0.5	105	6	290	16	30	64	0.5	0
Amygdalus armeniaca (apricot)	0.8	0.2	10.7	0.4	73.3	...	0	0	4	10	100	4	8	19	0.2	0
Anacardium occidentale (cashew nut)	0.162	0.5	9.75	1	0	0.4	...	...	372	...	...	5.4	...	21	0.7	...
Ananas comosus (pineapple)	0.7	0.3	11.6	0.6	5.1	0.14	0.04	0.3	165	1	40	18	14	8	0.3	1
Annona (atemoya) (atemoya)	...	...	...	...	0.005	0.1	0.13	0.9	37.4	...	...	26.2	...	42	0.8	...
Annona glabra (pond apple)	NA															
Annona muricata (soursop)	1.0	0.2	15.1	0.6	Trace	0.08	0.10	1.3	24	8	293	14	...	21	0.5	...
Annona reticulata (Bullock's heart)	2.4	0.2	18.5	0.9	...	0.1	0.1	...	15	...	...	18	...	15	0.4	...
Annona squamosa (sugar apple)	2.4	1.1	25	2.4	0	0	0.14	0	99	7	390	45	29	55	0.3	0
Armeniaca vulgaris (apricot)	3.5	5.2	84.7	0.5	0.5	0	0.18	0	0	93	64	83	13	88	0.8	1
Artocarpus altilis (breadfruit)	2.2	0.9	29.5	2.1	40	0.22	0.07	0.9	33	15	439	50	...	62	2.4	...

Scientific Name	Protein	Fat	Sugar	Fiber	Vitamins (mg)					Minerals (mg/100 g)						
					$A_{(RE)}$	B_1	B_2	B_6	C	Na	K	Ca	Mg	P	Fe	Zn
Artocarpus heterophyllus (marang, jackfruit)	0.8	0.4	22.7	1	6.5	0	0	0	0.6	11	120	118	9	10	0.2	0
Artocarpus lakoocha (monkey jack)	0.8	0.4	22.7	1	6.5	0	0	0	0.6	11	120	118	9	10	0.2	0
Averrhoa bilimbi (bilimbe)	0.61	...	...	0.6	0.035	0.01	0.026	0.3	15.5	...	...	3.4	...	11.1	1	...
Averrhoa carambola (carambola)	7.3	5.2	93.6	13.0	75	0.65	0.52	5.19	494	26.0	2350	104	...	195	15.6	...
Carica papaya (papaya)	1.0	0.1	6.2	0.9	15	0.02	0.03	0.3	40	7	215	38	12	20	0.3	0
Carissa grandiflora (carissa)	0.8	2.0	20.0	...	...	...	...	...	60	...	...	...	...	...	...	...
Casimiroa edulis (white sapote)	1.4	0.4	15.7	1.7	32	0.04	0.07	0.5	30	...	344	10	...	20	0.3	...
Castanea crenata (chestnut)	11.9	2.7	83.2	2.2	...	0.29	0.32	1.4	65	...	...	36	...	...	...	...
Castanea mollissima (Chinese chestnut)	4.2	0.8	46.3	3.2	7	0.23	0.14	0.6	25.9	2	534	30	60	118	1.1	1
Cerasus avium (Chinese cherry)	0.9	0.4	18	0.3	6	0.13	0.17	1.0	42	11	275	15	11	20	1.3	0
Citrullus vulgaris (watermelon)	10	8.9	86.5	25.7	47.8	0.63	0.78	2.70	125	13.5	1351	340	...	290	6.8	...
Citrus grandis (shaddock)	6.6	2.7	87.6	8.2	27.0	0.92	0.26	2.70	478	9	2117	342	...	290	5.2	...

Scientific Name	Protein	Fat	Sugar	Fiber	Vitamins (mg)					Minerals (mg/100 g)						
					$A_{(RE)}$	B_1	B_2	B_6	C	Na	K	Ca	Mg	P	Fe	Zn
Citrus limon (lemon)	1.1	0.8	8.8	0.9	14	0.6	0.02	0.1	53	4	138	41	...	19	0.7	...
Citrus medica (citron)	17.6	0	74.2	1.1	65	0.22	0.35	1.77	368	...	...	187	...	423	24.2	...
Citrus microcarpa (calamondin orange)	0.7	0.2	7.6	0.5	21.7	0	0	0	38	4	110	68	13	15	0.3	0
Citrus paradis (grapefruit)	0.7	0.3	7.8	0.3	46.7	0.1	0	0	38	7	60	21	9	17	0.1	0
Citrus reticulata (ponkan orange)	0.5	0.2	10.2	0.4	66.7	0.09	0.1	0.01	31	4	55	24	10	15	0.2	0.8
Citrus sinensis (sweet orange)	7.1	3.3	87.5	5.0	13.2	0.73	0.35	3.51	480	18	1427	293	12	175	5.7	0
Citrus tangelo "Murcott" (honey tangerine, tangerine)	6.2	2.2	89.5	4.3	40.8	0.79	0.36	3.51	368	15.4	1307	308	...	139	7.9	...
Citrus tankan (tankan)	1.8	0.8	21.9	3.7	260	0.07	0.1	0.5	150	12	70	21	13	20	0.5	0
Cocos nucifera (coconut)	4.5	41.6	13	3.6	Trace	0.5	0.03	0.8	7	7	190	10	4	24	1.7	0
Coffea arabica (coffee)	11.7	10.8	68.2	22.9	20	0.22	0.6	01.3	6.7	25	75	120	6	178	2.9	0
Cucumis sativus (cucumber)	18.4	2.6	73.9	16.3	30.6	0.79	1.05	6.12	304	342	4053	553	...	632	22.4	...

| Scientific Name | Protein | Fat | Sugar | Fiber | Vitamins (mg) | | | | | Minerals (mg/100 g) | | | | | | |
					$A_{(RE)}$	B_1	B_2	B_6	C	Na	K	Ca	Mg	P	Fe	Zn
Cyphomandra betacea (tree tomato)	15.6	6.4	83.8	24.3	32.6	0.71	0.28	8.51	206	…	…	578	…	340	5.7	…
Dillenia indica (elephant apple)	NA															
Diospyros kaki (persimmon)	3.3	1.9	89.6	7.4	52.8	0.23	0.25	0	123	12	813	27	8	49	15	0
Durio zibethinus (durian)	2.8	2	37.8	3	3.3	0	0.15	0.2	66	5	420	4	27	35	0.3	0
Elaeocarpus serratus (ceylon olive)	NA															
Eriobotrya japonica (loquat)	0.3	0.4	8.1	0.4	132	0	0.1	0	2	15	150	11	9	9	0.1	0
Eugenia jambos (rose apple)	0.5	0.2	8.6	0.6	0	0	0	0	17	7	70	4	8	10	0.1	0
Feijoa sellowiana (pineapple guava)	NA															
Ficus carica (common fig)	14.2	5.9	63.2	17.1	1.1	0.13	0.1	0.9	0.52	10	898	3160	96	160	4.5	1
Ficus pumila var. awkeotsang (moraceae)	…	…	0.4	…	…	…	…	…	0.01	13	167	…	2	…	…	…
Flacourtia inermis (lobi-lobi)	4.9	8.2	17.9	6.8	10	0.09	…	1.4	9	…	…	…	…	…	…	…

Scientific Name	Protein	Fat	Sugar	Fiber	Vitamins (mg)					Minerals (mg/100 g)						
					$A_{(RE)}$	B_1	B_2	B_6	C	Na	K	Ca	Mg	P	Fe	Zn
Fragaria ananassa (strawberry)	8.5	5.3	85	18.1	...	0.43	0.69	...	700	11	2053	290	...	319	10	...
Fragaria vesca (strawberry)	8.5	5.3	85	18.1	72.7	0.43	0.69	17.3	700	10.6	2053	290	...	...	10	...
Garcinia dulcis (mundo)	0.5	0.6	15.6	5.1	...	0	...	...	2	...	...	8	...	12	0.8	...
Garcinia mangostana (manggis)	3.2	1.9	93.6	31.8	0	0.19	0.13	3.82	25.5	6.4	860	63.7	23	63.7	3.2	0
Garcinia morella, G. xanthocymus (egg tree)	3.2	0.7	93.6	31.8	...	0.19	0.13	...	26	6	860	64	...	64	1.3	...
Ginkgo biloba (ginkgo)	10.2	3.1	83	1.3	...	0.52	0.26	...	54	15	1.1	11	...	327	2.6	...
Hibiscus sabdariffa (roselle)	1.9	0.1	12.3	2.3	30	0	0	0	14	12	12	1.72	2	57	2.9	0
Hylocereus undatus (triangular cactus)	1.1	0.2	12.5	1.2	0	0.17	0.45	1.2	54	16	190	4	31	27	0.3	1
Lansium domesticum (lansat)	22.9	16.4	18.5	...	863.2	181.2	...	...	305	...	550	381.4	...	...	14.4	...
Litchi chinensis (litchi)	4.5	0.6	90.5	0.6	...	0.12	0.18	...	279	16	939	30	...	139	1.7	...
Lucuma nervosa (egg fruit, canistel)	1.2	0.2	25.4	0.6	30	0	0	0	39	3	280	21	12	22	0.4	1
Malpighia glabra (acerola)	10.7	6.0	40.5	7.1	11.9	0.18	0.24	2.98	125	...	...	160.7	...	161	7.1	...

Scientific Name	Protein	Fat	Sugar	Fiber	Vitamins (mg)					Minerals (mg/100 g)						
					$A_{(RE)}$	B_1	B_2	B_6	C	Na	K	Ca	Mg	P	Fe	Zn
Mangifera indica (mango)	3.5	1.7	93.3	5.3	18.7	0.34	0.36	3.45	321	17.2	1230	140	...	129	7	...
Manilkara zapota (chicle)	0.6	0.8	20.5	1.9	3.3	0	0	0	39	10	250	18	10	10	0.2	0
Morus alba (mulberry)	0.8	2.1	13.8	1.0	140	0.08	0.06	0.5	28	...	...	26	...	31	2.2	...
Musa paradisiaca (banana)	96.5	1.2	93.9	3.9	22.5	0.69	0.25	2.88	58.1	14.9	1523	42.3	...	113	6.1	...
Musa sapientum (banana)	1.3	0.2	33.7	0.4	2.3	0	0	0	10	4	290	5	23	22	0.3	1
Myrciaria cauliflora (jaboticaba)	0.11	0	12.6	0.1	...	0	0	...	22.7	...	...	6.3	...	9.2	0.5	...
Nephelium lappaceum (rambutan)	1.2	1.2	17.4	0.5	0.5	0	0	0	8	16	160	17	15	27	0.7	0
Pachira macrocarpa (malabar chestnut)	NA															
Parmentiera edulis (guajilote tree)	0.8	0.2	10.2	0.4	340	0.1	0.4	0.6	54	...	...	21	...	19	0.3	...
Passiflora edulis (passion fruit)	28.8	2.8	85.1	6.2	16.8	0.14	0.52	6.02	121	112	1398	119	27	229	6.4	1
Persea americana (avocado)	8.1	86.4	62.9	10.6	26.9	0.42	0.77	0.77	99.4	15.4	323	96.4	...	234	7.1	...
Phyllanthus emblica (myrobalan)	NA															

Scientific Name	Protein	Fat	Sugar	Fiber	Vitamins (mg)					Minerals (mg/100 g)						
					$A_{(RE)}$	B_1	B_2	B_6	C	Na	K	Ca	Mg	P	Fe	Zn
Prunus avium (sweet cherry)	0.9	0.4	18	0.3	1.2	0	0.1	0	12	4	220	15	11	20	0.3	0
Prunus mume (Japanese apricot)	9.7	13	67.9	10.4	65	0.37	0.37	0	75	60	240	82	0	269	232	0
Prunus salicina (plum)	0.79	0.6	13	1.5	33.3	0	0.1	0	9.5	0	172	4	7	10	0.1	0
Psidium guajava (guava)	4.7	2.1	88.2	27.6	15	0.21	0.21	0	444	21	150	77	6	124	3.6	0
Punica granatum (pomegranate)	7.3	3.8	88.5	23.2	…	0.38	0.45	…	64	4.4	604	65	…	318	4.6	…
Pyrus betulaefolia (sand pear)	1.9	1.3	91.1	8.1	…	0.12	0.19	…	24	12	774	38	…	64	1.3	…
Pyrus serotina (sand pear)	0.4	0.3	10.1	0.7	0	0	0	0	5	12	110	3	5	11	0.2	0
Rollinia mucosa (borba)	2.8	0.2	…	1.3	…	0	0	…	33	…	…	24	…	26	1.2	…
Saccharum officinarum (sugarcane)	0.6	0.9	11.5	0.1	0	0	0	0	1.3	NA	NA	NA	NA	NA	NA	NA
Saccharum sinense (sugarcane)	5.3	1.5	82.9	35.9	…	…	…	…	…	…	…	…	…	…	…	…
Solanum nigrum (black nightshade)	3.2	0.4	6.4	1.1	…	0.12	0.24	…	61	…	…	199	…	88	9.9	…
Spondias dulcis (Tahitian quince)	1.3	1.0	15.1	…	…	…	…	…	…	…	…	25	…	41	…	…

Scientific Name	Protein	Fat	Sugar	Fiber	Vitamins (mg)					Minerals (mg/100 g)						
					$A_{(RE)}$	B_1	B_2	B_6	C	Na	K	Ca	Mg	P	Fe	Zn
Sterculia nobilis (ping-pong)	14.7	0.7	7.5	9.8	2	…	…	…	3	5	…	15.6	…	2.4	0	27
Synsepalum dulcificum (miracle fruit)	NA															
Syzygium samarangense (water wax apple, wax jumbo, java apple)	0.5	0.2	8.6	0.6	0	0	0	0	17	7	70	4	8	10	0.1	0
Tamarindus indica (tamarind)	2.3	0.2	56.7	1.9	1.0	0.22	0.08	1.10	3	3	570	81	…	86	1.3	…
Theobroma cacao (cacao tree)	12.0	46.3	34.7	8.6	0.3	0.17	0.14	1.7	3	…	…	106	…	537	3.6	…
Vaccinium corymbosum (highbush blueberry, blueberry)	0.7	0.5	62	…	100	0	0.1	0.84	14	1	81	15	…	13	1	…
Vitis labrusca (grape)	0.7	0.2	14.7	0.3	0	0	0.1	0	4	7	120	4	5	16	0.2	0
Vitis vinifera (grape)	0.6	0.4	15.8	2.0	Trace	0.05	0.04	0.5	3.0	…	…	21.0	…	19.0	0.8	…
Ziziphus mauritiana (Indian jujube)	1.2	0.2	11.1	0.5	5	0	0	0	45	7	200	8	7	20	0.2	0

Sources: Xue, C. X. 2001c. *The encyclopedia of vegetables and fruits in Taiwan.* Vol. 3. [In Chinese.] Taipei: Taiwan Pu-Lu Publ. Co.; Duke, J. A., and J. L. duCellier, eds. 1993. *CRC handbook of alternative cash crops.* Boca Raton, FL: CRC Press.

6 Vegetables and Fruits Used to Protect Health

Health Concerns	Vegetables Used to Protect Health	Special Crops	Fruits Used to Prevent Disorders
Aging	Soybean	...	Mulberry
Aphrodisiac	Chinese chive, Scallion, Pumpkin, Lotus, Great burdock, Celery, Coral flower, Cress, Sweet potato, Sweet potato vine	...	Apricot
Artery hardening	Sweet potato vine, Onion	...	Avocado, Acerola, Lemon
Assist urine	Watercress, Cucumber, Asparagus lettuce, Slender amaranth	Lemon grass, Screwpine	Carambola, Watermelon, Strawberry
Asthma	Chinese artichoke, Chinese radish, Ducks tongue grass, Horseradish, Lettuce, Indian lettuce, Parsnip, Pepper, Sweet basil, Watercress	...	Coffee
Bladder	Mustard cabbage, Thousand-veined mustard	...	...
Blood, blood circulation	Chicory, Chive, Gynura, Lima bean, Kidney bean, Rice, Bean, Brussels sprout, Ginger, Black nightshade, Bird-nest fern, Mu-erh	Green tea, Rosemary, Calamondin orange, Oval kumquat, Durian, White sapote, Grapefruit, Flowering quince	Plum, Common fig, Ping-pong, Litchi, Chinese jujube, Passion fruit, Avocado, Durian, Peach, Mulberry, Grape, Acerola, Chestnut, Passion fruit, Shaddock
Blood pressure	Celery, Chayote, Tomato, Broccoli, Prickly pear cactus, Yellow rattan palm, Rhubarb, Tomato	Hsien-t's ao, Grass jelly, Sugarcane, Comfrey, Common rue	Wax jumbo, Banana, Roselle, Water wax apple, Pineapple, Cantaloupe, Persimmon
Blood sugar	Carrot, Chinese wolfberry	...	Apple
Body weight	Chinese cabbage, Konjac, Kunichi cane	...	...
Bone density	Snake gourd	...	...

Health Concerns	Vegetables Used to Protect Health	Special Crops	Fruits Used to Prevent Disorders
Bronchitis	Chinese artichoke, Chinese spinach, Lettuce, Indian lettuce, Night-blooming cereus, Parsnip, Watercress	...	Caimito, Abiu
Cancer (prevention)	Ailanthus, Garlic, Tomato, Sweet corn, Water chestnut, Corn, Job's tears, Asparagus, Asparagus lettuce, Bitter gourd, Black nightshade, Carrot, Chicory, Chinese mustard, Chinese yam, Endive, Garlic, Ginger, Horseradish, Kidney bean, Konjac, Lettuce, Indian lettuce, Luffa, Pepper, Rhubarb, Thousand-veined mustard, Cauliflower	...	...
(A new study conducted by a research team [Ah-Ng and Tony Kong] at Rutgers has revealed that cauliflower, in particular, has natural ingredients that may reduce the risk of developing hereditary cancers [2006])	Angelica	Atemoya, Mango (not suitable for diabetic patient), Acerola, Triangular cactus	...
Chill feeling	Mustard, Japanese honeywort, Water celery	...	...
Cholesterol	Common bracken, Alfalfa sprout, Rhubarb	Tea, Grapefruit, Flowering quince	Triangular cactus, Avocado, Coffee, Apple, Grapefruit (not suitable for persons with high blood pressure and heart disease)

Health Concerns	Vegetables Used to Protect Health	Special Crops	Fruits Used to Prevent Disorders
Constipation	Swamp cabbage, Spinach, Chinese cabbage, Chinese mallow, Welsh onion, White mugwort, Carrot, Beet, Yacoa, Taro, Swlooen stemmed mustard, Sweet potato, Cassava, Elephant grass, Fireweed, Ma bamboo	Edible canna	Papaya, Peach, Apricot, Breadfruit, Triangular cactus, Shaddock, Persimmon. Honey tangerine. Egg fruit (canistel). Peach. Mango (not suitable for diabetic patient). Passion fruit, Ponkan orange, Sand pear
Cough	Taiwan velvet plant, Night-blooming cereus, Green bamboo. Arrowhead, Asparagus, Chinese radish, Lily bulb, Horseradish, Water spinach	...	Sand pear, Malabar chestnut, Moraceae, Carambola, Watermelon, Japanese apricot, Loquat, Mulberry, Ping-pong, Emblic, Myrobalan, Sweet orange, Persimmon, Pomegranate, Oval kumquat, Caimito, Calamondin orange
Diabetes	Carrot, Corn, Fenugreek, Garden pea, Hairy melon, Sweet corn, Winter melon	Stevia	Guava, Watermelon, Breadfruit, Avocado
Diarrhea	Chinese mahogany, Sorghum, Ducks tongue grass, Broad bean, Chinese radish, Garlic, Ginger, Hyacinth bean, Japanese honeywort, Lotus	Calamondin orange. Oval kumquat, Durian. White sapote, Grapefruit, Flowering quince, Ailanthus	Pineapple, Sugar apple, Pomegranate, Manggis, Rambutan, Carambola. Pineapple. Strawberry tree. Bay berry, Common fig. Apple, Atemoya, Avocado
Digestion	Chinese radish, Winged bean, Moso bamboo, Makino bamboo, Water chestnut, Sugarcane, Broad bean, Brussels sprout, Cabbage, Cauliflower, Chinese mustard, Ducks tongue grass, Endive, Fenugreek, Parsley, Spinach, Sweet basil	Ailanthus	Water wax apple, Pineapple, Papaya, Banana, Lemon, Cantaloupe, Peach, Strawberry tree, Bay berry, Jackfruit (not suitable for diabetic patient), Passion fruit, Shaddock, Sweet orange, Apple, Chinese olive, Oval kumquat

Health Concerns	Vegetables Used to Protect Health	Special Crops	Fruits Used to Prevent Disorders
Diuretic property, dysuria	Asparagus, Asparagus lettuce, Burdock, Carrot, Chinese mallow, Cress, Cucumber, Daylily, Globe artichoke, Hairy melon, Adzuki bean, Sunflower, Winter melon	...	Wax jumbo, Pineapple, Betel nut, Grape, Cantaloupe, Mango (not suitable for diabetic patient), Longan, Breadfruit, Triangular cactus, Avocado, Coffee, Sweet orange, Sand pear, Bullock's heart
Dysentery	Beet, Table beet, Black nightshade, Lotus	...	Water wax apple, Carambola, Atemoya
Energy	Chinese leek, Chinese artichoke, Buckwheat, Wheat, Cudweed, Chinese leek, Lily bulb	Lavender, Taiwan anoectochilus	Coconut, Longan, Indian Jujube, Cherry, Apricot, Lemon, Plum, Chicle, Litchi (not suitable for diabetic patient), Acerola, Chinese jujube
Eye problems	Endive, Laciniata, Winter mustard, Early dwarf pea	...	Mulberry
Flu	Parsley, Leek, Oriental pickling melon, Turnip	...	Emblic, Myrobalan, Pomegranate
Hemorrhoids	Mustard cabbage	...	Papaya, Loquat, Common fig
Hernia	Fennel, Chinese yam	...	Litchi, Ping-pong
Fever	Chinese spinach, Table beet (Swiss chard), Bitter gourd, White jute, Black nightshade, Fenugreek, Garden pea, Lily bulb, Oil vegetable, Parsnip, Sweet potato, Sweet potato vine, Turnip, Water dropwort	Honey tangerine (root), Manggis, Tankan (peel)	Emblic, Myrobalan, Malabar chestnut

Health Concerns	Vegetables Used to Protect Health	Special Crops	Fruits Used to Prevent Disorders
Inflammatory	Chinese kale, Winter pumpkin, Joined wax gourd, Broad bean, Eggplant, Purslane, Turnip, Yam, Bean, Adzuki bean, Mung bean, Lotus, Rapeseed, Coral flower, Black nightshade, Gooseweed, Broad bean, Celery, Chinese yam, Garlic, Luffa, Moso bamboo, Water chestnut, Yam	*Rhinacanthus nasutus*	Watermelon, Carambola, Guava, Water wax apple, Pepino, Melon pear, Mulberry, Mango (not suitable for diabetic patient), Chestnut, Kiwifruit, Moraceae
Intestinal disorder	Ceylon spinach, Lily bulb, Onion, Green onion, Rhubarb	...	...
Itch	...	Mint, Alpinia galanga	...
Kidney	Sword bean, Hyacinth bean (lablab), Pigeon pea, Red bean, Yam, Foxtail, Millet, Sesame, Fennel	Plina bristle grass, Chrysanthemum	Chestnut, Ceylon olive, Moraceae, Malabar chestnut
Leukemia	Cauliflower	...	...
Liver	Carambola	...	Ping-pong, Kiwifruit
Losing hair	Leaf lettuce	...	...
Lung	White-flowered gourd, Chinese wolfberry, watercress	...	...
Measles	...	...	Plum
Memory	Daylily, Soybean, Feather cooks comb	...	Longan
Menstrual, menstruation	Asiatic wormwood, Chinese mahogany, Japanese honeywort	Calamondin orange, Oval kumquat, Durian, White sapote, Wampi	...
Migraine	Bay laurel	...	Coffee, Shaddock
Mother's milk	Lettuce, Peanut	...	...
Obesity	...	...	Avocado, Coffee

Health Concerns	Vegetables Used to Protect Health	Special Crops	Fruits Used to Prevent Disorders
Nerve	Wasabi	⋮	⋮
Pain	Tobacco, Arabian jasmine	Rosemary	⋮
Parasites	Chili pepper	⋮	⋮
Phlegm	Garland chrysanthemum, Winter gourd	Betel pepper, Grapefruit, Flowering quince	Apricot, Betel nut, Watermelon, Sugarcane, Emblic, Myrobalan, Shaddock, Ponkan orange, Sweet orange, Persimmon, Oval kumquat, Calamondin orange
Skin	Bell pepper, Sunflower, Common bracken, Goa bean, Pigeon pea	Honey tangerine, Tankan (skin), Wampi	Water wax apple, Papaya (externally), Jackfruit, Sugar apple
Sleep (insomnia)	Lettuce, Indian lettuce	⋮	Kiwifruit
Stomach	Chinese mustard, Cabbage, Chinese kale, Coriander, White Dutch runner bean, Shallot, Asparagus bean, Vegetable soybean, Chinese radish, Potato, Rice, Bean, Ducks tongue grass, Ginger, Muskmelon, Mustard cabbage, Onion, Green onion, Perilla, Prickly pear cactus, Sweet potato, Sweet potato vine	Mint, Alpinia galanga	Sugarcane, Chicle, Strawberry tree, Grape, Ponkan orange, Sweet orange, Apple, Chinese olive, Tankan, Calamondin orange, Japanese apricot, Kiwifruit, Betel nut, Cantaloupe, Plum, Chestnut, Ceylon olive, Bullock's heart
Thirst	Water bamboo shoot	Grapefruit, Flowering quince	Loquat, Apricot, Ginkgo, Lobi-lobi, Coconut, Mango (not suitable for diabetic patient)

Health Concerns	Vegetables Used to Protect Health	Special Crops	Fruits Used to Prevent Disorders
Throat pain, swollen	Okra, Fenugreek, Prickly pear cactus, Snake gourd, Sweet potato, Sweet potato vine	…	Pineapple, Watermelon, Loquat, Strawberry tree, Bay berry, Litchi (not suitable for diabetic patient), Common fig, Emblic, Myrobalan, Persimmon, Chinese olive, Avocado
Tongue	…	Dwarf flowering cherry	Rambutan
Urinary infection, urination	Okra, Broad bean, Chicory, Endive, Garden pea	…	Japanese apricot, Litchi (not suitable for diabetic patient)
Vomiting, nausea	Ginger, Black nightshade, Bird-nest fern, Hyacinth bean, Perilla, Sweet potato, Sweet potato vine	…	Japanese apricot, Strawberry tree, Bay berry, Mango (not suitable for diabetic patient), Ponkan orange
Windpipe infection	Snake gourd	…	Loquat, Triangular cactus, Persimmon, Pomegranate

Note: This information should not be used for the diagnosis, treatment, or prevention of diseases in humans. The information contained herein is in no way intended to be a guide to medical practice or a recommendation that herbs be used for medicinal purposes. The information presented here is mainly for educational purposes and should not be used to promote the sale of any product or replace the services of a physician.

Appendix 1: Chemical Components and Their Sources

Component	Source
(+)-Catechin-pentaacetate	*Ginkgo biloba*
(+)-Gallocatechin-hexacetate	*Ginkgo biloba*
(+)-Nyasol	*Asparagus officinalis*
(()-Epicatechin-pentaacetate	*Ginkgo biloba*
(()-Epigallocatechin-hexacetate	*Ginkgo biloba*
α-aminodimethyl	*Asparagus officinalis*
α-amyrin	*Brassica oleracea* var. *botrytis, Cichorium endivia, Zea mays*
α-carotene	*Asparagus officinalis, Capsicum annum* var. *longum*
α-copaene	*Zea mays*
α-crytoxanthin	*Capsicum annum* var. *longum*
α-crytoxanthus	*Capsicum annum* var. *longum*
α-eleostearic acid	*Momordica charantia*
α-galactosidase	*Trigonella foenum-graecum*
α-guttiferin	*Garcinia morella, G. xanthocymus*
α-hydroxyeudesmol	*Arctium lappa*
α-linolenic acid	*Asparagus officinalis, Beta vulgaris, Brassica chinensis, B. oleracea* var. *capitata, Lactuca sativa*
α-phellandrene	*Foeniculum vulgare*
α-pinene	*Zea mays, Zingiber officinale*
α-sein	*Zea mays*
α-solanigrine	*Solanum nigrum*
α-spinasterol	*Medicago sativa*
α-terpinene	*Coriandrum sativum, Foeniculum vulgare*
α-tocopherol	*Beta vulgaris, Brassica chinensis, B. oleracea* var. *gemmifera, B. pekinensis, Lepidium sativum, Medicago sativa*
β-amyrin	*Artocarpus altilis, A. lakoocha, Brassica oleracea* var. *botrytis, Ficus carica, F. pumila* var. *awkeotsang, F. pyriformis, Zea mays*

Component	Source
β-carotene	*Allium tuberosum, Amaranthus gangeticus, Asparagus officinalis, Beta vulgaris, Brassica chinensis, B. oleracea* var. *capitata, B. oleracea* var. *gemmifera, B. rapa, Capsicum annum* var. *longum, Daucus carota subsp. sativus, Foeniculum vulgare, Laurus nobilis, Lepidium sativum, Manihot esculenta, Medicago sativa, Momordica charantia, Solanum nigrum, Trigonella foenum-graecum, Vicia faba*
β-copaene	*Zea mays*
β-cryptoxanthin	*Capsicum annum* var. *longum*
β-cyanoalanine	*Vicia faba*
β-cyclopyrethrosin	*Capsicum annum* var. *longum, Chrysanthemum coronarium*
β-D-glucoside	*Momordica charantia*
β-ecdysterone	*Chenopodium album*
β-elaterin	*Momordica charantia*
β-eudesmol	*Arctium lappa*
β-fenchene	*Zingiber officinale*
β-guttiferin	*Garcinia morella, G. xanthocymus*
β-lactucerol	*Lactuca sativa*
β-mannanon	*Trigonella foenum-graecum*
β-phellandrene	*Foeniculum vulgare*
β-pinene	*Coriandrum sativum, Foeniculum vulgare, Zingiber officinale*
β-selinene	*Apium graveolens, Zea mays*
β-sitosterol	*Asparagus officinalis, Beta vulgaris, Cichorium endivia, Foeniculum vulgare, Hemerocallis fulva, H. longituba, Lepidium sativum, Lycium chinese, Medicago sativa, Momordica charantia*
β-solanigrine	*Solanum nigrum*
β-zein	*Zea mays*
γ-terpinene	*Coriandrum sativum*
1,2-cyclopentandione	*Coffea arabica*
1,2-propanedione	*Coffea arabica*
1,3,4-trimethyl-2-orbicylcho	*Zingiber officinale*
1,3,4-trimethyltricyel	*Zingiber officinale*
1,8-cineole	*Foeniculum vulgare, Zingiber officinale*
11,13-dihydrotaraxine acid-1-O-β-D-glucopyranoside	*Taraxacum officinale*
16-alpha-hydroxyestrone	*Brassica oleracea* var. *capitata*
2-alpha-hydroxyestrone	*Brassica oleracea* var. *capitata*
2-hydroxypropylene	*Allium sativum*

Component	Source
2-methylpropanol	*Medicago sativa*
2-phenethyl isothiocyanate	*Brassica oleracea* var. *capitata*
22-deoxocucur bitacin D	*Benincasa hispida* var. *chieh-gua*
3-butenyl-isothiocyanates	*Lepidium sativum*
3-methoxycoumestrol	*Medicago sativa*
3-methylbutanol	*Medicago sativa*
3,5-dugkycisude	*Perilla frutescens*
3,5,6-trihydroxyl-7,3,4-trimethoxy-flavone	*Citrus medica* var. *sarcodactylis*
3-O-β-D-glucosyl-β-D-quercetin-xyloside	*Armoracia rusticana*
3-p-coumarylglycoside-5-glucoside	*Perilla frutescens*
4-O-methylcoumestrol	*Medicago sativa*
4-ethexyl-6-hydroxymethyl	*Opuntia dillenii*
4-vinylguaiacol	*Asparagus officinalis*
4-vinylphenol	*Asparagus officinalis*
5-hepten-2-one-6-methyl	*Zingiber officinale*
5-methoxy-methylfurfurol	*Asparagus officinalis*
5-methyl-1,2-dithio-3-cydopentene	*Allium sativum*
5,6,2(-trimethoxyflavone	*Casimiroa edulis*
6-methyl-1-thio-2,4-cyclohexadiene	*Allium sativum*
7-caffeyl-glucoside	*Perilla frutescens*
Abginine	*Beta vulgaris*
Abscisic acid	*Pisum sativum, Zea mays*
Acetamide	*Beta vulgaris*
Acetic acid	*Arctium lappa*
Acetogenin	*Annona glabra, A. muricata, A. reticulata*
Acetone	*Coriandrum sativum, Medicago sativa*
Acetophenone	*Cichorium intybus*
Acetylacrolein	*Coffea arabica, Trigonella foenum-graecum*
Acetylcholine	*Capsicum annum* var. *longum*
Achlorhydria	*Prunus mume*
Aconitic acid	*Beta vulgaris, Zea mays*
Acyclic diterpene	*Lycium chinese*
Adenine	*Amaranthus gangeticus, Chrysanthemum coronarium, Medicago sativa, Phaseolus vulgaris, Pisum sativum, Solanum melongena, Zea mays*
Adenosine	*Zea mays*
Aglycone	*Solanum nigrum*

Component	Source
Alanine	*Asparagus officinalis, Beta vulgaris, Brassica chinensis, B. oleracea* var. *gongylodes, B. rapa, Foeniculum vulgare, Lactuca sativa, Manihot esculenta, Trigonella foenum-graecum, Vicia faba*
Alantoinase	*Pisum sativum*
Albuminoids	*Eleocharis dulcis*
Alexiteric acid	*Deliciosa lablab*
Aliphatic hydrocarbons	*Theobroma cacao*
Alkaloids	*Lilium tigrinum*
Allantoin	*Allantoic acid, Beta vulgaris, Brassica rapa, Dioscorea alata, Zea mays*
Allicin	*Allium sativum, A. schoenoprasum, A. tuberosum*
Allistatin	*Allium chinese, A. fistulosum, A. sativum*
Alloaromadenerene	*Zingiber officinale*
Allomatatabiol	*Actinidia deliciosa*
Alloxurbasen	*Armoracia rusticana*
Allyl disulfide	*Allium cepa*
Allyl isothiocyanate	*Armoracia rusticana, Lepidium sativum*
Allyl methyl disulfide	*Allium sativum*
Allyl methyl pentasulfide	*Allium sativum*
Allyl methyl sulfide	*Allium sativum*
Allyl methyl trisulfide	*Allium sativum*
Allyl propyl disulfide	*Allium sativum*
Aluminum	*Armoracia rusticana, Beta vulgaris, Medicago sativa, Zea mays*
Ambonic acid	*Mangifera indica*
Amebic acid	*Hibiscus esculentus, H. syriacus*
Amino acid	*Asparagus officinalis, Canavalia gladiata, Zea mays*
Amygdalin	*Cerasus avium, Eriobotrya japonica, Malus domestica, Phaseolus lunatus, Prunus armeniaca, P. japonica, P. mume, P. persica, P. salicina*
Amylase	*Armoracia rusticana, Medicago sativa, Pisum sativum*
Amyrin	*Ficus carica, F. pyriformis*
Anacardic acid	*Anacardium occidentale*
Anacardol	*Anacardium occidentale*
Anasarca	*Tamarindus indica*
Anethole	*Foeniculum vulgare*
Anicetone	*Foeniculum vulgare*
Aniline	*Brassica oleracea* var. *capitata, B. oleracea* var. *gongylodes*
Anisaldehyde	*Foeniculum vulgare*
Anisic acid	*Foeniculum vulgare*

Component	Source
Annoglabasin A, B	*Annona glabra*
Anolide	*Lycium chinese*
Anolobine	*Magnolia acuminata*
Anthelmintic acid	*Asplenium nidus*
Anthocyanin	*Perilla frutescens*
Anthocyanosides	*Vaccinium corymbosum*
Anthraquinones	*Dillenia indica, Rheum rhaponticum*
Apigenin	*Apium graveolens, Perilla frutescens*
Apigravin	*Apium graveolens*
Apiin	*Apium graveolens*
Arabinogalactan	*Opuntia dillenii*
Arabinose	*Trigonella foenum-graecum*
Arachic acid	*Lepidium sativum*
Arachidic acid	*Brassica oleracea* var. *gemmifera, Zea mays*
Arbutin	*Vaccinium corymbosum*
Arctigenin	*Arctium lappa*
Arctin	*Arctium lappa*
Arctinol a, b, c	*Arctium lappa*
Arctinone a, b	*Arctium lappa*
Arecoline	*Areca catechu*
Areticin	*Annona reticulata*
Arginine	*Amaranthus gangeticus, Armoracia rusticana, Asparagus officinalis, Beta vulgaris, Brassica chinensis, B. oleracea* var. *capitata, B. oleracea* var. *gemmifera, B. oleracea* var. *gongylodes, B. rapa, Chenopodium album, Cichorium intybus, Cucumis sativus, Dioscorea alata, Foeniculum vulgare, Lactuca sativa, Manihot esculenta, Phaseolus vulgaris, Pisum sativum, Solanum melongena, Vicia faba, Zea mays*
Arsenic acid	*Armoracia rusticana, Brassica oleracea* var. *gongylodes, B. pekinensis, Lactuca sativa, Vicia faba*
Asaron	*Daucus carota subsp. sativus*
Ascaridole	*Chenopodium album*
Ascorbate	*Apium graveolens*

Component	Source
Ascorbic acid	*Allium tuberosum, Amaranthus gangeticus, Apium graveolens, Armoracia rusticana, Asparagus officinalis, Benincasa hispida* var. *chieh-gua, Beta vulgaris, Brassica chinensis, B. oleracea* var. *capitata, B. oleracea* var. *gemmifera, B. oleracea* var. *gongylodes, B. rapa, Chenopodium album, Chrysanthemum coronarium, Cichorium intybus, Foeniculum vulgare, Glycine max, Lactuca sativa, Laurus nobilis, Lepidium sativum, Manihot esculenta, Phaseolus angularis, Trigonella foenum-graecum, Vicia faba*
Asimicin	*Annona glabra*
Asparagine	*Asparagus officinalis, Capsicum annum, Hemerocallis fulva, H. longituba, Pisum sativum, Sagittaria sinensis*
Asparagome	*Armoracia rusticana, Asparagus officinalis*
Asparagosides a–h	*Asparagus officinalis*
Aspartic acid	*Asparagus officinalis, Brassica oleracea* var. *botrytis, B. oleracea* var. *capitata, Canavalia gladiata, Manihot esculenta, Trigonella foenum-graecum*
Asteroids A, B	*Lycium chinese*
Astragalin	*Zea mays*
Atemoyacin E	*Annona (atemoya)*
Auxin	*Ficus carica, F. pyriformis*
Barium	*Beta vulgaris*
Baurenyl acetate	*Cichorium endivia*
Behenic acid	*Capsicum annum* var. *longum, Lepidium sativum, Trigonella foenum-graecum*
Benzaldehyde	*Zea mays*
Benzoic acid	*Foeniculum vulgare*
Benzophenones	*Garcinia morella, G. xanthocymus*
Benzylamin	*Brassica oleracea* var. *capitata, B. oleracea* var. *gongylodes*
Benzyl isothiocyanate	*Lepidium sativum*
Berberine	*Zanthoxylum ailanthoides*
Bergapten	*Apium graveolens*
Betacyanin	*Portulaca oleracea*
Betaine acid	*Beta vulgaris, Lycium chinese, Pisum sativum, Stachys officinalis, S. sieboldii, Zea mays*
Betaonicine	*Chenopodium album, Stachys officinalis, S. sieboldii*
Betulinic acid	*Vicia faba*
Bile acids	*Medicago sativa*
Bilobetin	*Ginkgo biloba*
Biochanin A	*Medicago sativa*
Bioflavonoids	*Citrus limon*

Component	Source
Bisabol	*Daucus carota* subsp. *sativus*
Bisabolene	*Zingiber officinale*
Bis-tetrahydrofuran	*Annona (atemoya)*
Blanthraquinonyl	*Rheum rhaponticum*
Borneol	*Coriandrum sativum, Zingiber officinale*
Boron	*Brassica oleracea* var. *capitata, B. oleracea* var. *gemmifera*
Brassicasterol	*Brassica rapa*
Brassinin	*Brassica chinensis* var. *pekinensis, B. pekinensis, B. petsai*
Bromelin	*Ananas comosus*
Butanone	*Brassica rapa*
Butenyl-glucosinolate	*Brassica oleracea* var. *gongylodes*
Butin	*Brassica oleracea* var. *gemmifera*
Butyl-glucosinolate	*Brassica oleracea* var. *capitata, B. oleracea* var. *gongylodes*
Butylisothiocyanate	*Armoracia rusticana*
Butyric acid	*Arctium lappa, Trigonella foenum-graecum*
Butyrothetin	*Asparagus officinalis*
Cadmium	*Armoracia rusticana, Beta vulgaris, Lactuca sativa*
Caffeic acid	*Allium cepa, Arctium lappa, Beta vulgaris, Brassica oleracea* var. *botrytis, B. oleracea* var. *capitata, B. oleracea* var. *gemmifera, B. oleracea* var. *gongylodes, Cichorium intybus, Cucumis sativus, Cynara scolymus, Foeniculum vulgare, Glycine max, Lactuca sativa, Solanum melongena, Stachys officinalis, S. sieboldii, Zea mays*
Calcium	*Beta vulgaris, Chenopodium album, Coriandrum sativum, Laurus nobilis, Medicago sativa, Momordica charantia, Phaseolus angularis*
Campesterol	*Brassica rapa, Capsicum annum* var. *longum, Chenopodium album, Medicago sativa, Zea mays*
Camphene	*Coriandrum sativum, Zingiber officinale*
Camphor	*Coriandrum sativum*
Canaline	*Canavalia gladiata, Medicago sativa*
Canavanine	*Canavalia gladiata*
Capric acid	*Cocos nucifera, Cucumis melo*
Caprylic acid	*Cucumis melo, Ginkgo biloba*
Capsaicin	*Capsicum annum* var. *longum*
Capsanthin	*Asparagus officinalis, Capsicum annum* var. *longum*
Capsianoside A	*Capsicum annum* var. *longum*
Carbohydrates	*Arctium lappa, Beta vulgaris, Brassica oleracea* var. *capitata, B. oleracea* var. *gemmifera, Coriandrum sativum, Dolichos lablab, Lagenaria siceraria, Laurus nobilis, Medicago sativa, Momordica charantia*

Component	Source
Carotene	*Allium cepa, A. tuberosum, Chenopodium album, Lycium chinese, Toona sinensis*
Carotenoids	*Daucus carota subsp. sativus, Momordica charantia*
Carvacrol	*Zea mays*
Caryophyllene	*Zingiber officinale*
Casimiroin	*Casimiroa edulis*
Cellulose	*Malva verticillata* var. *crispa, Zea mays*
Cenzent	*Zingiber officinale*
Ceraldone	*Vicia faba*
Cerotic acid	*Artocarpus altilis, A. heterophyllus, A. lakoocha*
Ceryl alcohol	*Foeniculum vulgare, Lactuca indica, Taraxacum officinale*
Ceucocyanidin	*Zea mays*
Charantin	*Momordica charantia*
Chelidonic acid	*Asparagus officinalis, Zea mays*
Chenopodine	*Chenopodium album*
Chloride	*Perilla frutescens*
Chlorine	*Chrysanthemum coronarium, Trigonella foenum-graecum, Vicia faba*
Chlorogenic acid	*Arctium lappa, Beta vulgaris, Brassica oleracea* var. *capitata, B. oleracea* var. *gongylodes, Cucumis sativus, Glycine max, Stachys officinalis, S. sieboldii*
Chlorophyll a, b	*Spinacia oleracea*
Cholesterin	*Pisum sativum*
Choline	*Apium graveolens, Cichorium intybus, Foeniculum vulgare, Pisum sativum, Solanum melongena, Taraxacum officinale, Trigonella foenum-graecum, Zea mays*
Chromium	*Beta vulgaris, Phaseolus vulgaris, Trigonella foenum-graecum*
Chrysophenol	*Hemerocallis fulva, H. longituba*
Cichoric acid	*Cichorium intybus*
Cineole acid	*Daucus carota subsp. sativus, Zingiber officinale*
Cinerin I, II	*Chrysanthemum coronarium*
Cinnamic acid	*Brassica oleracea* var. *botrytis, Foeniculum vulgare, Lycium chinese, Perilla frutescens, Stachys officinalis, S. sieboldii*
cis-ajoene	*Allium sativum*
cis-β-sesquiphellandrol	*Zingiber officinale*
Citral	*Allium sativum, Manihot esculenta, Zanthoxylum ailanthoides, Zingiber officinale*
Citrate	*Allium cepa*

Component	Source
Citric acid	*Beta vulgaris, Brassica oleracea* var. *botrytis, B. oleracea* var. *capitata, B. oleracea* var. *gemmifera, B. oleracea* var. *gongylodes, Foeniculum vulgare, Lactuca indica, Medicago sativa, Solanum nigrum, Vicia faba*
Citronic acid	*Beta vulgaris*
Citrostadienol	*Capsicum annum* var. *longum*
Citrulline	*Cucumis sativus, Medicago sativa*
Clucoiberin	*Brassica oleracea* var. *capitata*
Cobalt	*Armoracia rusticana, Zea mays*
Colchicine	*Hemerocallis fulva, H. longituba, Lilium tigrinum*
Colmestrol	*Brassica oleracea* var. *capitata*
Concanavalin A, B	*Canavalia gladiata*
Coniferin	*Asparagus officinalis*
Copper	*Beta vulgaris, Phaseolus angularis*
Coriandrol	*Coriandrum sativum*
Cornevin	*Solanum nigrum*
Coumaric acid	*Allium cepa, Apium graveolens, Asparagus officinalis, Brassica oleracea* var. *gongylodes, Foeniculum vulgare*
Coumarin	*Trigonella foenum-graecum*
Coumetrol	*Brassica oleracea* var. *gemmifera, Medicago sativa*
Crocetin	*Brassica oleracea* var. *gongylodes*
Cryptochlorogenic acid	*Stachys officinalis, S. sieboldii*
Cryptotaenen	*Cryptotaenia canadensis*
Cryptoxanthin	*Momordica charantia, Zea mays*
Crystalline	*Taraxacum officinale*
Cubebenol	*Zea mays*
Cucurbitacin A, B, C, D, E	*Cucumis sativus, Lagenaria siceraria*
Curcumin	*Brassica oleracea* var. *botrytis*
Cyanidin	*Brassica oleracea* var. *capitata, Perilla frutescens, Zea mays*
Cyanidin 3-glucoside	*Malpighia glabra* var. *florida*
Cyanocobalamin	*Trigonella foenum-graecum*
Cyclopentanol	*Capsicum annum* var. *longum, Zea mays*
Cymene	*Allium sativum, Coriandrum sativum*
Cynaratriol	*Cynara scolymus*
Cynarin	*Cynara scolymus*
Cynaropicrin	*Cynara scolymus*
Cystine	*Chenopodium album, Phaseolus vulgaris*
Cytidine	*Zea mays*
Cytokinin	*Zea mays*
D-abscisin	*Dioscorea alata*

Component	Source
Daidzein	*Pueraria lobata, P. montana, Vicia faba*
Daidzin	*Medicago sativa, Pueraria lobata*
Daphnoretin	*Medicago sativa*
Daucic acid	*Beta vulgaris*
Daucosterine	*Daucus carota subsp. sativus*
D-borneol	*Zingiber officinale*
Decanal	*Coriandrum sativum*
Decanol	*Coriandrum sativum*
Decylic aldehyde	*Coriandrum sativum*
Dehydrocy-naropicrin	*Stachys officinalis, S. sieboldii*
Dehydrozacorbic acid	*Brassica oleracea* var. *capitata, B. oleracea* var. *gongylodes*
Delphinidin	*Medicago sativa*
Delphinidin 3-glucoside	*Solanum melongena*
Delphinidin-3,5,diglucoside	*Solanum melongena*
Delta-amino-levulinic acid	*Zea mays*
Delta-5-avenasterol	*Lactuca sativa*
Desacetyluvaricin	*Annona glabra*
Dextrin	*Manihot esculenta*
D-ferchone	*Foeniculum vulgare*
D-fructose	*Foeniculum vulgare*
D-galactose	*Foeniculum vulgare*
D-glucose	*Amorphophallus konjac*
D-glyceric acid	*Vicia faba*
D-hydroxylysine	*Vicia faba*
Diallyl sulfide	*Allium sativum*
Diallyl tetrasulfide	*Allium sativum*
Dicoumarol	*Medicago sativa*
Dictamine	*Zanthoxylum ailanthoides*
Diethyl sulfide	*Zingiber officinale*
Dihydrocapsaicin	*Capsicum annum* var. *longum*
Dihydronepetalactol	*Zea mays*
Dimethyl amine	*Brassica oleracea* var. *capitata, B. oleracea* var. *gongylodes*
Dimethyl disulfide	*Allium sativum*
Dimethyl sulfide	*Allium sativum*
Dimethyl trisulfide	*Allium sativum*
Dindolymethane	*Brassica oleracea* var. *capitata, B. oleracea* var. *gongylodes*
Diosbulbin A, B, C	*Dioscorea alata*
Dioscorecin	*Dioscorea alata*
Dioscorenin	*Dioscorea alata*

Component	Source
Diosgenin	*Asparagus officinalis, Dioscorea alata, D. batatas, Solanum melongena, S. nigrum, Trigonella foenum-graecum*
Dipentene	*Coriandrum sativum*
Disulfide	*Allium sativum*
Diterpenes	*Ginkgo biloba*
Dithiocydopentene	*Allium sativum*
Divinylsulfide	*Allium sativum*
D-limonene	*Apium graveolens*
D-linalool	*Coriandrum sativum*
D-mannose	*Amorphophallus konjac*
D-raffinose	*Sagittaria sinensis, S. trifolia* var. *sinensis*
D-sylose	*Lepidium sativum*
Duacine	*Daucus carota* subsp. *sativus*
D-verbascose	*Sagittaria sinensis, S. trifolia* var. *sinensis*
Eadesmol	*Zingiber officinale*
Egomaketone	*Perilla frutescens*
Elaterin	*Momordica charantia*
Ellagic acid	*Canarium album, Eriobotrya japonica, Rubus fruticosus, R. reflexus, Vitis vinifera*
Eremophilene	*Arctium lappa*
Erepsin	*Pisum sativum*
Ergosterol	*Lactuca indica, L. sativa, Zea mays*
Erucic acid	*Lepidium sativum, Raphanus sativus* var. *longipinnatus*
Essential oils	*Asparagus officinalis, Asplenium nidus, Brassica oleracea* var. *botrytis*
Estragol	*Brassica oleracea* var. *capitata*
Ethanol	*Zea mays*
Etheral oil	*Taraxacum officinale*
Ethylamine	*Brassica oleracea* var. *capitata*
Eugenol	*Zea mays*
Evobioside	*Lepidium sativum*
Evomonoside	*Lepidium sativum*
Farnasene	*Zingiber officinale*
Farnesol	*Beta vulgaris, Zingiber officinale*
Fatty acid	*Apium graveolens, Brassica rapa, Zea mays*
Fenchone	*Foeniculum vulgare*
Fenicularin	*Foeniculum vulgare*
Fermaldehyde	*Beta vulgaris*

Component	Source
Ferulic acid	*Allium cepa, Beta vulgaris, Brassica chinensis, B. oleracea* var. *capitata, B. oleracea* var. *gemmifera, B. oleracea* var. *gongylodes, Chenopodium album, Cichorium intybus, Glycine max, Lactuca sativa, Raphanus sativus* var. *longipinnatus, Vicia faba*
Fiber	*Asparagus officinalis, Brassica oleracea* var. *capitata, B. oleracea* var. *gongylodes, B. pekinensis, Chrysanthemum coronarium, Cichorium intybus, Foeniculum vulgare, Laurus nobilis, Lepidium sativum, Manihot esculenta, Medicago sativa, Phaseolus angularis, Pueraria lobata, Vicia faba*
Ficusin	*Ficus carica, F. pyriformis*
Filicic acid	*Asplenium nidus*
Fix oil	*Trigonella foenum-graecum*
Flavones	*Medicago sativa*
Flavonoids	*Apium graveolens, Asparagus officinalis, Lagenaria siceraria*
Fluorine	*Brassica oleracea* var. *capitata, B. oleracea* var. *gongylodes, B. rapa*
Flutathion	*Beta vulgaris, Brassica oleracea* var. *capitata, B. oleracea* var. *gongylodes, B. rapa*
Folacin	*Amaranthus gangeticus, Beta vulgaris, Brassica oleracea* var. *capitata, B. oleracea* var. *gongylodes, B. rapa, Trigonella foenum-graecum*
Folic acid	*Brassica oleracea* var. *italica, Phaseolus angularis, Trigonella foenum-graecum*
Formononetin	*Medicago sativa*
Friedelin	*Hemerocallis fulva, H. longituba*
Fructose	*Asparagus officinalis, Cichorium intybus, Medicago sativa, Pueraria lobata, Solanum nigrum, Trigonella foenum-graecum*
Fukinanolide	*Arctium lappa*
Fumaric acid	*Brassica oleracea* var. *gemmifera, Foeniculum vulgare, Medicago sativa, Vicia faba*
Funkioside	*Capsicum annum* var. *longum*
Furanocoumarin	*Apium graveolens*
Gadoleic acid	*Lepidium sativum*
Galactane	*Cucumis sativus*
Galactinol	*Trigonella foenum-graecum*
Galactomannan	*Trigonella foenum-graecum*
Galactosamine	*Capsicum annum* var. *longum*
Galactose	*Capsicum annum* var. *longum*
Gallic acid	*Toona sinensis*

Component	Source
Gamma-aminobutyric acid	*Trigonella foenum-graecum*
Gamma-fagarine	*Casimiroa edulis*
Gamma-hydroxycitrullin	*Vicia faba*
Genistein	*Medicago sativa, Pueraria lobata*
Gentianine	*Trigonella foenum-graecum*
Gentisic acid	*Foeniculum vulgare, Raphanus sativus* var. *longipinnatus*
Geosmin	*Zea mays*
Geranial	*Coriandrum sativum, Zanthoxylum ailanthoides, Zea mays*
Geraniol	*Allium sativum, Coriandrum sativum, Zanthoxylum ailanthoides, Zea mays, Zingiber officinale*
Gibberelin A	*Canavalia gladiata, Pisum sativum, Vicia faba*
Gingerol	*Zingiber officinale*
Ginkgetin	*Ginkgo biloba*
Globulin	*Phaseolus vulgaris, Zea mays*
Glucocochlearin	*Armoracia rusticana*
Glucoconringin	*Armoracia rusticana*
Glucoerucin	*Brassica oleracea* var. *botrytis*
Glucoiberin	*Brassica oleracea* var. *botrytis, B. oleracea* var. *gongylodes*
Glucomannan	*Amorphophallus konjac, Asparagus officinalis*
Glucoputranjivin	*Armoracia rusticana*
Glucoraphanin	*Brassica oleracea* var. *italica*
Glucose	*Asparagus officinalis, Cichorium intybus, Medicago sativa, Pueraria lobata, Sagittaria sinensis, S. trifolia* var. *sinensis, Solanum nigrum*
Glucosides	*Dioscorea alata, Solanum melongena*
Glucosinolates	*Brassica oleracea* var. *capitata, B. oleracea* var. *italica, B. rapa, Lepidium sativum*
Glucotropeolin	*Lepidium sativum*
Glucuronic acid	*Zea mays*
Glutamic acid	*Amaranthus gangeticus, Beta vulgaris, Brassica oleracea* var. *botrytis, B. oleracea* var. *capitata, Canavalia gladiata, Foeniculum vulgare, Litchi chinensis, Manihot esculenta, Prunus salicina, Trigonella foenum-graecum, Vicia faba*
Glutamine	*Asparagus officinalis, Pisum sativum*
Glutathione	*Asparagus officinalis, Brassica oleracea* var. *gongylodes*
Gluten	*Taraxacum officinale*
Glyceric acid	*Cynara scolymus, Vicia faba*
Glycerol	*Raphanus sativus* var. *longipinnatus*
Glycine	*Amaranthus gangeticus, Beta vulgaris, Brassica chinensis, Brassica oleracea* var. *capitata, Lactuca sativa, Medicago sativa, Trigonella foenum-graecum*

Component	Source
Glycoalkaloids	*Solanum nigrum*
Glycolic acid	*Asparagus officinalis, Cichorium intybus, Cynara scolymus, Foeniculum vulgare, Lycium chinese, Zea mays*
Glycosides	*Dioscorea alata*
Goitrin	*Brassica oleracea* var. *capitata*
Goryanu	*Stachys officinalis, S. sieboldii*
Graveobiosides A, B	*Apium graveolens*
Gringerol	*Zingiber officinale*
Grossheimin	*Stachys officinalis, S. sieboldii*
Guanidinobutyric acid	*Arctium lappa*
Gumarin	*Momordica charantia*
Gutta-percha	*Manihot esculenta*
Guttiferin	*Morus alba*
Gypsogenin	*Momordica charantia*
Helueticoside	*Lepidium sativum*
Hemaggluthins A, B	*Dolichos lablab*
Hemerocallin	*Hemerocallis fulva, H. longituba*
Hemicellulose	*Malva verticillata* var. *crispa*
Hemostatic acid	*Asplenium nidus*
Heptane	*Zingiber officinale*
Heptanol	*Zingiber officinale*
Hethylglyoxal	*Zingiber officinale*
Hexanoic acid	*Capsicum annum* var. *longum*
Histidine	*Asparagus officinalis, Beta vulgaris, Brassica chinensis, B. oleracea* var. *gemmifera, Canavalia gladiata, Cichorium intybus, Cucumis sativus, Manihot esculenta*
Homo-grecoline	*Trigonella foenum-graecum*
Homo-orientin	*Phaseolus vulgaris*
Homo-stachydrine	*Medicago sativa*
Homo-taraxasterol	*Taraxacum officinale*
Hypoglycemic acid	*Coriandrum sativum, Trigonella foenum-graecum*
Hydroxamic acid	*Zea mays*
Hydrocyanic acid	*Manihot esculenta*
Imidazolyle thylamine	*Solanum melongena*
Imulin	*Taraxacum officinale*
Indole-3-carbinol	*Brassica oleracea* var. *botrytis, B. oleracea* var. *gemmifera, B. oleracea* var. *italica*
Inosine	*Asparagus officinalis, Brassica chinensis, B. oleracea* var. *capitata, B. oleracea* var. *gemmifera, Coriandrum sativum, Laurus nobilis, Manihot esculenta, Momordica charantia, Zea mays*

Component	Source
Inositol	*Cichorium intybus, Medicago sativa, Zea mays*
Inulin	*Arctium lappa, Cichorium intybus, Cynara scolymus, Taraxacum officinale*
Inverstase	*Armoracia rusticana*
Irisolidone	*Pueraria lobata*
Iron	*Asparagus officinalis, Brassica chinensis, B. oleracea* var. *capitata, B. oleracea* var. *gemmifera, Chenopodium album, Coriandrum sativum, Laurus nobilis, Manihot esculenta, Momordica charantia, Phaseolus angularis, Zea mays*
Isoarctigenin	*Arctium lappa*
Isocytosine	*Asparagus officinalis, Brassica chinensis, B. oleracea* var. *capitata, B. oleracea* var. *gemmifera, Coriandrum sativum, Laurus nobilis, Manihot esculenta, Momordica charantia, Zea mays*
Isoegomaketon	*Perilla frutescens*
Isoflavonoid	*Glycine max, Medicago sativa*
Isoflavonoid glycoside	*Pueraria lobata*
Isolencine	*Trigonella foenum-graecum*
Isoleucine	*Amaranthus gangeticus, Asparagus officinalis, Beta vulgaris, Brassica chinensis, B. rapa, Canavalia gladiata, Chenopodium album, Foeniculum vulgare*
Isoliensinine	*Nelumbo nucifera*
Isomangiferolic acid	*Mangifera indica*
Isomenthol	*Brassica oleracea* var. *capitata*
Isomesityl oxide	*Cryptotaenia canadensis*
Isomultiflorenyl acetate	*Benincasa hispida* var. *chieh-gua*
Isopimpinellin	*Casimiroa edulis, Zanthoxylum ailanthoides*
Isopropyl isothiocyanate	*Armoracia rusticana*
Isoquercitrin	*Cucumis sativus*
Isorhamnetin	*Zea mays*
Isothiocyanates	*Lepidium sativum*
Jaboticabin	*Myrciaria cauliflora*
Jamogenin	*Asparagus officinalis*
Kaempferitrin	*Asparagus officinalis, Beta vulgaris, Brassica oleracea* var. *capitata, B. oleracea* var. *gongylodes, Cichorium intybus, Foeniculum vulgare, Vicia faba, Zea mays*
Kaempferol	*Armoracia rusticana*
Kaempferol glucoside	*Allium cepa, Trigonella foenum-graecum*
Ketone	*Cryptotaenia canadensis, Zingiber officinale*
Kiganen	*Cryptotaenia canadensis*
Kiganol	*Cryptotaenia canadensis*

Component	Source
Kinetin	*Zea mays*
Kukoamines	*Lycium chinese*
Lactic acid	*Zea mays*
Lactones	*Chrysanthemum coronarium*
Lactuce-roltaraxacin	*Taraxacum officinale*
Lactucin	*Cichorium intybus, Lactuca sativa*
Lactucopicrin	*Cichorium intybus*
Lactucopictin	*Lactuca sativa*
Lagenaria D	*Lagenaria siceraria*
Lanostenol	*Capsicum annum* var. *longum, Zea mays*
Lanthanum	*Lactuca sativa*
Lappaol	*Arctium lappa*
Lappaphen A, B	*Arctium lappa*
L-arabinose	*Beta vulgaris*
L-aspariginase	*Capsicum annum* var. *longum*
Lauric acid	*Asparagus officinale, Manihot esculenta*
Laurifoline	*Zanthoxylum ailanthoides*
Lecithin	*Pisum sativum, Trigonella foenum-graecum*
Leucine	*Beta vulgaris, Brassica chinensis, B. oleracea* var. *capitata, B. oleracea* var. *gemmifera, Canavalia gladiata, Pisum sativum, Trigonella foenum-graecum, Vicia faba, Zea mays*
Levulin	*Chenopodium album, Taraxacum officinale*
Lignin	*Arctium lappa, Malva verticillata* var. *crispa, Trigonella foenum-graecum*
Limonene acid	*Apium graveolens, Armoracia rusticana, Coriandrum sativum, Daucus carota subsp. sativus, Foeniculum vulgare, Medicago sativa, Zea mays, Zingiber officinale*
Linalool	*Allium sativum, Coriandrum sativum, Foeniculum vulgare, Medicago sativa, Zea mays, Zingiber officinale*
Linalyl acetate	*Zanthoxylum ailanthoides*
Linoleic acid	*Benincasa hispida* var. *chieh-gua, Chrysanthemum coronarium, Trigonella foenum-graecum*
Linolenic acid	*Asparagus officinalis, Beta vulgaris, Brassica chinensis, B. oleracea* var. *botrytis, B. oleracea* var. *gemmifera, B. oleracea* var. *gongylodes, B. rapa, Cichorium intybus, Cucumis sativus, Foeniculum vulgare, Lepidium sativum, Lycium chinese, Perilla frutescens, Vicia faba, Zea mays*
Lipase	*Pisum sativum*
Lithium	*Beta vulgaris, Brassica oleracea* var. *capitata, B. oleracea* var. *gongylodes, B. pekinensis, Capsicum annum* var. *longum*
Louric acid	*Cocos nucifera*

Component	Source
L-perillaldehyde	*Perilla frutescens*
L-stachydrine	*Medicago sativa*
Lucernol	*Medicago sativa*
Lupeol	*Capsicum annum* var. *longum*
Lutein	*Brassica oleracea* var. *capitata, B. oleracea* var. *gongylodes, Capsicum annum* var. *longum, Medicago sativa*
Luteolin	*Perilla frutescens, Trigonella foenum-graecum*
Lyciumin A, B	*Lycium chinese*
Lycopene	*Brassica rapa*
Lysine	*Amaranthus gangeticus, Asparagus officinalis, Beta vulgaris, Brassica chinensis, B. oleracea* var. *botrytis, B. oleracea* var. *capitata, B. oleracea* var. *gemmifera, Canavalia gladiata, Chenopodium album, Cichorium intybus, Cucumis sativus, Manihot esculenta, Phaseolus vulgaris, Pisum sativum, Trigonella foenum-graecum, Vicia faba*
Magnesium	*Asparagus officinalis, Beta vulgaris, Brassica oleracea* var. *capitata, Coriandrum sativum, Manihot esculenta, Pueraria lobata*
Magnoflorine	*Zanthoxylum ailanthoides*
Malate	*Allium cepa*
Maleic acid	*Brassica oleracea* var. *gemmifera, Coriandrum sativum, Lactuca indica, Medicago sativa, Zea mays*
Malonic acid	*Medicago sativa, Zea mays*
Maltase	*Pisum sativum*
Malvidin	*Medicago sativa*
Manganese	*Beta vulgaris, Brassica oleracea* var. *capitata, Medicago sativa, Phaseolus angularis*
Manihotin	*Manihot esculenta*
Mannan	*Dioscorea alata*
Mannite	*Cichorium intybus, Manihot esculenta*
Mannitol	*Cichorium intybus*
Mannose	*Cucumis sativum*
Margaric acid	*Capsicum annum* var. *longum*
Matai-resinol	*Arctium lappa*
Maysin	*Zea mays*
Medicagenic acid	*Asparagus officinalis*
Menthene	*Zingiber officinale*
Menthol	*Brassica oleracea* var. *capitata, Zea mays*
Mercury	*Beta vulgaris*
Mesityl oxide	*Cryptotaenia canadensis*

Component	Source
Methanethiol	*Asparagus officinalis*
Methanol	*Brassica oleracea* var. *botrytis*
Methionine	*Amaranthus gangeticus, Asparagus officinalis, Benincasa hispida* var. *chieh-gua, Brassica chinensis, B. oleracea* var. *capitata, B. oleracea* var. *gongylodes, Trigonella foenum-graecum*
Methyl chavicol	*Foeniculum vulgare*
Methyl cinnamate	*Zanthoxylum ailanthoides*
Methyl disulfide	*Allium cepa*
Methyl heptenone	*Zingiber officinale*
Methyl isobutyl	*Cryptotaenia canadensis*
Methyl lamine	*Zea mays*
Methyl n-nonyl ketone	*Zanthoxylum ailanthoides*
Methyl phenylacetate	*Zea mays*
Methyl propyl trisulfide	*Allium sativum*
Mevalonic acid	*Brassica oleracea* var. *capitata, B. oleracea* var. *gongylodes*
Miacin	*Lepidium sativum*
Minerals	*Chrysanthemum coronarium*
Molybdenum	*Armoracia rusticana, Asparagus officinalis, Brassica oleracea* var. *gemmifera, Chenopodium album*
Momordic acid	*Beta vulgaris, Brassica oleracea* var. *botrytis, B. oleracea* var. *capitata, B. oleracea* var. *gongylodes, B. pekinensis, B. rapa, Capsicum annum* var. *longum*
Momordicine	*Momordica charanti*
Monounsaturated fatty acid	*Glycine max*
Morellic acid	*Garcinia morella, G. xanthocymus*
Morellin	*Morus alba*
Mucilage	*Arctium lappa, Foeniculum vulgare, Zea mays*
Myrcene	*Capsicum annum* var. *longum, Coriandrum sativum, Medicago sativa, Zingiber officinale*
Myrosin	*Armoracia rusticana*
Naringin	*Citrus grandis, C. limon, C. paradis, C. reticulata*
Nasunin	*Solanum melongena*
Neochlorogenic acid	*Brassica oleracea* var. *capitata, B. oleracea* var. *gongylodes, Stachys officinalis, S. sieboldii*
Neoglucobrassicin	*Brassica oleracea* var. *botrytis*
Neral	*Zingiber officinale*
Nerolidol	*Zingiber officinale*

Component	Source
Niacin	*Allium tuberosum, Amaranthus gangeticus, Apium graveolens, Armoracia rusticana, Asparagus officinalis, Benincasa hispida* var. *chieh-gua, Beta vulgaris, Brassica chinensis, B. oleracea* var. *capitata, B. oleracea* var. *gemmifera, Chrysanthemum coronarium, Cichorium intybus, Foeniculum vulgare, Laurus nobilis, Manihot esculenta, Phaseolus angularis, Trigonella foenum-graecum*
Nicotinic acid	*Solanum nigrum, Trigonella foenum-graecum*
Nonanal	*Coriandrum sativum*
Nonylaldehyde	*Zingiber officinale*
Nuclease	*Pisum sativum*
Obtusifolin	*Hemerocallis fulva, H. longituba*
Obtusifoliol	*Capsicum annum* var. *longum*
Octacosanyl acetate	*Chenopodium album*
Octadecadienoic acid	*Zea mays*
Octanal	*Zingiber officinale*
Oleanene	*Asparagus officinalis*
Oleanoic acid	*Chenopodium album*
Oleic acid	*Asparagus officinalis, Brassica chinensis, B. oleracea* var. *capitata, B. oleracea* var. *gemmifera, B. rapa, Cichorium intybus, Cucumis sativum, Hemerocallis fulva, Lepidium sativum, Manihot esculenta, Taraxacum officinale, Trigonella foenum-graecum, Vicia faba*
Ononitol	*Medicago sativa*
Ornithine	*Beta vulgaris*
Osthenol	*Apium graveolens*
Oxalate	*Brassica oleracea* var. *capitata*
Oxalic acid	*Beta vulgaris, Chenopodium album, Coriandrum sativum, Lactuca indica, Manihot esculenta, Medicago sativa, Vicia faba*
Oxycitronic acid	*Beta vulgaris*
Palmitic acid	*Arctium lappa, Asparagus officinalis, Benincasa hispida* var. *chieh-gua, Beta vulgaris, Brassica oleracea* var. *gemmifera, Chrysanthemum coronarium, Cucumis sativus, Foeniculum vulgare, Lepidium sativum, Trigonella foenum-graecum, Vicia faba*
Palmitoleic acid	*Asparagus officinalis, Brassica oleracea* var. *botrytis, B. oleracea* var. *capitata, B. oleracea* var. *gemmifera, B. rapa, Lactuca sativa, Manihot esculenta, Vicia faba*
Pantothenic acid	*Beta vulgaris, Brassica oleracea* var. *botrytis, B. oleracea* var. *capitata, B. oleracea* var. *gongylodes, B. rapa, Lactuca sativa*

Component	Source
Paolinitic acid	*Lepidium sativum*
P-coumaric acid	*Beta vulgaris, Brassica pekinensis, Lactuca sativa, Pueraria lobata, Vicia faba*
Pectic acid	*Lactuca indica, Malus domestica, M. pumila*
Pectin	*Arctium lappa, Cichorium intybus, Foeniculum vulgare, Medicago sativa, Raphanus sativus* var. *longipinnatus*
Pelargonidin	*Zea mays*
Pentosans	*Beta vulgaris*
Pepsin	*Pisum sativum*
Peptidase	*Asparagus officinalis, Cucumis sativus, Lycium chinese*
Perilla ketone	*Perilla frutescens*
Perillaldehyde	*Perilla frutescens*
Peroxidase	*Armoracia rusticana, Medicago sativa, Solanum melongena, Zea mays*
Petasitolone	*Arctium lappa*
Petroselic acid	*Cryptotaenia canadensis*
Petunidin	*Medicago sativa*
Phasedunatin	*Phaseolus vulgaris*
Phellandrene	*Coriandrum sativum, Zingiber officinale*
Phellopterin	*Casimiroa edulis*
Phenol	*Asparagus officinalis, Brassica oleracea* var. *capitata*
Phenylalanine	*Canavalia gladiata, Beta vulgaris, Brassica chinensis, B. rapa, Zea mays*
Phenylethylamine	*Amaranthus gangeticus, Brassica oleracea* var. *capitata, Canavalia gladiata, Capsicum annum* var. *longum*
Phenylethyl-isothiocyanate	*Armoracia rusticana*
Philothion	*Asparagus officinalis*
Phonethyl isothiocyanate	*Brassica oleracea* var. *botrytis*
Phosphatide	*Vicia faba*
Phosphatidyl glycerides	*Zea mays*
Phosphorus	*Asparagus officinalis, Phaseolus angularis, Pueraria lobata*
Phthalides	*Apium graveolens, Cucumis sativus*
P-hydroxybenzoic acid	*Armoracia rusticana, Brassica oleracea* var. *botrytis, Vicia faba*
Physalin	*Lycium chinensis*
Phytagglutinin	*Pisum sativum*
Phytic acid	*Dioscorea alata*
Phytin	*Dolichos lablab, Pisum sativum*
Phytoalexin	*Apium graveolens*
Phytoestrogens	*Medicago sativa*

Component	Source
Phytosterol	*Asparagus officinalis, Brassica oleracea* var. *botrytis, B. oleracea* var. *capitata, B. oleracea* var. *gemmifera*
Pinene acid	*Daucus carota subsp. sativus*
Plastoquinone	*Vicia faba*
Podophyllin	*Arctium lappa*
Polypeptide	*Momordica charantia*
Polyphenol	*Brassica oleracea* var. *capitata, B. oleracea* var. *italica, Glycine max, Lagenaria siceraria*
Polypodine B	*Chenopodium album*
Polysaccharides	*Allium cepa, Amorphophallus konjac, Asparagus officinalis, Lilium tigrinum, Lycium chinese*
Polyunsaturated fatty acid	*Perilla frutescens*
Pomolic acid	*Malus domestica, M. pumila*
Potassium	*Amaranthus gangeticus, Brassica oleracea* var. *capitata, Coriandrum sativum, Medicago sativa, Momordica charantia, Phaseolus angularis, Pueraria lobata, Trigonella foenum-graecum*
Progoitrin	*Brassica oleracea* var. *capitata*
Proline	*Amaranthus gangeticus, Asparagus officinalis, Brassica chinensis* var. *longum, Capsicum annum, Chenopodium album, Lactuca sativa, Manihot esculenta*
Propenylcysteine sulfoxide	*Allium schoenoprasum, A. tuberosum*
Propion aldehyde	*Zingiber officinale*
Propionic acid	*Arctium lappa*
Protein	*Brassica oleracea* var. *gemmifera, Canavalia gladiata, Chrysanthemum coronarium, Dioscorea alata, Glycine max, Lagenaria siceraria, Medicago sativa, Pueraria lobata, Sagittaria sinensis, Solanum nigrum, Trigonella foenum-graecum*
Protopectin	*Allium chinese, A. fistulosum*
Provitamin A	*Laurus nobilis*
Proximate principles	*Canavalia gladiata*
Psoralen	*Casimiroa edulis*
Psyllic acid	*Lycium chinese*
Puerarin	*Pueraria lobata*
Putin	*Taraxacum officinale*
Pyrethrin I, II	*Chrysanthemum coronarium*
Pyrethrol	*Chrysanthemum coronarium*
Pyrethrosin	*Chrysanthemum coronarium*
Pyrrolidine	*Capsicum annum* var. *longum, Daucus carota subsp. sativus*

Component	Source
Quercetin	*Allium cepa, Asparagus officinalis, Beta vulgaris, Brassica oleracea* var. *botrytis, B. oleracea* var. *capitata, B. oleracea* var. *gemmifera, Cichorium intybus, Pueraria lobata, Trigonella foenum-graecum, Vicia faba, Zea mays*
Quinic acid	*Brassica oleracea* var. *botrytis, B. oleracea* var. *capitata, B. oleracea* var. *gemmifera, Medicago sativa, Zea mays*
Raffinose	*Beta vulgaris*
Raphanin	*Raphanus sativus* var. *longipinnatus*
Raphanol	*Beta vulgaris*
Rhamnose	*Asparagus officinalis*
Rhein	*Hemerocallis fulva, H. longituba, Rheum rhaponticum*
Rheumatoid	*Nasturtium officinale, Rorippa nasturtium-aquaticum, Solanum melongena*
Riboflavin	*Allium tuberosum, Amaranthus gangeticus, Apium graveolens, Benincasa hispida* var. *chieh-gua, Beta vulgaris, Brassica chinensis, B. oleracea* var. *gemmifera, B. rapa, Chenopodium album, Chrysanthemum coronarium, Cichorium intybus, Foeniculum vulgare, Laurus nobilis, Lepidium sativum, Manihot esculenta, Phaseolus angularis, Pueraria lobata, Solanum nigrum*
Ricinoleic acid	*Zea mays*
Robinin	*Pueraria lobata*
Rutin	*Amaranthus gangeticus, Asparagus officinalis*
Rutoside	*Armoracia rusticana*
Sabinene	*Coriandrum sativum, Zanthoxylum ailanthoides*
Salicylic acid	*Beta vulgaris, Zea mays*
Santalol	*Zingiber officinale*
Saponin	*Asparagus officinalis, Medicago sativa, Solanum nigrum, Taraxacum officinale, Vicia faba, Zea mays*
Sarasapogenin	*Asparagus officinalis*
Sativol	*Asparagus officinalis, Medicago sativa, Solanum nigrum, Vicia faba, Zea mays*
Scopoletin	*Capsicum annum* var. *longum, Cichorium intybus*
Sedanolide	*Apium graveolens*
Sedanonic anhydride	*Apium graveolens*
Selenium	*Armoracia rusticana, Asparagus officinalis, Beta vulgaris, Brassica oleracea* var. *botrytis, B. oleracea* var. *capitata, B. oleracea* var. *gemmifera, B. oleracea* var. *gongylodes, Medicago sativa, Trigonella foenum-graecum, Lactuca sativa*
Selinene	*Apium graveolens, Trigonella foenum-graecum*

Component	Source
Serine	*Amaranthus gangeticus, Beta vulgaris, Brassica chinensis, Chenopodium album, Manihot esculenta, Vicia faba*
Seselin	*Apium graveolens*
Sesquilignins	*Arctium lappa*
Sesquiterpene alcohols	*Apium lapa*
Sesquiterpene lactones	*Stachys officinalis, S. sieboldii*
Shisonin	*Solanum melongena*
Shogaol	*Zingiber officinale*
Sialic acid	*Medicago sativa*
Silica	*Pueraria lobata*
Sinalbin	*Lepidium sativum*
Sinapate	*Raphanus sativus* var. *longipinnatus*
Sinapic acid	*Allium cepa, Armoracia rusticana, Brassica oleracea* var. *capitata, B. oleracea* var. *gongylodes, B. pekinensis, Lepidium sativum*
Sinapine	*Raphanus sativus* var. *longipinnatus*
Sirconium	*Capsicum annum* var. *longum*
Sitosterol	*Ficus carica, F. pumila* var. *awkeotsang, F. pyriformis, Ipomoea aquatica, Lactuca sativa*
Skimmianine	*Zanthoxylum ailanthoides*
Sodium	*Brassica oleracea* var. *botrytis, B. rapa, Medicago sativa*
Solamargine	*Solanum melongena, S. nigrum*
Solandine	*Solanum melongena*
Solanine	*Solanum melongena, S. muricatum, S. verbascifolium, S. xanthocarpum*
Soyasapogenols	*Medicago sativa*
Spinacin	*Spinacia oleracea*
Spinosterol	*Cucumis melo* var. *conomon*
Squamocin	*Annona glabra*
Stachydrine	*Chrysanthemum coronarium*
Starch	*Apium lappa, Pueraria lobata, Sagittaria sinensis*
Stearic acid	*Benincasa hispida* var. *chieh-gua, Lactuca sativa, Trigonella foenum-graecum*
Stereoisomer	*Arctium lappa*
Steroidal sapogenin	*Asparagus officinalis, Solanum nigrum, Trigonella foenum-graecum*
Steroids	*Capsicum annum* var. *longum, Solanum melongena, S. nigrum*
Sterol	*Lagenaria siceraria, Medicago sativa, Toona sinensis*
Stigmasterol	*Brassica oleracea* var. *botrytis, Chenopodium album, Lactuca sativa, Pisum sativum*

Component	Source
Stizolamine	*Vicia faba*
Strontium	*Asparagus officinalis, Beta vulgaris*
Strophanthidine	*Lepidium sativum*
Succinates	*Manihot esculenta*
Succinic acid	*Asparagus officinalis, Brassica oleracea* var. *botrytis, B. oleracea* var. *capitata, B. oleracea* var. *gemmifera, Pisum sativum*
Sucrose	*Arctium lappa, Medicago sativa, Pueraria lobata*
Sulforaphane	*Brassica oleracea* var. *italica*
Sulforaphen	*Raphanus sativus* var. *longipinnatus*
Sulfur dioxide	*Allium sativum*
Tannic acid	*Coriandrum sativum*
Tannin	*Arctium lappa, Asplenium nidus, Cichorium intybus, Stachys officinalis, S. sieboldii, Taraxacum officinale, Zea mays*
Tarasacerine	*Taraxacum officinale*
Taraxacin	*Taraxacum officinale*
Taraxasterol	*Cichorium intybus, Taraxacum officinale*
Taraxerin	*Taraxacum officinale*
Taraxerol	*Taraxacum officinale*
Taraxerone	*Cichorium endivia*
Tectoridin	*Pueraria lobata*
Terpenes	*Apium graveolens*
Terpenes limonene	*Apium graveolens*
Terpinene	*Coriandrum sativum*
Terpineol	*Zingiber officinale*
Terpinolene	*Capsicum annum* var. *longum, Coriandrum sativum, Cryptotaenia canadensis*
Tetramethylpyrazine	*Capsicum annum* var. *longum*
Thamin	*Cichorium intybus, Foeniculum vulgare, Laurus nobilis*
Thatglycosides	*Stachys sieboldii*
Thiamine	*Benincasa hispida* var. *chieh-gua, Beta vulgaris, Chenopodium album, Chrysanthemum coronarium, Manihot esculenta*
Thiosulfinates	*Allium cepa*
Threonine	*Amaranthus gangeticus, Asparagus officinalis, Brassica chinensis, B. oleracea* var. *botrytis, B. oleracea* var. *capitata, B. Rapa, Cichorium intybus, Manihot esculenta, Vicia faba*
Thujene	*Zingiber officinale*
Thymine	*Allium cepa*
Thymohydroquinone	*Foeniculum vulgare*

Component	Source
Tiglic acid	*Arctium lappa, Daucus carota subsp. sativus*
Tigogenin	*Solanum melongena, S. nigrum*
Tocopherol	*Asparagus officinalis, Canavalia gladiata, Glycine max*
Toosendanin	*Toona sinensis*
Trans-ajone	*Allium sativum*
Trans-beta-ocimene	*Cryptotaenia canadensis*
Tre-halase	*Hemerocallis fulva, H. longituba*
Triacontanol	*Medicago sativa*
Tricarballyl acid	*Beta vulgaris*
Tricin	*Medicago sativa*
Tricyclene	*Zingiber officinale*
Trigofoenosides	*Trigonella foenum-graecum*
Trigoforin	*Trigonella foenum-graecum*
Trigonelline acid	*Medicago sativa, Monochoria vaginalis, Pisum sativum, Solanum melongena, Trigonella foenum-graecum*
Trigonellosides	*Trigonella foenum-graecum*
Trigonenine	*Chenopodium album, Phaseolus vulgaris*
Trisulfide	*Allium cepa*
Triterpene	*Dioscorea alata*
Tryptophan	*Amaranthus gangeticus, Asparagus officinalis, Benincasa hispida* var. *chieh-gua, Brassica chinensis, B. oleracea* var. *capitata, B. oleracea* var. *gemmifera, B. oleracea* var. *longum, B. rapa, Cucumis sativus, Lactuca sativa, Manihot esculenta, Medicago sativa, Phaseolus vulgaris, Pisum sativum, Vicia faba*
Trysin	*Pisum sativum*
Tyrosine	*Amaranthus gangeticus, Asparagus officinalis, Beta vulgaris, Brassica chinensis, B. oleracea* var. *capitata, B. oleracea* var. *gongylodes, B. rapa, Canavalia gladiata, Chenopodium album, Lactuca sativa, Manihot esculenta, Trigonella foenum-graecum, Vicia faba*
Uglic acid	*Arctium lappa*
Umbelliferone	*Apium graveolens, Cichorium intybus*
Uranic acid	*Lucuma nervosa, Pouteria campechiana*
Urease	*Cucumis sativus, Pisum sativum*
Uric acid	*Lepidium sativum*
Valine	*Amaranthus gangeticus, Asparagus officinalis, Brassica chinensis, B. oleracea* var. *gemmifera, B. rapa, Canavalia gladiata, Capsicum annum* var. *longum, Chenopodium album, Cichorium intybus, Lactuca sativa, Manihot esculenta, Pisum sativum, Trigonella foenum-graecum, Vicia faba*

Component	Source
Vanadium	*Asparagus officinalis, Brassica oleracea* var. *capitata*
Vanillic acid	*Armoracia rusticana, Beta vulgaris, Brassica oleracea* var. *botrytis, Chenopodium album, Cichorium intybus*
Vanilloyl glucose	*Capsicum annum* var. *longum*
Vernin	*Medicago sativa, Pisum sativum*
Vicenin	*Trigonella foenum-graecum*
Vicine	*Vicia faba*
Violaxanthin	*Brassica oleracea* var. *capitata, B. oleracea* var. *gongylodes*
Vitamin A	*Allium schoenoprasum, A. tuberosum, Asparagus officinalis, Brassica oleracea* var. *capitata, Cichorium intybus, Cucumis sativus, Dolichos lablab, Hemerocallis fulva, Lepidium sativum, Manihot esculenta, Medicago sativa, Pisum sativum, Solanum nigrum, Taraxacum officinale*
Vitamin B	*Brassica oleracea* var. *capitata, Canavalia gladiata, Cucumis sativus, Dolichos lablab, Hemerocallis fulva, H. longituba, Medicago sativa, Pisum sativum, Sagittaria sinensis, Toona sinensis*
Vitamin B1	*Allium tuberosum, Lycium chinese, Momordica charantia, Phaseolus angularis, Pueraria lobata*
Vitamin B2	*Allium tuberosum, Momordica charantia, Phaseolus angularis*
Vitamin B3	*Allium tuberosum, Momordica charantia, Phaseolus angularis*
Vitamin B6	*Brassica oleracea* var. *capitata, Lactuca sativa, Phaseolus angularis*
Vitamin B12	*Lycium chinese*
Vitamin C	*Allium tuberosum, Apium graveolens, Asparagus officinalis, Benincasa hispida* var. *chieh-gua, Brassica oleracea* var. *capitata, Cichorium intybus, Cucumis sativus, Dolichos lablab, Hemerocallis fulva, Laurus nobilis, Lepidium sativum, Lycium chinese, Medicago sativa, Momordica charantia, Pisum sativum, Raphanus sativus* var. *longipinnatus, Solanum nigrum, Taraxacum officinale, Toona sinensis*
Vitamin D	*Medicago sativa*
Vitamin E	*Brassica oleracea* var. *capitata, Lactuca sativa, Medicago sativa*
Vitamin G	*Lactuca sativa*
Vitamin K	*Canavalia gladiata, Lactuca sativa, Medicago sativa*
Xanthophyll	*Capsicum annum* var. *longum, Medicago sativa, Taraxacum officinale, Trigonella foenum-graecum*
Xanthotoxin	*Chenopodium album*
Xenognosin	*Pisum sativum*

Component	Source
Xylose	*Beta vulgaris, Medicago sativa, Trigonella foenum-graecum*
Yamogenin	*Trigonella foenum-graecum*
Zapotin	*Casimiroa edulis*
Zeatin	*Zea mays*
Zeaxanthin	*Asparagus officinalis, Capsicum annum* var. *longum, Medicago sativa, Zea mays*
Zinc	*Asparagus officinalis, Beta vulgaris, Brassica oleracea* var. *capitata, Manihot esculenta, Medicago sativa, Phaseolus angularis, Trigonella foenum-graecum*
Zingerone	*Zingiber officinale*
Zingiberene	*Zingiber officinale*
Zirconium	*Asparagus officinalis, Beta vulgaris, Brassica oleracea* var. *capitata, B. oleracea* var. *gongylodes, Zea mays*
Z-methoxy-obtusifolin	*Hemerocallis fulva, H. longituba*

Appendix 2: List of English and Scientific Names: Vegetables

English Name	Scientific Name
Adzuki bean	*Phaseolus calcaratus, P. angularis*
Ailanthus	*Zanthoxylum ailanthoides*
Alfalfa	*Medicago sativa*
Alfalfa sprout	*Medicago sativa*
Arrowhead	*Sagittaria sinensis, S. trifolia* var. *sinensis*
Asparagus	*Asparagus officinalis*
Asparagus bean	*Vigna sesquipedalis*
Asparagus lettuce	*Asparagus officinalis*
Bay laurel	*Laurus nobilis*
Bean (tao-tou)	*Canavalia ensiformis, C. gladiata*
Beet	*Beta vulgaris*
Bell pepper	*Capsicum annuum* var. *longum*
Bird-nest fern	*Asplenium nidus*
Bitter gourd	*Momordica charantia*
Black nightshade	*Solanum nigrum*
Bottle gourd	*Lagenaria leucantha, L. siceraria, L. vulgaris*
Broad bean	*Vicia faba*
Broccoli	*Brassica oleracea* var. *italica*
Brussels sprouts	*Brassica oleracea* var. *gemmifera*
Burdock	*Arctium lappa*
Cabbage	*Brassica oleracea* var. *capitata*
Carrot	*Daucus carota* var. *sativa*
Cassava	*Manihot esculenta*
Cauliflower	*Brassica oleracea* var. *botrytis*
Celery, leaf celery	*Apium graveolens* var. *dulce*
Celery cabbage	*Brassica chinensis* var. *pekinensis, B. pekinensis, B. petsai*
Celery seeds	*Apium graveolens* var. *dulce*
Chicory	*Cichorium intybus*
Chili pepper	*Capsicum annuum* var. *longum*
Chinese artichoke	*Stachys officinalis, S. sieboldii*
Chinese basil, perilla	*Perilla frutescens*
Chinese broccoli	*Brassica oleracea* var. *capitata*
Chinese cabbage	*Brassica chinensis*

English Name	Scientific Name
Chinese chive	*Allium tuberosum, A. schoenoprasum*
Chinese kale	*Brassica oleracea*
Chinese leek	*Allium tuberosum*
Chinese mahogany	*Toona sinensis*
Chinese mallow	*Malva verticillata* var. *crispa*
Chinese mustard	*Brassica chinensis*
Chinese radish	*Raphanus sativus* var. *longipinnatus*
Chinese spinach	*Amaranthus mangostanus, A. mangosteens, A. tricolor*
Chinese wolfberry	*Lycium chinese*
Chinese yam	*Dioscorea alata, D. batatas*
Chive	*Allium schoenoprasum*
Common bracken	*Anisogonium esculentum, Diplazium esculentum*
Coral flower	*Talinum paniculatum*
Coriander	*Coriandrum sativum*
Corn	*Zea mays*
Cress	*Lepidium sativum*
Cucumber	*Cucumis sativus*
Dandelion	*Taraxacum officinale*
Dasheen	*Colocasia esculenta*
Daylily	*Hemerocallis fulva*
Decorative kale	*Brassica oleracea*
Ducks tongue grass	*Monochoria vaginalis*
Edamame	*Glycine max*
Eggplant	*Solanum melongena*
Endive	*Cichorium endivia*
Fennel	*Foeniculum vulgare*
Fenugreek	*Trigonella foenum-graecum*
Garden cress	*Lepidium sativum*
Garden pea, pea	*Pisum sativum*
Garland chrysanthemum	*Chrysanthemum coronarium*
Garlic	*Allium sativum*
Ginger	*Zingiber officinale*
Globe artichoke	*Cynara scolymus*
Goa bean	*Psophocarpus tetragonolobus*
Gourd	*Lagenaria leucantha, L. siceraria, L. vulgaris*
Great burdock	*Arctium lappa*
Green onion	*Allium cepa* var. *aggregatum*
Gynura	*Gynura formosana*
Hairy melon	*Benincasa hispida* var. *chieh-gua*

English Name	Scientific Name
Horseradish	*Armoracia rusticana*
Hyacinth bean	*Dolichos lablab*
Indian lettuce	*Lactuca indica*
Japanese honeywort	*Cryptotaenia canadensis* var. *japonica, C. japonica*
Kidney bean	*Phaseolus vulgaris*
Kohlrabi	*Brassica oleracea* var. *caulorapa*
Konjac	*Amorphophallus konjac, A. rivieri*
Kudzu	*Pueraria lobata, P. montana*
Lamb's quarter	*Chenopodium album*
Leaf-beet	*Beta vulgaris* var. *cicla*
Leaf celery	*Apium graveolens* var. *dulce*
Leaf mustard	*Brassica juncea*
Leek	*Allium porrum*
Lettuce	*Lactuca sativa*
Lily bulb	*Lilium tigrinum*
Lima bean	*Phaseolus limensis, P. lunatus*
Lotus	*Nelumbo nucifera*
Luffa	*Luffa aculangula*
Ma bamboo	*Dendrocalamus latiflorus*
Makino bamboo	*Phyllostachys makinoi*
Malabar chestnut	*Pachira aquatica, P. macrocarpa*
Malabar spinach	*Anredera cordifolia*
Mint	*Mentha arvensis*
Mitsuba	*Cryptotaenia canadensis* var. *japonica, C. japonica*
Moso bamboo	*Phyllostachys bambusoides, P. pubescens*
Mu-erh	*Auricularia auricula-judae*
Mung bean	*Phaseolus sureus*
Mung bean sprout	*Phaseolus sureus*
Muskmelon	*Cucumis melo*
Mustard cabbage	*Brassica juncea* var. *sareptona*
Night-blooming cereus	*Hylocereus undatus*
Oil vegetable	*Brassica chinensis* var. *utilis*
Okra	*Hibiscus esculentus, H. syriacus*
Onion, green onion	*Allium cepa* var. *aggregatum*
Oriental pickling melon	*Cucumis melo* var. *conomon*
Parsley	*Apium petroselinum*
Parsnip	*Peucedanum sativum, Pustinaca sativa*
Pea	*Pisum sativum*
Pepper	*Capsicum annuum* var. *longum*

English Name	Scientific Name
Perilla	*Perilla frutescens*
Pigeon pea	*Cajanus cajan*
Pumpkin	*Cucurbita pepo*
Purslane	*Portulaca oleracea*
Red bean	*Phaseolus calcaratus, P. angularis*
Rhubarb	*Rheum rhaponticum*
Scallion	*Allium chinese, A. fistulosum*
Shan-Chiai-Ts'ai	*Rorippa indica*
Shepherd's purse	*Capsella bursa-pastoris* var. *auriculata*
Slender amaranth	*Amaranthus viridis*
Snake gourd	*Trichosanthes anguina*
Soybean	*Glycine max*
Soybean sprout	*Glycine max*
Spinach	*Spinacia oleracea*
Sugarcane	*Saccharum officinarum, S. sinense*
Sunflower	*Helianthus annuus*
Sweet basil	*Ocimum basilicum*
Sweet corn	*Zea mays* var. *rugosa*
Sweet potato	*Ipomoea batatas*
Sweet potato vine	*Ipomoea batatas*
Sword bean	*Canavalia ensiformis, C. gladiata*
Table beet	*Beta vulgaris*
Taiwan velvet plant	*Gynura formosana*
Tao-tou	*Canavalia gladiata*
Taro	*Colocasia antiquorum* var. *esculenta*
Thousand-veined mustard	*Brassica juncea* var. *multiseps*
Tomato	*Lycopersicon esculentum*
Turnip	*Brassica rapa* var. *rapa*
Vegetable soybean	*Glycine max*
Vegetable sponge	*Luffa cylindrica*
Wasabi	*Wasabia japonica*
Water bamboo shoot	*Zizania aquatica*
Water celery	*Oenanthe javanica*
Water chestnut	*Eleocharis plantaginea*
Watercress	*Nasturtium officinale, Rorippa nasturtium-aquaticum*
Water dropwort	*Oenanthe stolonifera*
Water spinach	*Ipomoea aquatica*
White Dutch runner bean	*Phaseolus coccineus* var. *albanians*

English Name	Scientific Name
White jute	*Corchorus capsularis*
Winter melon	*Benincasa hispida, Lagenaria dasistemon*
Yam	*Dioscorea alata, D. batatas, D. opposilla*

Appendix 3:
List of Scientific and English
Names: Vegetables

Scientific Name	English Name
Allium cepa var. *aggregatum*	Onion, green onion
Allium chinese	Scallion
Allium fistulosum	Scallion
Allium porrum	Leek
Allium sativum	Garlic
Allium schoenoprasum	Chive
Allium tuberosum	Chinese chive, Chinese leek
Amaranthus mangostanus	Chinese spinach
Amaranthus mangosteens	Chinese spinach
Amaranthus tricolor	Chinese spinach
Amaranthus viridis	Slender amaranth
Amorphophallus konjac	Konjac
Amorphophallus rivieri	Konjac
Anisogonium esculentum	Common bracken
Anredera cordifolia	Malabar spinach
Apium graveolens var. *dulce*	Celery, celery seeds
Apium petroselinum	Parsley
Arctium lappa	Great burdock
Armoracia rusticana	Horseradish
Asparagus officinalis	Asparagus, asparagus lettuce
Asplenium nidus	Bird-nest fern
Auricularia auricula-judae	Mu-erh
Benincasa hispida	Winter melon
Benincasa hispida var. *chieh-gua*	Hairy melon
Beta vulgaris	Beet, table beet
Beta vulgaris var. *cicla*	Leaf-beet
Brassica chinensis	Chinese cabbage, Chinese mustard
Brassica chinensis var. *pekinensis*	Celery cabbage
Brassica chinensis var. *utilis*	Oil vegetable
Brassica juncea	Leaf mustard
Brassica juncea var. *multiseps*	Thousand-veined mustard
Brassica juncea var. *sareptona*	Mustard cabbage
Brassica oleracea	Chinese kale, decorative kale

Scientific Name	English Name
Brassica oleracea var. *botrytis*	Cauliflower
Brassica oleracea var. *capitata*	Cabbage, Chinese broccoli
Brassica oleracea var. *caulorapa*	Kohlrabi
Brassica oleracea var. *gemmifera*	Brussels sprouts
Brassica oleracea var. *italica*	Broccoli
Brassica pekinensis	Celery cabbage
Brassica petsai	Celery cabbage
Brassica rapa var. *rapa*	Turnip
Cajanus cajan	Pigeon pea
Canavalia ensiformis	Bean (tao-tou), sword bean
Canavalia gladiata	Bean (tao-tou), sword bean
Capsella bursa-pastoris var. *auriculata*	Shepherd's purse
Capsicum annuum var. *longum*	Bell pepper, chili pepper
Chenopodium album	Lamb's quarter
Chrysanthemum coronarium	Garland chrysanthemum
Cichorium intybus	Chicory
Colocasia antiquorum var. *esculenta*	Taro
Colocasia esculenta	Dasheen
Corchorus capsularis	White jute
Coriandrum sativum	Coriander
Cryptotaenia canadensis var. *japonica*	Japanese honeywort, Mitsuba
Cryptotaenia japonica	Japanese honeywort, Mitsuba
Cucumis melo	Muskmelon
Cucumis melo var. *conomon*	Oriental pickling melon
Cucumis sativus	Cucumber
Cucurbita pepo	Pumpkin
Cynara scolymus	Globe artichoke
Daucus carota var. *sativa*	Carrot
Dendrocalamus latiflorus	Ma bamboo
Dioscorea alata	Chinese yam, yam
Dioscorea batatas	Chinese yam, yam
Dioscorea opposilla	Yam
Diplazium esculentum	Common bracken
Dolichos lablab	Hyacinth bean
Eleocharis plantaginea	Water chestnut
Foeniculum vulgare	Fennel
Glycine max	Soybean, soybean sprout, vegetable soybean
Gynura formosana	Gynura, Taiwan velvet plant
Helianthus annuus	Sunflower
Hemerocallis fulva	Daylily
Hibiscus esculentus	Okra
Hibiscus syriacus	Okra
Hylocereus undatus	Night-blooming cereus

Scientific Name	English Name
Ipomoea aquatica	Water spinach
Ipomoea batatas	Sweet potato, sweet potato vine
Lactuca indica	Indian lettuce
Lactuca sativa	Lettuce
Lagenaria dasistemon	Winter melon
Lagenaria leucantha	Bottle gourd, gourd
Lagenaria siceraria	Bottle gourd, gourd
Lagenaria vulgaris	Bottle gourd, gourd
Laurus nobilis	Bay laurel
Lepidium sativum	Garden Cress
Lilium tigrinum	Lily bulbs
Luffa aculangula	Luffa
Luffa cylindrica	Vegetable sponge
Lycium chinese	Chinese wolfberry
Lycopersicon esculentum	Tomato
Malva verticillata var. *crispa*	Chinese mallow
Manihot esculenta	Cassava
Medicago sativa	Alfalfa, alfalfa sprout
Mentha arvensis	Mint
Momordica charantia	Bitter gourd
Monochoria vaginalis	Ducks tongue grass
Nasturtium officinale	Watercress
Nelumbo nucifera	Lotus
Ocimum basilicum	Sweet basil
Oenanthe javanica	Water celery
Oenanthe stolonifera	Water dropwort
Perilla frutescens	Perilla
Peucedanum sativum	Parsnip
Phaseolus angularis	Adzuki bean, red bean
Phaseolus calcaratus	Adzuki bean, red bean
Phaseolus coccineus var. *albanians*	White Dutch runner bean
Phaseolus limensis	Lima bean
Phaseolus lunatus	Lima bean
Phaseolus angularis	Adzuki bean
Phaseolus sureus	Mung bean, mung bean sprout
Phaseolus vulgaris	Kidney bean
Phyllostachys bambusoides	Moso bamboo
Phyllostachys makinoi	Makino bamboo
Phyllostachys pubescens	Moso bamboo
Pisum sativum	Pea
Portulaca oleracea	Purslane
Psophocarpus tetragonolobus	Goa bean
Pueraria lobata	Kudzu

Scientific Name	English Name
Pueraria montana	Kudzu
Pustinaca sativa	Parsnip
Raphanus sativus	Chinese radish
Raphanus sativus var. *longipinnatus*	Chinese radish
Rheum rhaponticum	Rhubarb
Rorippa indica	Shan-Chiai-Ts'ai
Roripa nasturtium-aquaticum	Watercress
Saccharum officinarum cv. *betala*	Sugarcane
Sagittaria sinensis	Arrowhead
Sagittaria trifolia var. *sinensis*	Arrowhead
Solanum melongena	Eggplant
Spinacia oleracea	Spinach
Stachys officinalis	Chinese artichoke
Stachys sieboldii	Chinese artichoke
Talinum paniculatum	Coral flower
Taraxacum officinale	Dandelion
Toona sinensis	Chinese mahogany
Trichosanthes anguina	Snake gourd
Trigonella foenum-graecum	Fenugreek
Vicia faba	Broad bean
Vigna sesquipedalis	Asparagus bean
Wasabia japonica	Wasabi
Zanthoxylum ailanthoides	Ailanthus
Zea mays	Corn
Zea mays var. *rugosa*	Sweet corn
Zingiber officinale	Ginger
Zizania aquatica	Water bamboo shoot

Appendix 4:
List of English and
Scientific Names: Fruits

English Name	Scientific Name
Abiu	*Pouteria caimito*
Acerola	*Malpighia emarginata, M. glabra* var. *florida*
Apple	*Malus domestica*
Apricot	*Armeniaca armeniaca, A. vulgaris, P. armeniaca*
Atemoya	*Annona (atemoya)*
Avocado	*Persea americana*
Banana	*Musa sapientum, Musa (paradisiaca)*
Barbados cherry	*Malpighia emarginata, M. glabra* var. *florida*
Batoko plum	*Flacourtia inermis, F. rukam*
Betel nut	*Areca catechu*
Bilimbe	*Averrhoa bilimbi, A. carambola*
Biriba	*Rollinia mucosa*
Bitter orange	*Citrus aurantium*
Black nightshade	*Solanum nigram*
Blueberry	*Vaccinium corymbosum*
Breadfruit	*Artocarpus altilis*
Bullock's heart	*Annona reticulata*
Cacao tree	*Theobroma cacao*
Caimito	*Pouteria caimito*
Calamondin orange	*Citrus microcarpa*
Cantaloupe	*Cucumis melo, C. sativus*
Carambola	*Averrhoa carambola*
Carissa	*Carissa grandiflora, C. carandas*
Cashew nut	*Anacardium occidentale*
Ceylon olive	*Elaeocarpus serratus, E. grandiflorus*
Chestnut	*Castanea crenata*
Chicle	*Manilkara kauki, M. zapota*
Chinese bayberry	*Myrica rubra*
Chinese cherry	*Cerasus avium, Prunus avium*
Chinese gooseberry	*Actinidia deliciosa*
Chinese jujube	*Zizyphus vulgaris* var. *inermis*

English Name	Scientific Name
Chinese olive	*Canarium album*
Citron	*Citrus medica*
Coconut	*Cocos nucifera*
Coffee	*Coffea arabica*
Common fig	*Ficus carica, F. pyriformis*
Cucumber tree	*Magnolia acuminata*
Custard apple	*Annona reticulata*
Durian	*Durio oxleyanus, D. zibethinus*
Dwarf flowering cherry	*Prunus japonica*
Egg fruit (canistel)	*Lucuma nervosa, Pouteria campechiana*
Egg tree	*Garcinia morella, G. xanthocymus*
Elephant apple	*Dillenia indica*
European blackberry	*Rubus fruticosus, R. japonica, R. reflexus*
Fiji longan	*Pometia pinnata*
Fingered citron	*Citrus medica* var. *sacrodactylis*
Flowering quince	*Chaenomeles speciosa*
Ginkgo	*Ginkgo biloba*
Grape	*Vitis labrusca, V. vinifera*
Grapefruit	*Citrus paradis*
Guajilote tree	*Parmentiera edulis*
Guava	*Psidium guajava*
Highbush blueberry	*Vaccinium corymbosum*
Honey tangerine	*Citrus tangelo "Murcott"*
Indian dillenia	*Dillenia indica*
Indian jujube	*Zizyphus mauritiana*
Jaboticaba	*Myrciaria cauliflora*
Jackfruit	*Artocarpus heterophyllus, A. odoratissimus*
Japanese apricot	*Prunus mume*
Java apple	*Syzygium malaccense, S. samarangense*
Jujuba	*Zizyphus jujuba*
Kiwifruit	*Actinidia deliciosa, A. chinensis, A. latifolia*
Lansat	*Lansium domesticum*
Lemon	*Citrus limon*
Litchi	*Litchi chinensis*
Lobi-lobi	*Flacourtia inermis, F. rukam*
Longan	*Dimocarpus longan*
Loquat	*Eriobotrya japonica*
Malabar chestnut	*Pachira aquatica, P. macrocarpa*
Manggis	*Garcinia mangostana*

English Name	Scientific Name
Mango	*Mangifera indica*
Marang	*Artocarpus odoratissimus, A. heterophyllus*
Mazzard cherry	*Cerasus avium, prunus avium*
Miracle fruit	*Synsepalum dulcificum*
Monkey jack	*Artocarpus lakoocha*
Moraceae	*Ficus pumila* var. *awkeotsang*
Mulberry	*Morus alba*
Mundo	*Garcinia dulcis*
Murcott	*Citrus tangelo "Murcott"*
Myrobalan	*Phyllanthus emblica*
Papaya	*Carica papaya*
Paradise apple	*Malus pumila*
Passion fruit	*Passiflora edulis, P. foetida*
Peach	*Amygdalus persica, Prunus persica*
Pepino	*Solanum melongena, S. muricatum, S. verbascifolium, S. xanthocarpum*
Persimmon	*Diospyros kaki*
Phoenix eye	*Sterculia nobilis*
Pineapple	*Ananas comosus*
Pineapple guava	*Feijoa sellowiana*
Ping-pong	*Sterculia nobilis*
Pitanga	*Eugenia uniflora, E. urceolata*
Plum	*Prunus salicina*
Pomarrosa	*Eugenia jambos*
Pomegranate	*Punica granatum*
Pomelo	*Citrus grandis*
Pond apple	*Annona glabra*
Ponkan orange	*Citrus reticulata*
Prickly pear cactus	*Opuntia dillenii*
Rambutan	*Nephelium lappaceum*
Rose apple	*Eugenia jambos*
Roselle	*Hibiscus sabdariffa, H. schizopetalus, H. tiliaceus*
Round kumquat	*Fortunella japonica*
Sand pear	*Pyrus betulaefolia, P. serotina, P. sinensis*
Santol	*Sandoricum koetjape*
Shaddock	*Citrus grandis*
Soursop	*Annona muricata*
Strawberry	*Fragaria ananassa, F. vesca*
Strawberry guava	*Psidium cattleianum*
Strawberry tree	*Myrica rubra*

English Name	Scientific Name
Sugar apple	*Annona squamosa*
Sugarcane	*Saccharum officinarum, S. sinense*
Sweet cherry	*Cerasus avium, Prunus avium*
Sweet orange	*Citrus sinensis*
Tahitian quince	*Spondias dulcis*
Tamarillo	*Cyphomandra betacea*
Tamarind	*Tamarindus indica*
Tankan	*Citrus tankan*
Tava	*Pometia pinnata*
Tobacco nightshade	*Solanum melongena, S. muricatum, S. verbascifolium, S. xanthocarpum*
Tree tomato	*Cyphomandra betacea*
Triangular cactus	*Hylocereus undatus*
Wampi	*Clausena lansium*
Water cherry	*Syzygium aqueum*
Watermelon	*Citrullus lanatus, C. vulgaris*
Water wax apple	*Syzygium malaccense, S. samarangense*
Wax jumbo	*Syzygium aqueum, S. malaccense, S. samarangense*
White sapote	*Casimiroa edulis*

Appendix 5: List of Scientific and English Names: Fruits

Scientific Name	English Name
Actinidia chinensis	Chinese gooseberry, kiwifruit
Actinidia deliciosa	Chinese gooseberry, kiwifruit
Actinidia latifolia	Chinese gooseberry, kiwifruit
Amygdalus armeniaca	Apricot
Amygdalus persica	Peach
Anacardium occidentale	Cashew nut
Ananas comosus	Pineapple
Annona (atemoya)	Atemoya
Annona glabra	Pond apple
Annona muricata	Soursop
Annona reticulata	Bullock's heart, custard apple
Annona squamosa	Sugar apple
Areca catechu	Betel nut
Armeniaca armeniaca	Apricot
Armeniaca vulgaris	Apricot
Artocarpus altilis	Breadfruit
Artocarpus heterophyllus	Jackfruit, Marang
Artocarpus lakoocha	Monkey jack
Artocarpus odoratissimus	Jackfruit, Marang
Averrhoa bilimbi	Bilimbe, cucumber tree
Averrhoa carambola	Bilimbe, carambola, cucumber tree
Canarium album	Chinese olive
Carica papaya	Papaya
Carissa carandas	Carissa
Carissa grandiflora	Carissa
Casimiroa edulis	White sapote
Castanea crenata	Chestnut
Cerasus avium	Chinese cherry, sweet cherry, Mazzard cherry
Chaenomeles speciosa	Flowering quince
Citrullus lanatus	Watermelon
Citrullus vulgaris	Watermelon
Citrus aurantium	Bitter orange
Citrus grandis	Pomelo, shaddock

Scientific Name	English Name
Citrus limon	Lemon
Citrus medica	Citron
Citrus medica var. *sacrodactylis*	Fingered citron
Citrus microcarpa	Calamondin orange
Citrus paradis	Grapefruit
Citrus reticulata	Ponkan orange
Citrus sinensis	Sweet orange
Citrus tangelo "Murcott"	Honey tangerine, Murcott
Citrus tankan	Tankan
Clausena lansium	Wampi
Cocos nucifera	Coconut
Coffea arabica	Coffee
Cucumis melo	Cantaloupe
Cucumis sativus	Cantaloupe
Cyphomandra betacea	Tamarillo, tree tomato
Dillenia indica	Elephant apple, Indian dillenia
Dimocarpus longan	Longan
Diospyros kaki	Persimmon
Durio oxleyanus	Durian
Durio zibethinus	Durian
Elaeocarpus grandiflorus	Ceylon olive
Elaeocarpus serratus	Ceylon olive
Eriobotrya japonica	Loquat
Eugenia jambos	Pomarrosa, rose apple
Eugenia uniflora	Pitanga
Eugenia urceolata	Pitanga
Feijoa sellowiana	Pineapple guava
Ficus carica	Common fig
Ficus pumila var. *awkeotsang*	Moraceae
Ficus pyriformis	Common fig
Flacourtia inermis	Batoko plum, lobi-lobi
Flacourtia rukam	Batoko plum, lobi-lobi
Fortunella japonica	Round kumquat
Fragaria ananassa	Strawberry
Fragaria vesca	Strawberry
Garcinia dulcis	Mundo
Garcinia mangostana	Manggis
Garcinia morella	Egg tree
Garcinia xanthocymus	Egg tree

Scientific Name	English Name
Ginkgo biloba	Ginkgo
Hibiscus sabdariffa	Roselle
Hibiscus schizopetalus	Roselle
Hibiscus tiliaceus	Roselle
Hylocereus undatus	Triangular cactus
Lansium domesticum	Lansat
Litchi chinensis	Litchi
Lucuma nervosa	Egg fruit (canistel)
Magnolia acuminata	Cucumber tree
Malpighia emarginata	Acerola, Barbados cherry
Malpighia glabra cv. *florida*	Acerola, Barbados cherry
Malus domestica	Apple
Malus pumila	Paradise apple
Mangifera indica	Mango
Manilkara kauki	Chicle
Manilkara zapota	Chicle
Morus alba	Mulberry
Musa (paradisiaca)	Banana
Musa sapientum	Banana
Myrciaria cauliflora	Jaboticaba
Myrica rubra	Chinese bayberry, strawberry trees
Nephelium lappaceum	Rambutan
Opuntia dillenii	Prickly pear cactus
Pachira aquatica	Malabar chestnut
Pachira macrocarpa	Malabar chestnut
Parmentiera edulis	Guajilote tree
Passiflora edulis	Passion fruit
Passiflora foetida	Passion fruit
Persea americana	Avocado
Phyllanthus emblica	Myrobalan
Pometia pinnata	Fiji longan, Tava
Pouteria caimito	Abiu, caimito
Pouteria campechiana	Egg fruit (canistel)
Prunus armeniaca	Apricot
Prunus avium	Chinese cherry, sweet cherry, Mazzard cherry
Prunus japonica	Dwarf flowering cherry
Prunus mume	Japanese apricot
Prunus persica	Peach
Prunus salicina	Plum

Scientific Name	English Name
Psidium cattleianum	Strawberry guava
Psidium guajava	Guava
Punica granatum	Pomegranate
Pyrus betulaefolia	Sand pear
Pyrus serotina	Sand pear
Pyrus sinensis	Sand pear
Rollinia mucosa	Biriba
Rubus fruticosus	European blackberry
Rubus japonica	European blackberry
Rubus reflexus	European blackberry
Saccharum officinarum	Sugarcane
Saccharum sinense	Sugarcane
Sandoricum koetjape	Santol
Solanum melongena	Pepino, tobacco nightshade
Solanum muricatum	Pepino, tobacco nightshade
Solanum nigram	Black nightshade
Solanum verbascifolium	Pepino, tobacco nightshade
Solanum xanthocarpum	Pepino, tobacco nightshade
Spondias dulcis	Tahitian quince
Sterculia nobilis	Ping-pong, phoenix eye
Synsepalum dulcificum	Miracle fruit
Syzygium aqueum	Water cherry
Syzygium malaccense	Java apple, water wax apple, wax jumbo
Syzygium samarangense	Java apple, water wax apple, wax jumbo
Tamarindus indica	Tamarind
Theobroma cacao	Cacao tree
Vaccinium corymbosum	Blueberry, highbush blueberry
Vitis labrusca	Grape
Vitis vinifera	Grape
Zizyphus jujuba	Jujuba
Zizyphus mauritiana	Indian jujube
Zizyphus vulgaris var. *inermis*	Chinese jujube

References

Abascal, K., and E. Yamell. 2005. Using bitter melon to treat diabetes. *Altern. Complement Ther.* 11 (4): 179–84.

Adab, M. J., P. Bermejo, A. Villar, and S. Sanchez-Palomino. 1998. Antiviral activity of medicinal plant extracts. *Phytother. Res.* 11 (3): 198–202.

Ahmed, M. S., A. A. Seida, N. D. El-Tanbouly, W. T. Islam, A. A. Sleem, and A. S. El-Senousy. 2005a. Antihyperglycemic effect and nutritive value of *Opuntia dillenii. Bull. Nat. Res. Centre, Cairo* 30 (2): 159–77.

Ahmed, M. S., N. D. El-Tanbouly, W. T. Islam, A. A. Sleem, and A. S. El-Senousy. 2005b. Antiinflammatory flavonoids from *Opuntia dillenii* flowers growing in Egypt. *Phytother. Res.* 19 (9): 807–9.

Akihisa, T., N. Shimizu, P. Ghosh, S. Thakur, F. U. Rosenstein, T. Tamura, and T. Matsumoto. 1987. Sterols of the Cucurbitaceae. *Phytochemistry* 26: 1693–1706.

Al-Saikhan, S., L. R. Howard, and J. C. Miller Jr. 1995. Antioxidant activity and total phenolics in different genotypes of potato (*Solanum tuberosum* L.). *J. Food Sci.* 60: 341–3.

Ameer, B., and R. A. Weintraub. 1997. Drug interactions with grapefuit juice. *Clin. Pharmacokinet.* 33 (2): 103–21.

Anderson, R. A., J. A. Hart, G. Kracoff, and S. Ottariono. 2002. Grape seed. University of Maryland Medical Center, Center for Integrative Medicine, Baltimore, MD. http://www.umm.edu/altmed/articles/grape-seed-000254.htm.

Andreana, L., L. Ososki, P. Lohr, and M. Reiff. 2002. Ethnobotanical literature survey of medicinal plants in the Dominican Republic used for women's health conditions. *J. Ethnopharmacol.* 79: 285–98.

Arias, Pimentel. 1989. *Regalo de la naturalexa medicinario casero.* Santo Domingo, Dominican Republic: Impresora Valdez.

Arthur, H., and T. Cheung. 1960. A phytochemical survey of the Hong Kong medicinal plants. *J. Pharm. Pharmacol.* 12: 567–70.

Awad, A. B., and C. S. Fink. 2000. Phytosterols and anticancer dietary components: Evidence and mechanism of action. *J. Nutr.* 130: 2127–30.

Babu, P. S., and K. Srinivasam. 1997. Influence of dietary capsaicin and onion on the metabolic abnormalities associated with streptozotocin induced diabetes mellitus. *Molecular Cell. Biochem.* 175: 49–57.

Baggett, S., P. Protiva, E. P. Mazzola, H. Yang, E. T. Ressler, M. J. Basile, I. B. Weinstein, and E. J. Kennelly. 2005. Bioactive benzophenones from *Garcinia xanthochymus* fruits. *J. Nat. Prod.* 68 (3): 354–60.

Basch, E., C. Ulbricht, G. Kuo, P. Szapary, and M. Smith. 2003. Therapeutic applications of fenugreek. *Alternative Med. Rev.* 8: 20–27.

Bathory, M., I. Toth, K. Szendrei, and J. Reisch. 1982. Ecdysteroids in *Spinacia oleracea* and *Chenopodium bonus-henricus. Phytochemistry* 21: 236–8.

Beecher, M.M., 1994. Cancer preventive properties of varieties of *Brassica oleracea*: A review. *Am. J. Clin. Nutr.* 59 (5 supp.): 1166S–70S.

Beers, M. H., ed. 2004. *The Merck manual of medical information.* 2nd home edition. Whitehouse Station, NJ: Merck and Co.

Belen-Camacho, D. R., E. D. Sanchez, D. Garcia, M. J. Moreno-Alvarez, and O. Linares. 2004. Physicochemical characteristics and fatty acid composition of oil from tree tomato (*Cyphomandra betacea* sendt) seeds. *Grass-y-Aceites-Sevilla* 55 (4): 428–33.

Berg, P., and P. T. Daniel. 1988. Effects of flavonoid compounds on the immune response. In *Plant flavonoids in biology and medicine*, ed. A. R. Liss, 2: 157–71. New York: Alan R. Liss.

Bermejo, J., E. Hernando, and J. Leon, eds. 1994. *Neglected crops: 1492 from a different perspective.* Plant Production Series 26, 181–91. Rome: FAO.

Bisset, N. G., and M. Wichtl. 1994. *Herbal drugs and phytopharmaceuticals: A handbook for practice on a scientific basis.* Boca Raton, FL: CRC Press.

Blazso, G., and M. Gabor. 1994. Evaluation of the anti-oedematous effects of some H1-receptor antagonists and methysergide in rats. *Pharmazie* 49 (7): 540–1.

Bliss, B. 1973. *Chinese medicinal herbs.* San Francisco: Georgetown Press.

Block, G., B. Patterson, and A. Subar. 1992. Fruits, vegetables, and cancer prevention: A review of the epidemiological evidence. *Nutr. Cancer* 18: 1–29.

Blumenthal, M. 1998. *The complete German Commission e-monographs: Therapeutic guide to herbal medicines.* Trans S. Klein. Boston: American Botanical Council.

Boik, J. 1996. *Cancer and natural medicine.* Princeton, MN: Oregon Medical Press.

Bombardelli, E., and P. Morazzoni. 1997. *Cucurbita pepo* L. *Fitoterapia* 68 (4): 291–302.

Bomser, J., D. L. Madhavi, K. Singletary, and M. A. Smith. 1996. In vitro anticancer activity of fruit extracts from *Vaccinium* species. *Planta Med.* 62: 212–6.

Bourdy, G., C. Francois, C. Andary, and M. Boucard. 1996. Maternity and medicinal plants in Vanuatu; Part 2: Pharmacological screening of five selected specis. *J. Ethnopharmacol.* 52 (3): 139–43.

Bown, D. 1995. *Encyclopedia of herbs and their uses.* New York: DK Publishing.

Brinker, F. 1998. *Herb contraindications and drug interactions.* 2nd ed. Sandy, OR: Eclectic Medical Publications.

Brown, A. C., and R. D. Ana Valiere. 2004. The medicinal uses of poi. *Nutr. Clin. Care* 7 (2): 69–74.

Brown, A. C., J. E. Reiitzenstein, J. Liu, and M. R. Jadus. 2005. The anti-cancer effect of *Colocasia esculenta* on colonic adenocarcinoma cells in vitro. *Phytother. Res.* 19 (9): 767–71.

Buckmire, R. E., and F. J. Francis. 1976. Anthocyanins and flavonols of miracle fruit, *Synsepalum dulcificum. J. Food Sci.* 41 (6): 1363–5.

Bunney, S. 1992. *The illustrated encyclopedia of herbs: Their medicinal and culinary uses.* London: Chancellor Press.

Butland, B. K., A. M. Fehily, and P. C. Elwood. 2000. Diet, lung function, and lung function decline in a cohort of 2,512 middle aged men. *Thorax* 55 (2): 102–108.

Caceres, A., N. Menendez, E. Mendez, E. Cohobon, B. E. Samayoa, E. Jaurequi, E. Peralta, and G. Carrillo. 1995. Anti-gonorrhoeal activity of plants used in Guatemala for the treatment of sexually transmitted diseases. *J. Ethnopharmacol.* 48 (2): 85-88.

Camplimi, P., A. Sertoli, P. Fabbri, and E. Panconesi. 1978. Alantolactone sensitivity in chrysanthemum contact dermatitis. *Contact Dermatitis* 4 (2): 93–102.

Cantwell, M., X. Nie, R. J. Aang, and M. Yamaguchi. 1996. Asian vegetables: Selected fruit and leafy types. In *Progress in new crops*, ed. J. Janick, 488–95. Arlington, VA: ASHA Press.

Cao, G., E. Sofic, and R. L. Prior. 1996. Antioxidant capacity of tea and common vegetables. *J. Agric. Food Chem.* 44: 3426–31.

Carpenter, D. O. 2001. *Nursing herbal medicine handbook.* Springhouse, PA: Springhouse Corp.

Cassidy, A., P. Albertazzi, and I. L. Nielsen. 2006. Critical review of health effects of soybean phyto-oestrogens in post-menopausal women. *Proc. Nutr. Soc.* 65: 76–92.

Castilho, R. O., R. B. da Costa, A. Pott, V. J. Pott, G. N. Scheidt, and M. da Silva Batista. 2005. Medicinal plants used by the Kaiwa and Guarani indigenous populations in the Caarapo Reserve, Mato Crosso do Sul, Brazil. *Acta Bot. Bras.* 19 (1): 39–44.

Chadwick, A. 1985. The production of watercress in Great Britain. *Herbs Spices Med. Plants* 3: 3-4.

Chan, W. K., L. T. Nguyen, V. P. Miller, and R. Z. Harris. 1998. Mechanism-based inactivation of human cytochrome P450 3A4 by grapefruit juice and red wine. *Life Sci.* 62: 135–42.

Chandrika, U. G., E. R. Jansz, S. M. D. Nalinie Wickramasinghe, and N. D. Wamasuriya. 2003. Carotenoids in yellow- and red-fleshed papayas (*Carica papaya*). *J. Sci. Food Agric.* 83 (12): 1279–82.

Chandrika, U. G., E. R. Jansz, and N. D. Wamasuriya. 2004. Analysis of carotenoids in ripe jackfruit kernel and study of their bioconversion in rats. *J. Sci. Food Agric.* 85 (2): 186–90.

Chang, F. R., J. L. Chen, H. F. Chiu, M. J. Wu, and Y. C. Wu. 1998a. Acetogenins from seeds of *Annona reticulata*. *Phytochemistry* 47 (6): 1057–61.

Chang, F. R., P. Y. Yang, J. Y. Lin, K. H. Lee, and Y. C. Wu. 1998b. Bioactive kaurane diterpenoids from *Annona glabra*. *J. Nat. Prod.* 61 (4): 437–39.

Chang, S. C., M. S. Lee, C. J. Lin, and M. L. Chen. 1998. Dietary fiber content and composition of fruits in Taiwan. *Asia Pacific J. Clin. Nutr.* 7 (3/4): 206–10.

Chang, Y. X. 2000. *Taiwan native medicinal plants.* Taipei, Taiwan: Committee on Chinese Medicine and Pharmacy, Dept. Health, Executive Yuan.

Chao-Ming, L., T. Ning-Hua, M. Qing, Z. Hui-Lan, H. Xiao-Jiang, W. Yu, and Z. Jun. 1997. Cyclopeptide from seeds of *Annona* species. *Phytochemistry* 45 (3): 521–3.

Charoenkiatkul, S., A. Valyasevi, and K. Tontisirin. 1985. Dietary approaches to the prevention of vitamin A deficiency. *Food Nutr. Bull.* 7: 72–6.

Chau, C. F., Peter C. K. Cheung, and Y. S. Wong. 1998. Hypocholesterolemic effects of protein concentrates from three Chinese indigenous legume seeds. *J. Agric. Food Chem.* 46 (9): 3698–701.

———. 1999. Effects of cooking on content of amino acids and anti-nutrients in three Chinese indigenous legume seeds. *J. Sci. Food Agric.* 75 (4): 447–52.

Chauhan, N. S. 1999. *Medicinal and aromatic plants of Himachal Pradesh.* New Delhi: Indus. Publ.

Chen, B. H., J. R. Chuang, J. H. Lin, and C. P. Chiu. 1995. Quantification of provitamin A compounds in Chinese vegetables by high-performance liquid chromatography. *J. Food Prot.* 56: 51–4.

Chen, B., and S. Yang. 1992. An improved analytical method for the determination of carotenes and xanthophylls in dried plant materials and mixed feeds. *Food Chem.* 44: 61–6.

Chen, C. C., I. M. Liu, and J. T. Cheng. 2006. Improvement of insulin resistance by miracle fruit (*Synsepalum dulcificum*) in fructose-rich chow-fed rats. *Phytother. Res.* 20 (11): 987–92.

Chen, F. C. 1997. *Active ingredients and identification in common Chinese herbs.* Beijing: People Health Publ.

Chen, H. 2006. Chives. In *Handbook of herbs and spices*, ed. K. V. Peter, 3: 337–46. Cambridge, England: Woodhead Publ.

Chen, J. 2005. Medicinal food in China. *Nutrition Advocate* 3 (9). http://www.nutritionadvocate.com/story/medicinalfoodinchina.html.

Chen, Q., and E. T. S. Li. 2005. Bitter melon reduces fat accumulation in rats. *Br. J. Nutr.* 93 (5): 747–54.

Chen, X., and R. Ran. 1996. Rhubarb decoction prevents intestinal bacterial translocation during necrotic pancreatitis. *Hua Xi Yi Ke Da Xue Xue Bao* 27: 418–21.

Chen, Y. H., H. Y. Chen, C. L. Hsu, and G. C. Yen. 2007. Induction of apoptosis by the *Lactuca indica* in human leukemia cell line and its active components. *J. Agric. Food Chem.* 55 (5): 1743–9.

Cheng, H. Y., T. C. Lin, K. Ishimaru, C. M. Yang, K. C. Wang, and C. C. Lin. 2003. In vitro antiviral activity of prodel phinidin B-2 3.3-di-0-gallate from *Myrica rubra*. *Planta Medica* 69 (10): 953–6.

Chevallier, A. 1996. *The encyclopedia of medicinal plants.* London: Dorling Kindersley.

Chiej, R. 1984. *Encyclopaedia of medicinal plants.* London: MacDonald.

Chiu, C. 1955. Abstracts of scientific researches on Chinese medicine. In *A new manual of Chinese materia medica*, ed. Chung Yao Hsin Pien. Shanghai.

Chiu, N., and Chang, K. 1995a. *The illustrated medicinal plants in Taiwan.* Vol. 1. Taipei, Taiwan: SMC Publ.

———. 1995b. *The illustrated medicinal plants in Taiwan.* Vol. 2. Taipei, Taiwan: SMC Publ.

———. 1995c. *The illustrated medicinal plants in Taiwan.* Vol. 4. Taipei, Taiwan: SMC Publ.

———. 1995d. *The illustrated medicinal plants in Taiwan.* Vol. 5. Taipei, Taiwan: SMC Publ.

Cho, E. J., Y. A. Lee, H. H. Yoo, and T. Yokozawa. 2006. Protective effects of broccoli (*Brassica oleracea*) against oxidative damage in vitro and in vivo. *Nutr. Sci. Vitaminol. (Tokyo)* 52 (6): 437–44.

Chopra, R. N., S. L. Nayar, and I. C. Chopra. 1982. *Glossary of Indian medicinal plants.* New Delhi: Council of Scientific and Industrial Research.

———. 1986. *Glossary of Indian medicinal plants.* New Delhi: Council of Scientific and Industrial Research.

Chung, Y. S., C. T. Chien, K. Y. Teng, and S. T. Chou. 2006. Antioxidative and mutagenic properties of *Zanthoxylum ailanthoides* Sieb. and Zucc. *Food Chem.* 97 (3): 418–25.

Cichewicz, R. H., and P. A. Thorpe. 1996. The antimicrobial properties of chile peppers (*Capsicum* species) and their uses in Mayan medicine. *J. Ethnopharmacol.* 52: 61–70.

Colker, C. M., D. S. Kalman, G. C. Torina, T. Perlis, and C. Street. 1999. Effects of *Citrus aurantium* extract, caffeine, and St. John's wort on body fat loss, lipid levels, and mood states in overweight healthy adults. *Curr. Ther. Res.* 60 (3): 121–53.

Colodny, L. R., A. Montgomery, and M. Houston. 2001. The role of ester in processed alfalfa saponins in reducing cholesterol. *J. Am. Nutraceutical Assoc.* 3: 6–15.

Cook, N. C., and S. Samman. 1996. Flavonoids: Chemistry, metabolism, cardioprotective effects, and dietary sources. *J. Nutr. Biochem.* 7: 66–76.

Cordell, G. A., Telma L. G. Lemos, Francisco J. Q. Monte, and Marcos C. de Mattos. 2007. Vegetables as chemical reagents. *J. Nat. Prod.* 70: 478–92.

Cousin, P. J., and K. Hartvig. 2006. *The complete guide to nutritional health.* London: Duncan Baird Publishers.

Criqui, M. H., and B. I. Ringel. 1994. Does diet or alcohol explain the French paradox? *Lancet* 344: 1719–23.

Dalessandrik, K. M., and K. Boor. 1994. World nutrition, the great breadfruit source. *Ecol. Food Nutr.* 33 (1/2): 131–4.

Dalimov, D. N., G. N. Dalimova, and M. Bhatt. 2004. Chemical composition and lignins of tomato and pomegranate seeds. *Chem. Nat. Comp.* 39 (1): 37–40.

Datta, P. K., P. S. Basu, and T. K. Datta. 1988. Purification of human erythrocyte-specific lectins from *Phaseolus calcaratus* (red bean or rice bean) by high performance liquid chromatography. *J. Chromatogr.* 431 (1): 37–44.

Deachathai, S., W. Mahabusarakam, S. Phongpaichit, W. C. Taylor, Y. J. Zhang, and C. R. Yang. 2006. Phenolic compounds from the flowers of *Garcinia dulcis*. *Phytochemistry* 67 (5): 464–9.

Dekkers, R. 1999. Apple juice and the chemical-contact softening of gallstones. *Lancet* 354 (9196): 2171.

Delaquis, P. J., and G. Mazza. 1995. Antimicrobial properties of the isothiocyanates and their role in food preservation. *Food Tech.* 49: 73–84.

Dhawan, K., S. Kumar, and A. Shama. 2003. Evaluation of central nervous system effect of *Passiflora incarnate* in experimental animal. *Pharm. Biol.* 41 (2): 87–91.

Dobelis, I. N., ed. 1986. *Magic and medicine of plants.* Pleasantville, NY: Reader's Digest Association.

Du, H., S. Yuan, and P. Jiang. 1998. Chemical constituents of *Cichorium intybus* L. *Zhongguo Zhong Yao Za Zhi* 23: 682–3.

Duh, P. D., P. C. Du, and G. C. Yen. 1999. Action of methanolic extract of mung bean hulls as inhibitors of lipid peroxidation and non-lipid oxidative damage. *Food Chem. Toxicol.* 37: 1055–61.

Duke, J. A. 1981. *Handbook of legumes of world economic importance.* New York: Lenum Press.

———. 1984. *Handbook of medicinal herbs.* Boca Raton, FL: CRC Press.

———. 1997. *The green pharmacy.* Emmaus, PA: Rodale Press.

———. 2001. *Handbook of phytochemical constituents of GRAS herbs and other economic plants.* Boca Raton, FL: CRC Press.

Duke, J. A., and A. A. Atchley. 1994. Proximate analysis chapter, submitted to CRC Press, Boca Raton, FL.

Duke, J. A., and E. S. Ayensu. 1985. *Medicinal plants of China.* 2 vols. Algonac, MI: Reference Publications.

Duke, J. A., and J. L. duCellier, eds. 1993. *CRC handbook of alternative cash crops.* Boca Raton, FL: CRC Press.

Duke, J. A. and Wain, K. K. 1981. Medicinal plants of the world. Computer index of more than 85,000 entries. 3 vols. 1654 p.

Easdown, W., and T. Kalb. 2004. Antioxidant capacities and daily antioxidant intake from vegetables consumed in Taiwan. AVRDC progress report. Shanhua, Taiwan: Asian Vegetable Research and Development Center.

Edenharder, R., P. Kurz, K. John, S. Burgard, and K. Seeger. 1994. In vitro effect of vegetable and fruit juices on the mutagenicity of 2-amino-3-methylimidazo (4,5)quinoline, 2-amino-3,4-dimethylimidazo(4,5-f) quinoline and 2-amino-3,8-dimethylimidazo(4,5-f)quinoxaline. *Food Chem. Toxicol.* 32: 443–59.

Einbond, L. S., K. A. Reynertson, X. D. Luo, M. J. Basile, and E. J. Kennelly. 2004. Anthocyanin antioxidants from edible fruits. *Food Chem.* 84: 23–28.

Ernst, E., and M. H. Pittler. 2000. Efficacy of ginger for nausea and vomiting: A systematic review of randomized clinical trials. *Br. J. Anaesthesia* 84: 367–71.

Estevez, M. A., and M. Baez. 1998. *Plantas curativas: Uso populares cientificos.* Caribe Soy, Santo Domingo, Dominican Republic.

Etoh, S., I. Keiko, T. Toshiyuki, Y. Kohji, S. Kazuki, and K. Masuko. 2002. Bitter gourd induces apoptosis in cancer cell lines. *Nippon-Shokuhin-Kagaku-Kogaku-Kaishi* 49: 250–6.

Facciola, S. 1990. *Cornucopia: A source book of edible plants.* Vista, CA: Kampong Publication.

Fang, Q. 1980. Some current study and research approaches relating to the use of plants in the traditional Chinese medicine. *J. Ethnopharmacol.* 2: 57–63.

Fang, T. T., and J. H. Huang. 1999. Extraction, fractionation, and identification of bitter oligopeptides and amino acids in mume fruits. *J. Beijing For. Univ.* 21: 61–71.

Farrell, K. T. 1985. *Spices, condiments, and seasonings.* Westport, CT: AVI Publ.

Fenwick, G. R., R. K. Heaney, and W. J. Mullin. 1983. Glucosinolates and their breakdown products in food and food plants. *CRC Crit. Rev. Food Sci. Nutr.* 18: 123–201.

Ferguson, A. R., and L. R. Ferguson. 2003. Are kiwifruit really good for you? *ISHS Acta Hort.* 610.

Fernandez, M. L., E. C. Lin, A. Trejo, and D. J. McNamara. 1994. Prickly pear (*Opunita* sp.): Pectin alters hepatic cholesterol metabolism without affecting cholesterol absorption in guinea pigs fed a hypercholesterolemic diet. *J. Nut.* 124 (6): 617–24.

Fife, B. 2005. *Coconut cures: Preventing and treating common health problems with coconut.* Colorado Springs, CO: Piccadilly Books.

Figueiredo, S. F. L., V. R. C. Viana, C. Simoes, N. Albarello, L. C. Trugo, M. A. C. Kaplan, and W. R. Krul. 1999. Lignans from leaves, seedlings, and micropropagated plant of *Rollinia mucosa*. *Plant Cell. Tissue Organ Culture* 56 (2): 121–4.

Forastiere, F., R. Pistelli, and P. Sestini. 2000. Consumption of fresh fruit rich in vitamin C and wheezing symptoms in children. *Thorax* 55: 283–8.

Foster, S. 1993. *Herbal renaissance.* Layton, UT: Peregrine Smith Books.

Foster, S., and J. A. Duke. 1999. *A field guide to medicinal plants and herbs of Eastern and Central North America.* Boston: Houghton Mifflin.

Foster, S., and V. E. Tyler. 1999. *Tyler's honest herbal.* 4th ed., Binghamton, NY: Haworth Herbal Press.

Frati-Munari, A. C. 1989. Hypoglycemic action of *Opuntia streptacantha* Lemaire: Study using raw extracts. *Arch. Invest. Med.* 20 (4): 321–5.

Frei, B., B. Stocker, and B. N. Ames. 1988. Antioxidant defenses and lipid peroxidation in human blood plasma. *Proc. Natl. Acad. Sci. USA* 85: 9748–52.

Fuju, Y., S. S. Parvez, M.M. Parvez, Y. Ohmae, and O. Iida. 2003. Screening of 239 medicinal plant species for allelopathic activity using the sandwich method. *Weed Biol. Manage.* 3: 233–41.

Fukuda, K., T. Ohta, and Y. Oshima. 1997. Specific CYP3A4 inhibitors in grapefruit juice: Furocoumarin dimers as components of drug interaction. *Pharmacogenetics* 7 (5): 391–6.

Gao, X. X., and X. Q. Liu. 1979. *Radix puerariae* in migraine. *Chin. Med. J.* 93: 815–22.

Garcia, D., M. Escalante, R. Delgado, F. M. Ubeira, and J. Leiro. 2003. Anthelminthic and anti-allergic activities of *Mangifera indica* stem bark components vimang and mangiferin. *Phytother. Res.* 17 (10): 1203–8.

Garden, J. 1989. Sunflower hull anthocyanins: Varietal comparisons, characterization, and selected stability properties. M.S. thesis, North Dakota State Univ.

Gazzani, G., A. Papetti, G. Massolini, and M. Daglia. 1998. Anti- and prooxidant activity of water soluble components of some common diet vegetables and the effect of thermal treatment. *J. Agric. Food Chem.* 46: 4118–22.

Gelenberg, A. J., J. D. Wojcik, and W. E. Falk. 1990. Tyrosine for depression: A double-bind trial. *J. Affect. Disord.* 19: 125–32.

Geng, T. L., W. X. Li, Y. Y. Chen, and L. H. Wei. 1996. The hepatoprotective actions of nine compounds isolated from the leaves of *Clausena lansium*. *Adv. Chin. Med.* 39 (2): 174–8.

Ghayur, M. N., A. H. Gilani, A. Khan, E. C. Armor, I. M. Villasefior, and M. I. Choudhary. 2006. Presence of calcium antagonist activity explains the use of *Syzygium samarangense* in diarrhoea. *Phytother. Res.* 20 (1): 49–52.

Ghule, B. V., M. H. Ghante, A. N. Saoji, and P. G. Yeole. 2006. Hypolipidemic and antihyperlipidemic effect of *Lagenaria siceraria* fruit extracts. *Indian J. Exp. Biol.* 44 (11): 905–9.

Goda, Y., S. Sakai, T. Nakamura, K. Kondo, H. Akiyama, and M. Toyoda. 1998a. Determination of digitoxigenin glycosides in moroheiya (*Corchorus olitorius*) and its products by HPLC. *J. Food Hyg. Soc. Jpn.* 39: 415–20.

———. 1998b. Identification and analyses of main cardiac glycosides in *Corchorus olitorius* seeds and their acute oral toxicity to mice. *J. Food Hyg. Soc. Jpn.* 39: 256–65.

Goldman, I. L., and I. Li. 2002. Forgotten and future vegetable phytoceuticals. In *Trends in new crops and new uses*, 484–90. Eds. J. Janick and A. Whipkey. Alexandria, VA: ASHS Press.

Grams, G. W., C. W. Blessin, and G. E. Inglett. 1970. Distribution of tocopherols within the corn kernel. *J. Am. Oil Chemists' Soc.* 47: 357–9.

Grant, G., L. More, N. H. McKenzie, J. C. Stewart, and A. Pusztai. 1983. A survey of the nutritional and haemagglutination properties of legume seeds generally available in the U.K. *Br. J. Nutr.* 50 (2): 207–14.

Grieve, M. 1971. *A modern herbal.* 2 vols. http://botanical.com.

Grindley, P. B., F. O. Omoruyi, H. N. Asemota, and E. St. A. Morrison. 2001. Effect of yam and dasheen extracts on the kidney of streptozotocin-induced diabetic rats. *J. Food Sci. Nutr.* 52 (5): 429–33.

Grivetti, L. E. 1978. Nutritional success in a semi-arid land: Examination of Tswana agro pastoralists of eastern Kalahari, Botswana. *J. Clin. Nutr.* 31: 1204–20.

Gruenwald, J. 1998. *PDR for herbal medicines.* 1st ed. Montvale, NJ: Medical Economics.

Gucla, K., M. Altun, M. Ozyurek, S. E. Karademir, and R. Apak. 2006. Antioxidant capacity of fresh, sun- and sulphited-dried malatya apricot (*Prunus armeniaca*) assayed by CRPRAC, ABTS/TEAC, and folin method. *Int. J. Food Sci. Technol.* 41 (1): 76.

Guenther, E. 1950. *The essential oils.* 4: 241–56, 634–45. New York: Van Nostrand.

Guerra, M. C., E. Speroni, M. Broccoli, and M. Cangini. 2000. Comparison between Chinese medicine herb *Pueraria lobata* crude extract and its main isoflavone puerarin antioxidant properties and effects on rat liver CYP-catalysed drug metabolism. *Life Sci.* 67 (24): 2997–3006.

Guimaraes, P. R., A. M. P. Galvao, C. M. Batista, G. S. Azevedo, R. D. Ohverira, and R. P. Lamounier. 2000. Eggplant (*Solanum melongena*) infusion has a modest and transitory effect on hypercholesterolemic subjects. *Braz. J. Med. Biol. Res.* 33 (9): 1027–36.

Guney, S., and W. W. Nawar. 1977. Seed lipids of the micracle fruit (*Synsepalum dulcificum*). *J. Food Biochem.* 1 (2): 173–84.

Guo, C., J. Yang, J. Wei, Y. Li, X. Jing, and Y. Jiang. 2003. Antioxidant activities of peel, pulp, and seed fractions of common fruits as determined by FRAP assay. *Nutr. Res.* 23 (12): 1719–26.

Gupta, R. K., A. N. Kesari, G. Watal, P. S. Murthy, R. Chandra, and V. Tandon. 2005. Nutritional and hypoglycemic effect of fruit pulp of *Annona squamosa* in normal healthy and alloxan-induced diabetic rabbits. *Ann. Nutr. Metab.* 49: 407–13.

Gupta, R. S., R. Sharma, A. Sharma, R. Chaudhudery, A. K. Bhatnager, M. P. Dobhal, Y. C. Joshi, and M. C. Sharma. 2002. Antispermatogenic effect and chemical investigation of *Opuntia dillenii. Pharm. Biol.* 40 (6): 411–5.

Hakkinen, S. H., and A. R. Torronen. 2000. Content of flavonols and selected phenolic acids in strawberries and *Vaccinium* species: Influence of cultivar, cultivation site, and technique. *Food Res. Int.* 33 (6): 517–24.

Halpin, A. M., ed. 1978. *Unusual vegetables.* Emmaus, PA: Rodals Press.

Han, J., S. Kang, R. Choue, H. Kim, K. Leem, S. Chung, C. Kim, and J. Chung. 2002. Free radical scavenging effect of *Diospyros khaki, Laminaria japonica,* and *Undaria pinnatifide. Fitoterapia* 73 (7/8): 710–2.

Hanamura, T., C. Mayoma, H. Aoki, Y. Hiravama, and M. Shimizu. 2006. Antihyperglycemic effect of polyphenols from acerola (*Malpighia emarginata*). *Biosci. Biotechnol. Biochem.* 70 (8): 1813–20.

Hannan, J. M., L. Marenah, L. Ali, B. Rokeya, P. R. Flatt, and Y. H. Abdel-Wahab. 2007. Insulin secretory actions of extracts of *Asparagus racemosus* root in perfuse pancreas isolated islets and clonal pancreatic beta-cells. *J. Endocrinol.* 192 (1): 159–68.

Harrington, G. 1978. *Grow your own Chinese vegetables.* New York: MacMillan.

Hartwell, J. L. 1971. Plants used against cancer: A survey. *Lloydia* 34: 103–60.

Hayase, F., and H. Kato. 1984. Antioxidative components of sweet potatoes. *J. Nutr. Sci. Vitaminol.* 30: 37–46.

Heinrich, M. 2000. Ethnobotany and its role in drug development. *Phytother. Res.* 14 (7): 479–488.

Ho, P. C., K. Ghose, D. Saville, and S. Wenwimolruk. 2000. Effect of grapefruit juice on pharmacokinetics and pharmacodynamics of verapamil enantiomers in healthy volunteers. *Eur. J. Clin. Pharmacol.* 56: 693–8.

Hoe, V. B., and K. H. Siong. 1999. The nutritional value of indigenous fruits and vegetables in Sarawak. *Asia Pac. J. Clin. Nutr.* 8 (1): 24.

Horigone, T., E. Sakaguchi, and C. Kishimoto. 1992. Hypocholesterolaemic effect of banana (*Musa sapientum* L. var. *cavendishii*) pulp in the rat fed on a cholesterol-containing diet. *Br. J. Nutr.* 68 (1): 231–44.

Hou, W. C., R. D. Lin, T. H. Lee, Y. H. Huang, F. L. Hsu, and M. H. Lee. 2004. The phenolic constituents and free radical scavenging activities of *Gynura formosana* Kiamnre. *J. Sci. Food Agric.* 85 (4): 615–21.

Howell, A.B., N. Vorsa, and L. Y. Foo. 1998. Inhibition of the adherence of p-fimbriated *Escherichia coli* to uroepithelial-cell surfaces by proanthocyanidin extracts from cranberries. *N. Engl. J. Med.* 339: 1085–6.

Hsu, S. Y. 1982. *Treating cancer with Chinese herbs.* Los Angeles: Oriental Healing Arts Institute.

Huang, K. C. 1999. *The pharmacology of Chinese herbs.* 2nd ed. Boca Raton, FL: CRC Press.

Hutchens, A. R. 1991. *Indian Herbalogy of North America.* Boston: Shambhala Publications.

Hwang, E. S., and P. E. Bowen. 2002. Can the consumption of tomatoes or lycopene reduce cancer risk? *Integrative Cancer Therapies* 1: 121–32.

Ibrahim, N. A., S. E. El-Gengaihi, A. Elhamid, S. Bashandy, and K. P. Svohoda. 1995. Chemical and biological evaluation of *Tamarindus indica* L. growing in Sudan. *Acta Hort.* 390: 51–7.

Iinuma, M., T. Ito, H. Tosa, T. Tanaka, and S. Riswan. 1996. Antibacterial activity of xanthones from guttiferaeous plants against metticillin-resistant staphylococcus aureus. *J. Nat. Prod.* 59 (5): 472–5.

Inoue, T., Y. Arai, and M. Nagai. 1984. Diary heptanoids in the bark of *Myrica rubra* Sieb et Zucc. *Yakuqaku Zasshi* 101 (1): 37–41.

Ioanna, G. B., and H. K. Berthold. 2002. Healthy volunteers and patients with type II hypercholesterolemia. *Am. Heart J.* 143 (2): 356–65.

Ishiwa, J., T. Sato, and Y. Mimaki. 2000. A citrus flavonoid, nobiletin, suppresses production and gene expression of matrix metalloproteinase 9/gelatinase B in rabbit synovial fibroblasts. *J. Rheumatol.* 27 (1): 20–5.

Ismail, I. S., H. Ito, T. Mukainaka, and H. Higashihara. 2003. Ichthyotoxic and anti-carcinogenic effects of triterpenoids from *Sandoricum koetjape* bark. *Biological Pharm. Bull.* 26 (9): 1351.

Istam, R., D. K. Paul, and R. K. Shada. 2004. Nutritional importance of some leafy vegetables available in Bangladesh, Pakistan. *J. Biological Sci.* 7 (8): 1380–4.

Ito, A., L. A. Shamon, B. Yu, E. Mata-Greewond, and S. K. Lee. 1998. Antimutagenic constituents of *Casimiroa edulis* with potential cancer chemopreventive activity. *J. Agric. Food Chem.* 46 (9): 3509–16.

Jacobsen, S. E., A. Mujica, and R. Ortiz. 2003. The global potential for quinoa and other Andean crops. *Food Rev. Int.* 19 (1/2): 139–48.

Je, Y. B. 1999. Pharmacological action and application of anti-cancer traditional Chinese medicine. Heilongjiang, China: Heilongjiang Science and Technology Publishing House.

Jellin, J. M., P. J. Gregory, F. Batz, and K. Hitchens. 2003. *Pharmacist's letter/prescriber's letter: Natural medicines comprehensive database.* 5th ed. Stockton, CA: Therapeutic Research Faculty.

Jeong, J. T., J. H. Moon, K. H. Park, and C. S. Shin. 2006. Isolation and characterization of a new compound from *Prunus mume* fruit that inhibits cancer cells. *J. Agric. Food Chem.* 54 (6): 2123–8.

Jiangsu New Medical College. 1979. *Dictionary of Chinese traditional medicine*. 3 vols. Shanghai: Shanghai Sci Tech. Publ.

Johnson, E. 2002. The role of carotenoids in human health. *Nutr. Clin. Care* 5: 56–65.

Johnston, J. C., R. C. Wetch, and G. L. K. Hunter. 1980. Volatile constituents of litchi (*Litchi chinensis* Sonn.). *J. Agric. Food Chem.* 28: 859–61.

Jolliff, G. C., and S. S. Snapp. 1988. New crop development: Opportunity and challenges. *J. Prod. Agric.* 1: 83–89.

Kahkonen, M. P., A. I. Hopia, H. J. Vuorela, J. P. Rauha, K. Pihlaja, T. S. Kujala, and M. Heinonen. 1999. Antioxidant activity of plant extracts containing phenolic compounds. *J. Agric. Food Chem.* 47: 3954–62.

Kariyone, T., and S. Y. Kimura. 1949. *Japanese-Chinese medicinal plants (their constituents and medicinal uses)*. 2nd ed.

Kaufman, P. B., J. A. Duke, H. Brielmann, J. Boik, and J. E. Hoyt. 1997. A comparative survey of leguminous plants as sources of the isoflavones genistein and daidzein: Implications for human nutrition and health. *J. Altern. Complement Med.* 3 (1): 7–12.

Kawaii, S., and E. P. Lansky. 2004. Differentiation-promoting activity of pomegranate fruit extracts in HL-60 human promyelocytic leukemia cells. *J. Medicinal Food* 7 (1): 13–8.

Kernaleguen, A., R. A. Smith, and C. W. Yong. 1989. Acute mustard seed toxicosis in beef cattle. *Can. Vet. J.* 30: 524.

Kerr, L. A., B. J. Johnson, and G. E. Burrows. 1986. Intoxication of cattle by *Perilla frutescens* (purple mint). *Ver. Hum. Toxicol.* 28: 412–6.

Keys, J. D. 1976. *Chinese herbs: Their botany, chemistry, and pharmacodynamics*. North Clarendon, VT: Charles E. Tuttle.

Khatoon, N., and J. Prakash. 2004. Nutritional quality of microwave-cooked and pressure-cooked legumes. *Int. J. Food Sci. Nutr.* 55 (6): 441–8.

Kikuzaki, H., Y. Kawasaki, and N. Nakatani. 1994. Structure of the antioxidative compounds in ginger. In *Food phytochemicals for cancer prevention; 2: Teas, spices, and herbs*. ACS Symposium Series No. 547, eds. C. T. Ho, T. Osawa, M. T. Huang, and R. T. Rosen, 237–47. Washington, DC: ACS Press.

Kim, M., H. J. Park, M. S. Hong, H. Park, M. Kim, K. Leem, J. Kim, Y. Kim, and H. Kim. 2005. *Citrus reticulata* Blanco induces apoptosis in human gastric cancer SUN-668. *Nutr. Cancer* 51 (1): 78–82.

Kimata, H. 2006. Improvement of atopic dermatitis and reduction of skin allergic responses by oral intake of konjac ceramide. *Pediatr. Dermatol.* 23 (4): 386–9.

Kolesnik, A. A., V. N. Golubev, and A. A. Gadzhieva. 1992. Lipids of the fruit of *Feijoa sellowiana*. *Chem. Nat. Compd.* 27 (4): 400–7.

Kolonel, L. 2007. Flavonoids and pancreatic cancer risk: The multiethnic cohort study. Abstract 856. Paper presented at AACR annual meeting, April 14–18, Los Angeles.

Kolonel, L. N., J. H. Hankin, A. S. Whittemore, A. H. Wu, R. P. Gallagher, L. R. Wilkens, E. M. John, G. R. Howe, D. M. Dreon, D. W. West, and R. S. Paffenbarger Jr. 2000. Vegetables, fruits, legumes, and prostate cancer: A multiethnic case-control study. *Cancer Epidemiol. Biomarkers Prev.* 9: 795–804.

Komatsu, M., I. Yokoe, Y. Shirataki, and T. Tomimori. 1982. Studies on the constituents of *Talinum paniculatum* Gaertner. *Yakuqaku Zasshi* 102 (5): 499–502.

Kooiman, D. 1972. Structures of the galactomannans from seeds of *Annona muricata, Arenga saccharifera, Cocos nucifera, Convolvulus tricolor*, and *Sophora japonica*. *Carbohydr. Res.* 20: 329.

Kowalchuk, J. 1976. Antiviral activity of fruit extract. *J. Food Sci.* 41: 1013–7.

Kowalska, M. T., and D. Puett. 1990. Potential biomedical applications for tropical fruit products. *Tropical Garden Fruit World* 1 (4): 126–7.

Kristal, A. R. 2002. Brassica vegetables and prostate cancer risk: A review of the epidemiologic evidence. *Pharm. Biol.* 40 (supp.): 55–8.

———. 2007. Flavonols and pancreatic cancer risk: The multiethnic cohort study. Abstract 856. Paper presented at AACR annual meeting, April 14–18, Los Angeles.

Kuebel, K. R., and A. O. Tucker. 1988. Vietnamese culinary herbs in the United States. *Econ. Bot.* 42: 413–9.

Kumamoto, H., Y. Matsubaray, Y. Izukay, and K. Okamoto. 1996. Hypotensive effect of flavonoid glycosides in *Citrus sinensis* peelings. *Agric. Biological Chem.* 50 (3): 781–3.

Kuo, P. L., Y. L. Hsu, and C. C. Lin. 2005. The chemopreventive effects of natural products against human cancer cells. *Int. J. Appl. Sci. Eng.* 3 (3): 203–14.

Kurilich, A. C., and J. A. Juvik. 1999. Quantification of carotenoid and tocopherol antioxidants in Zea mays. *J. Agric. Food Chem.* 47: 1948–55.

Kuroda, K., and M. Aleo. 1981. Antitumor and antiintoxication activities of fumaric acid in cultured cells. *Gan* 72(5), 777–778.

Kuusi, T., H. Pyysalo, and K. Autio. 1985. The bitterness properties of dandelion; 2: Chemical investigations. Lebensm. Wiss. Technol. (Zurich) 18: 349.

Lacuna-Richman, C. 2002. The socio-econonic significance of subsistence non-wood forest products in Leyte, Philippines. *Environ. Conserv.* 29 (2): 253–62.

Lakhanpal, T. N., and R. Monika. 2005. Medicinal and nutraceutical genetic resources of mushrooms. *Plant Genetic Resources: Characterization Utilization* 3 (2): 288–303.

Lamont, S. M. 1977. The fishermen of Slave Lake and their environment: A story of floral and faunal resources. M.Sc. thesis, Dept. Plant Ecology, University of Saskatchewan, Saskatoon.

Larkcom, J. 1984. *The salad garden*. New York: Viking Press.

———. 1991. *Oriental vegetables: The complete guide for kitchen and garden*. Tokyo: Kodansha Intl. In *Progress in new crops*, ed. J. Janick, 55–6. Alexandria, VA: ASHS Press.

Lawrence, B. M. 1992. Chemical components of Labiatae oils and their exploitation. In *Advances in labiate science*, eds. R. M. Harley and T. Reynolds, 399–436. Kew, U.K.: Royal Botanic Gardens.

Leakey, R. R. B. 1998. Potential for novel food products from agroforestry trees: A review. *Food Chem.* 66: 1–14.

Lee, J. I., E. Han, H. W. Park, and J. K. Bang. 1989. Review of the research results on Perilla and its prospects in Korea. In *Proceedings of National Symposium on Oil Crop Production and Its Utilization*, 40–52. Suwon, Korea: Crop Experiment Station, Rural Development Administration.

Lee, J. S., Y. S. Cho, E. J. Park, K. J. Oh, W. K. Lee, and J. S. Ahn. 1998. Phospholipase C gamma I inhibitory principles from the sarcotestas of *Ginkgo biloba*. *J. Nat. Prod.* 61: 867–71.

Lee, R., and M. J. Balick. 2001. Health benefits of chocolate. *Alternative Therapies* 7 (5): 120–2.

Lee, S. H., S. Y. Choi, H. Kim, J. S. Hwang, B. G. Lee, J. J. Gao, and S. Y. Kin. 2002. Mulberroside F isolated from the leaves of *Morus alba* inhibits melanin biosynthesis. *Biol. Pharm. Bull.* 25 (8): 1045–8.

Leighton, A. L. 1985. Wild plant use by the Wood Cree (Nihithawak) of east-central Saskatchewan. Canadian Ethnology Service paper No. 101. National Museum of Man, Mercury Series. Ottawa, ON: National Museums of Canada.

Le Marchand, I., S. P. Murphy, and J. H. Hankin. 2000. Intake of flavonoids and lung cancer. *J. Nat. Cancer Inst.* 92 (2): 154–60.

Leung, A. Y. 1980. *Encyclopedia of common natural ingredients used in food, drugs, and cosmetics*. New York: John Wiley and Sons.

Leung, A. Y., and S. Foster, eds. 1996. *Encyclopedia of common natural ingredients used in food, drugs, and cosmetics*. 2nd ed. New York: John Wiley and Sons.

Lewis, Y. S. 1984. *Spices and herbs for the food industry*. Orpington, U.K.: Food Trade Press.

Li, C., J. Zhou, P. Gui, and X. He. 2001. Protective effect of rhubarb on endotoxin-induced acute lung injury. *J. Tradit. Chin. Med.* 21: 54–8.

Li, T. S. C. 2000. *Medicinal plants: Culture, utilization, and phytopharmacology.* Lancaster, PA: Technomic.

———. 2002. *Chinese and related North American herbs.* New York: CRC Press.

———. 2003. The range of medicinal plants influencing mental and physical performance. In *Performance functional foods*, ed. D. H. Watson, 38–60. New York: CRC Press.

———. 2006. *Taiwanese native medicinal plants: Phytopharmacology and therapeutic values.* New York: CRC Press.

Li, X. M., Y. L. Ma, and X. J. Liu. 2007. Effect of the *Lycium barbarum* polysaccharides on age-related oxidative stress in aged mice. *J. Ethnopharmacol.* 111 (3): 504–11.

Li, Y., H. Liu, X. Ji, and J. Li. 2000. Optimized separation of pharmacologically active anthraquinones in rhubarb by capillary electrochromatography. *Electrophoresis* 21: 3109–3015.

Likhitwitayawuid, K., W. Chanmahasathien, N. Ruangrungsi, and J. Krungkral. 1998. Xanthones with antimalarial activity from *Garcinia dulcis. Planta-Medica* 64 (3): 281–2.

Lin, B. F., and R. F. Lin. 1999. Effect of Chinese stir-fry cooking on folate contents of vegetables. *J. Chin. Agric. Chem. Soc.* 37: 443–54.

Lin, C. C., S. J. Wu, J. S. Wang, J. J. Yang, and C. H. Chang. 2001. Evaluation of antioxidant activity of legumes. *Pharm. Biol.* 39 (4): 300–4.

Lin, H. M., H. C. Tseng, C. J. Wang, C. C. Chyau, K. K. Liao, P. L. Peng, and F. P. Chou. 2007. Induction of autophagy and apoptosis by the extract of *Solanum nigrum* Linn in HepG2 cells. *J. Agric. Food Chem.* 55: 3620–8.

Lin, K. H. 1998a. *Chinese medicinal herbs of Taiwan.* Vol. 1. [In Chinese.] Taipei, Taiwan: How Xiong Di Publ.

———. 1998b. *Chinese medicinal herbs of Taiwan.* Vol. 2. [In Chinese.] Taipei, Taiwan: How Xiong Di Publ.

———. 1998c. *Chinese medicinal herbs of Taiwan.* Vol. 3. [In Chinese.] Taipei, Taiwan: How Xiong Di Publ.

———. 1998d. *Chinese medicinal herbs of Taiwan.* Vol. 4. [In Chinese.] Taipei, Taiwan: How Xiong Di Publ.

———. 1998e. *Chinese medicinal herbs of Taiwan.* Vol. 5. [In Chinese.] Taipei, Taiwan: How Xiong Di Publ.

———. 1998f. *Chinese medicinal herbs of Taiwan.* Vol. 6. [In Chinese.] Taipei, Taiwan: How Xiong Di Publ.

———. 1998g. *Chinese medicinal herbs of Taiwan.* Vol. 7. [In Chinese.] Taipei, Taiwan: How Xiong Di Publ.

Lin, R. C. 1998. Effects of isoflavones on alcohol pharmacokinetics and alcohol-drinking behavior in rats. *Am. J. Clin. Nutr.* 68 (supp.): 1512S–5S.

Lockett, C. T., C. C. Calvert, and L. E. Grivetti. 2002. Energy and micronutrient composition of dietary and medicinal wild plants consumed during drought. *J. Food Sci. Nutr.* 51 (3): 195–208.

Lu, W., T. Ogata, S. Sato, K. Unoura, and J. I. Onodera. 2001. Superoxide scavanging activities of sixty Chinese medicines determined by an ESR spin-trapping method using electrogenerated superoxide. *Yakugaku Zasshi* 121 (4): 265–7.

Lu, Y., C. Zhang, P. Bucheli, and D. Wei. 2006. Citrus flavonoids in fruit and traditional Chinese medicinal food ingredients in China. *J. Plant Food Hum. Nutr.* 61 (2): 55–63.

Lukas, S. E., D. Penetar, and J. Berko. 2005. Kudzu extract found to reduce alcohol consumption in heavy drinkers. *Alcohol Clin. Exp. Res.* 29 (5): 756–62.

Lust, J. 1979. *The Herb Book.* London: Bantam Press.

Luximon-Ramma, A., T. Bahorun, and A. Crozier. 2003. Antioxidant actions and phenolic and vitamins contents of common Mauritian exotic fruits. *J. Sci. Food Agric.* 83 (5): 496–502.

Mackeen, M. M., A. M. Ali, S. H. El-Sharkawy, M. Y. Manap, K. M. Salleh, N. H. Lajis, and K. Kawazu. 1997. Antimicrobial and cytotoxic properties of some Malaysian traditional vegetables. *Pharm. Biol.* 35 (3): 174–8.

Malhotra, S. K. 2006. Celery. In *Handbook of herbs and spices*, ed. K. V. Peter, 3: 317–36. Cambridge, England: Woodhead Publishing.

Mandel, H., N. Levy, S. Izkovitch, and S. H. Korman. 2005. Elevated plasma citrulline and arginine due to consumption of *Citrullus vulgaris*. *J. Inherit. Metab. Dis.* 28 (4): 467–72.

Mani, U. V., M. Sharma, K. Waghray, U. Tyer, and I. Mani. 2005. Effect of Colocasia leaves (*Colocasia antiquorum*) on serum and tissue lipids in cholesterol-fed rats. *Plant Foods Hum. Nutr.* 39 (3): 245–55.

Mannan, N., B. J. Boucher, and S. J. W. Evans. 2000. Increased waist size and weight in relation to consumption of *Areca catechu* (betel nut): A risk factor for increased glycaemia in Asians in East London. *Br. J. Nutr.* 83 (3): 267–75.

Manousos, O. N. E., D. Day, D. Trichopoulos, F. Gerovassilis, A. Tnazou, and A. Polychronopoulos. 1983. Diet and colorectal cancer: A case control study in Greece. *Int. J. Cancer* 32: 1–5.

Mansell, R. L., and C. A. McIntosh. 1991. Citrus species: In vitro culture and the production of limon. In *Biotechnology in agriculture and forestry*, vol. 15. *Medicinal and aromatic plants*, 3rd, ed. Y. P. S. Bajaj, 193–210. New York: Springer-Verlag.

Mantena, S. K., J. S. R. Badduri, K. B. Siripurapu, and M. K. Unnikrishnan. 2003. In vitro evaluation of antioxidant properties of *Cocos nucifera* Linn. *Nahrung/Food* 47 (2): 126–31.

Manzi, F., V. Flood, K. Webb, and P. Mitchell. 2002. The intake of carotenoids in an older Australian population: The blue mountains eye study. *Public Health Nutr.* 5: 347–52.

Marles, R. J., C. Clavelle, L. Monteleone, N. Tays, and D. Burns. 2000. *Aboriginal plant use in Canada's northwest boreal forest*. Vancouver: UBC Press.

Marshall, D. E. 1988. A bibliography of rhubarb and Rheum species. *Bibliogr. Lit. Agric.* 62. USDA Agricultural Research Service. Supplement, July 12, 1995. Washington, DC: National Agricultural Library.

Martin, E. B. 1986. *Laurus nobilis*: bay tree. *Herbarist* 52: 25–7.

Martin, S. R. 2002. The extraction of medicinal compounds from fruits and vegetables. http://grouppekurosawa.com.

Martinez, M., L. G. Leon-de-Pinto, L. Sanabria, O. Beltran, J. M. Igartuburu, and A. Bahsas. 2003. Structural features of an arabinogalactan gum exudates from *Spondias dulsis* (Anacardiaceae). *Carbohydr. Res.* 338 (7): 619–24.

Masuda, R. 1991. Quality requirement and improvement of vegetable soybean. In *Vegetable soybean: Research needs for production and quality improvement*, ed. S. Shanmugasundaram. Taiwan: Asian Vegetable Res. Dev. Center.

Mazza, G. 1984. Volatiles in distillates of fresh, dehydrated, and freeze dried horseradish. *Can. Inst. Food Sci. Technol. J.* 17: 18–23.

Mehta, R. G., J. F. Liu, A. Constantinou, C. F. Thomas, M. Hawthorn, M. You, C. Gerhauser, J. M. Pezzuto, R. C. Moon, R. M. Moriaty, J. F. Liu, and M. You. 1995. Cancer chemopreventive activity of brassinin, a phytoalexin from cabbage. *Carcinogenesis* 16: 399–404.

Mentreddy, S. R., A. L. Mohamed, N. Joshee, and A. K. Yadav. 2002. Edamame: A nutritious vegetable crop. In *Trends in new crops and new uses*, eds. J. Janick and A. Whipkey, 432–8. Alexandria, VA: ASHS Press.

Messina, M. 2001. An overview of the health effects of soyfoods and soybean isoflavones. In *Proceedings of 2nd international vegetable soybean conference*, eds. T. A. Lumkin and S. Shanmugasundaram, 117–22. Pullman, WA.

Messina, M., and S. Barnes. 1991. The role of soy products in reducing risk of cancer. *J. Natl. Cancer Inst.* 83: 541–6.

Meyer, A. S., O. S. Yi, and D. A. Pearson. 1997. Inhibition of human low-density lipoprotein oxidation in relation to composition of phenolic antioxidants in grapes (*Vitis vinifera*). *J. Agric. Food Chem.* 45, 1638–43.

Michnovicz, J. J. 1998. Increased estrogen 2-hydroxylation in obese women using oral indole-3-carbinol. *Int. J. Obes. Relat. Metab. Disord.* 22: 227–9.

Misaki, A., T. Ito, and T. Harada. 1972. Constitutional studies on the mucilage of "yamano-imo" *Dioscorea batatas* Decne. Forma isukune: Isolation and structure of mannan. *Agric. Biol. Chem.* 36: 761–71.

Miyazawa, M., H. Kinoshita, and Y. Okuno. 2003. Antimutagenic activity of sakuranetin from *Prunus Jamasakura*. *J. Food Sci.* 68 (1): 52–6.

Mohamed, A., M. S. S. Rao, and T. Mebrahtu. 2001. Nutritional and health benefits of vegetable soybean: Beyond protein and oil. In *Proceedings 2nd Int. Vegetable Soybean Conf.*, eds. T. A. Lumkin and S. Shanmugasundaram, 131–34. Pullman, WA.

Mongeau, R., I. R. Siddiqui, J. Emery, and R. Brassard. 1990. Effect of dietary fiber concentrated from celery, parsnip, and rutabaga on intestinal functions, serum cholesterol, and blood glucose response in rats. *J. Agric. Food Chem.* 38: 195–200.

Morton, J. F. 1976. *Herbs and spices*. New York: Golden Press.

———. 1981. *Atlas of medicinal plants of Middle America*. Springfield, IL: Charles C. Thomas.

———. 1987a. Avocado. In *Fruits of warm climates*, 91–102. Miami: Florida Flair Books.

———. 1987b. Banana. In *Fruits of warm climates*, 29–46. Miami: Florida Flair Books.

———. 1987c. Biriba. In *Fruits of warm climates*, 88–90. Miami: Florida Flair Books.

———. 1987d. Citron. In *Fruits of warm climates*, 179–82. Miami: Florida Flair Books.

———. 1987e. Lucuma. In *Fruits of warm climates*, 405–6. Miami: Florida Flair Books.

———. 1987f. Indian jujube. In *Fruits of warm climates*, 272–5. Miami: Florida Flair Books.

———. 1987g. Jaboticaba. In *Fruits of warm climates*, 371–4. Miami: Florida Flair Books.

———. 1987h. Jackfruit. In *Fruits of warm climates*, 58–64. Miami: Florida Flair Books.

———. 1987i. Sapodilla. In *Fruits of warm climates*, 393–8. Miami: Florida Flair Books.

Mosig, A., and S. G. Schramm. 1955. Der Arzneipflanzen und Drogenschatz Chinas und die Bedeutung des Pen-ts'ao Kang-mu als: Standardwerk der Chinensischen Materia Medica. *Beih. Pharmazie Heft* 4: 1–71.

Mossman, J. 2005. Dietary supplements for diabetes. *Pharmacist* 30: 11.

Naim, M., B. Gestetner, S. Zilkah, Y. Birk, and A. Bondi. 1974. Soybean isoflavones, characterization, determination, and antifungal activity. *J. Agric. Food Chem.* 22: 806–10.

Newall, C. A., L. A. Anderson, and J. D. Philpson. 1996. *Herbal medicine: A guide for healthcare professionals*. London: Pharmaceutical Press.

Newman, Jacqueline M. 2000. Fruits and food as medicine, part 2. *Flavor Fortune* 7 (3).

Niazi, S. K. 2002. Pharmaceutical composition for the prevention and treatment of scar tissue. U.S. Patent 6,447,820.

Nishizawa, M., M. Emura, H. Yamada, M. Shiro, Y. Chairul-Hayashi, and H. Tokuda. 1989. Isolation of a new cycloartanoid triterpene from leaves of *Lansium domesticum*. *Tetrahedron Lett.* 30 (41): 5615–8.

Noble, R. 2000. *Physicians desk reference for herbal medicines*. 2nd ed. Toronto: Thomson Publ.

Noel, P. H., J. A. Pugh, A. C. Lame, and G. Marsh. 1997. The use of traditional plant medicines for non-insulin dependent diabetes mellitus in south Texas. *Phytother. Res.* 11 (7): 512–7.

Oberlies, N. H., L. L. Rogers, J. M. Martin, and J. L. McLaughlin. 1998. Cytotoxic and insecticidal constituents of unripe fruit of *Persea americana*. *J. Nat. Prod.* 61 (6): 781–5.

Obiajunwa, E. I., A. C. Adebajo, and O. R. Omobuwajo. 2002. Essential and trace element contents of some Nigerian medicinal plants. *J. Radioanal. Nucl. Chem.* 252 (3): 473–6.

Obukowicz, M. G., and S. L. Hummert. 2004. EP Patent 1,401,461. http://freepatentsonline.com.

Ogle, B. M., H. T. A. Dao, G. Mulokozi, and L. Hambraeus. 2001. Micro-nutrient composition and nutritional importance of gathered vegetables in vienan. *Int. J. Food Sci. Nutr.* 52 (6): 485–99.

Ohr, L. M. 2002. A growing arsenal against cancer. *Food Technol.* 56: 67–71.

Ohsawa, K., S. Atsuzawa, T. Mitaui, and I. Yamamoto. 1991. Isolation and insecticidal activity of three acetogenins from seeds of pond apple, *Annona glabra* L. *J. Pest. Sci.* 16 (1): 93–6.

Ojeda, M., B. Schaffer, and S. Frederick. 2004. Root and leaf ferric chelate reductase activity in pond apple and soursop. *J. Plant Nutr.* 27 (8): 1381–93.

Opticantha. 2000. http://opticantha.com/ataglance html.

Ordonez, R. M., A. A. L. Ordonez, J. E. Sayago, M. I. Nieva-Moreno, and M. I. Isla. 2006. Antimicrobial activity of glycosidase inhibitory protein isolated from *Cyphomandra betacea* Sandt. *Peptides* 27 (6): 1187–91.

Osman, H. E., N. Maalej, D. Shanmuganayagam, and J. D. Folts. 1998. Grape juice but not orange or grapefruit juice inhibits platelet activity in dogs and monkeys. *J. Nutr.* 128 (2): 2307–12.

Osman, M. A., M. A. M. Kicka, and M. B. A. El-Samei. 1979. Chemical composition and hypotensive activity of *Cucurbita pepo* seeds. *Res. Bull. Ain. Shams. U.* 1146: 14.

Palada, M. C., and S. M. A. Crossman. 1999. Evaluation of tropical leaf vegetables in the Virgin Islands. In *Perspectives on new crops and new uses*, ed. J. Janick, 388–93. Proceedings of fourth national symposium on new crops and new uses, Phoenix, AZ, Nov. 8–11, 1998.

Panday, B. P. 1990. *Spices and condiments*. New Delhi: Shree Publishing House.

Passalacqua, N. G., P. M. Guarrera, and G. De fine. 2007. Contribution to the knowledge of the folk plant medicine in Calabia region (Southern Italy). *Fitoterapia* 78 (1): 52–68.

Patwardhan, V. N. 1962. Pulses and beans in human nutrition. *Am. J. Clinical Nutr.* 11: 12–30.

Pedras, M. S., Q. A. Zheng, and R. S. Gadaqi. 2007. The first naturally occurring aromatic isothiocyanates rapalexins A and B are cruciferous phytoalexins. *Chem. Commun. (Camb.)* 2007 (4): 368–70.

Peirce, A. ed. 1999. *The American Pharmaceutical Association practical guide to natural medicines*. New York: William Morrow and Co.

Pellicciari, R., 1972. Triterpenes from *Pouteria caimito*. *Planta Med.* 22: 196–200.

Pereira, M. A., E. D. Parker, and A. R. Folsom. 2007. Coffee consumption and risk of type 2 diabetes mellitus. *Arch. Intern. Med.* 166: 1311–6.

Perez, R. M., C. Perez, M. A. Zavala, S. Perez, H. Hernandez, and F. Lagunes. 2000. Hypoglycemic effects of lactucin-8-0-methylacrylate of *Parmentiera edulis* fruit. *J. Ethnopharmacol.* 71 (3): 391–4.

Perez, C., J. R. Canal, J. E. Campillo, A. Romero, and M. D. Torres. 1999. Hypotriglyceridaemic activity of *Ficus carica* leaves in experimental hypertriglyceridaemic rats. *Phytother. Res.* 13: 188–91.

Perez, G. R. M., S. R. Vargas, and H. Y. D. Ortiz. 2005. Wound healing properties of *Hylocereus undatus* on diabetic rats. *Phytother. Res.* 19 (8): 665–8.

Perez, R. M., C. Perez, M. A. Zavala, S. Perez, H. Hernandez, and F. Lagunes. 2000. Hypoglycemic effects of lactucin-8-O-methylacrylate of *Parmentiera edulis* fruit. *J. Ethnopharmacol.* 71 (3): 391–4.

Perry, L. M. 1980. *Medicinal plants of east and southeast Asia*. Cambridge, MA: MIT Press.

Perry, L. M., and J. Metzger. 1980. Medicinal plants of East and Southeast Asia. Cambridge, MA: MIT Press.

Peterson, J. J., G. R. Beecher, S. A. Bhagwat, and J. T. Dwyer. 2006. Flavanones in grapefruit, lemons, and limes: A compilation and review of the data from the analytical literature. *J. Food Composition Anal.* 19, 874–80.

Pieroni, A. 2000. Medicinal plants and food medicines in the folk traditions of the upper Lucca Province, Italy. *J. Ethnophamacol.* 70: 235–73.

Pinto, A. C., M. C. R. Cordeiro, and S. R. M. de Andrade. 2005. *Annona species: International Center for underutilized crops.* Southampton, U.K.: Univ. Southampton.

Plumb, G. W., N. Lambert, S. J. Chambers, S. Wanigatunga, R. K. Heaney, J. A. Plumb, O. I. Aruoma, B. Halliwell, N. J. Miller, and G. Williamson. 1996. Are whole extracts and purified glucosinodates from cruciferous vegetables antioxidants? *Free Rad. Res.* 25: 75–86.

Poulsen, N. 1990. Chives, *Allium schoenoprasum* L. In: *Onions and allied crops*, vol. 3 of *Biochemistry, food science, and minor crops*, ed. J. L. Brewster and H. D. Rabinowitch, 231–50. Boca Raton, FL: CRC Press.

Prasad, K., V. A. Laxdal, M. Yu, and B. L. Raney. 1995. Antioxidant activity of allicin, an active principle in garlic. *Mol. Cell. Biochem.* 148: 183–189.

Pratt, D. E., and P. M. Birac. 1979. Source of antioxidant activity of soybeans and soy products. *J. Food Sci.* 44: 1720–2.

Pratt, D. E., and B. M. Watts. 1964. The antioxidant activity of vegetable extracts, 1: Flavone aglycones. *J. Food Sci.* 29: 27–33.

Prohens, J., and F. Nuez. 2000. The tamarillo (*Cyphomandra betacea*): A review of a promising small fruit crop. *Small Fruits Rev.* 1 (2): 43–68.

Purseglove, J. W., E. G. Brown, C. L. Green, and S. R. Robbins. 1981. *Spices.* 2 vols. New York: Longman.

Qian, H., and N. Venant. 2004. Antioxidant power of photochemical from *Psidium guajava* leaf. *J. Zhejiang Univ. Sci.* 3 (6): 676–83. http://www.zju.edu.cn/jzus.

Radha, A. K. Gopi. 2006. Medicinal values of common fruits in Siddha system of medicine. New Delhi: National Informatics Centre (NIC). http://openmed.nic.in/1778/.

Ragone, D. 1997. *Breadfruit* (Artocarpus altilis): *Promoting the conservation and use of underutilized and neglected crops.* Rome: Gaterleben/International Plant Genetic Resources Institute.

Rajaram, N., and K. Janardhanan. 1992. Nutritional and chemical evaluation of raw seeds of *Canavalia gladiata*, the under-utilized food and fodder crops in India. *Plant Foods Hum. Nutr.* 42 (4): 329–336.

Raju, K., G. Anbuganapathi, V. Gokulakrishnan, and B. Rajkapoor. 2003. Effect of dried fruits of *Solanum nigrum* Linn. against CCl_4-induced hepatic damage in rats. *Biological Pharm. Bull.* 26 (11): 1618.

Ramulu, P., and P. U. Rao. 2003. Total insoluble and soluble dietary fiber contents of Indian fruit. *J. Food Composition Anal.* 16: 677–85.

Rangkadilok, N., L. Worasuttayangkun, R. N. Bennett, and J. Satayavivad. 2005. Identification and quantification of polyphenolic compounds in longan (*Euphoria longana* Lam.) fruit. *J. Agric. Food Chem.* 53 (5): 1387–92.

Reid, D. P. 1993. *Chinese herbal medicine.* Boston: Shambhala Publications.

Reinten, E., and J. H. Coetzee. 2002. Commercialization of South African indigenous crops: Aspects of research and cultivation of products. In *Trends in new crops and new uses*, eds. J. Janick and A. Whipkey, 76–80. Alexandria, VA: ASHS Press.

Reynertson, K. A. 2006. Bioactive depsides and anthocyanins from Jaboticaba (*Myrciaria cauliflora*). *J. Nat. Prod.* 69 (8): 1228–30.

Rieger, M., 2006. *Introduction to fruit crops.* New York: Food Products Press/Haworth Press.

Rimando, A. M., W. Kalt, J. B. Magoe, J. Dewey, and J. R. Ballington. 2004. Resveratrol, pterostilbene, and piceatannol in Vaccinium berries. *J. Agric. Food Chem.* 52 (15): 4713–9.

Rinzler, C. A. 1990. *The complete book of herbs, spices, and condiments.* New York: Facts On File.

Robards, K., X. Li, M. Antolovich, and S. Boyol. 1999. Characterization of citrus by chromatographic analysis of flavonoids. *J. Sci. Food Agric.* 75 (1): 87–101.

Robbers, J. E., and V. E. Tyler. 1999. *Tyler's herbs of choice: The therapeutic use of phytomedicinals.* New York: Haworth Herbal Press.

Roberts, K. L. 1995. A comparison of chilled cabbage leaves and chilled gelpaks in reducing breast engorgement. *J. Hum. Lact.* 11: 17–20.

Roberts, K. L., M. Reiter, and D. Schuster. 1995. A comparison of chilled and room temperature cabbage leaves in treating breast engorgement. *J. Hum. Lact.* 11: 191–4.

———. 1998. Effects of cabbage leaf extract on breast engorgement. *J. Hum Lact.* 14: 231–6.

Rodriguez, D. B., L. C. Raymundo, T. C. Lee, K. L. Simpson, and C. O. Chichester. 1976. Carotenoid pigment changes in ripening *Momordica charantia* fruits. *Ann. Bot.* 40: 615–24.

Rogers, R. D. 1997. *Sundew, moonwart, medicinal plants of the prairies.* 2 vols. Edmonton, AB.

Roi, J. 1955. Traite des plantes medicinales chinoises. *Encyc. Biol.* 47: 1–500.

Ruiz, A. N., B. E. B. Ramirez, J. G. Estrada, P. G. Lopez, and P. Garzon. 1995. Anticonvulsant activity of *Casimiroa edulis* in comparision to phenytoin and phenobarbital. *J. Ethnopharmacol.* 45 (3): 199–206.

Ryan-Borchers, T. A., J. S. Park, B. P. Chew, M. K. McGuire, L. R. Fournier, and K. A. Beerman. 2006. Effects of soy isoflavones on immune function and oxidative stress in postmenopausal women. *Am. J. Clin. Nutr.* 83: 1118–25.

Saewan, N., J. D. Sutherland, and K. Chantrapromma. 2006. Antimalarial tetranortriterpenoids from the seeds of *Lansium domesticum. Phytochemistry* 67 (20): 2288–93.

Saito, S. 1990. Chinese chives: *Allium tuberosum* Rottl. In *Onions and allied crops,* vol. 3 of *Biochemistry, food science, and minor crops,* eds. J. L. Brewster and H. D. Rabinowitch, 219–30. Boca Raton, FL: CRC Press.

Salah-Abbes, J. B., S. Abbes, Z. Ouanes, Z. Houas, M. A. Abodel-Wahhab, H. Bacha, and R. Oueslati. 2007. Tunish radish (*Taphanus sativus*) extract enhances the antioxidant status and protects against oxidative stress induced by zearalenone in bulb/c mice. *J. Appl. Toxicol.* vol. 27(2): 103–200. 2007 Mar. 27.

Saleh, N. A. M., A. E. A. El Sherbeiny, and H. I. El Sissi. 2005. Local plants as potential sources of tannins in Egypt: Part 7. *Plant Foods Hum. Nutr.* 20 (4): 311–28.

Sang, W. C., J. C. Fun, Y. H. Tae, and H. C. Kyoung. 1997. Antioxidative activity of acylated anthocyanin isolated from fruits and vegetables. *J. Food Sci. Nutr.* 2: 191–6.

Sasek, T. W., and B. R. Strain. 1988. Effects of carbon dioxide enrichment on the growth and morphology of kudzu (*Pueraria lobata*). *Weed Sci.* 36: 28–36.

Schmandke, H. 2004. Urosolic acid and its derivatives with antitumor activity in berries of *Vaccinium* species. *Ernahrungs-Umschau* 51 (6): 235–7.

Schulz, V., R. Hansel, and V. E. Tyler. 1998. *Rational phytotherapy: A physician's guide to herbal medicine.* 3rd ed. Trans. Terry C. Telger. Berlin: SGER Springer.

Sena, L. P., D. J. Vanderjagt, C. Rivora, A. Pastuszyn, and R. H. Glew. 2004. Analysis of nutritional components of eight famine foods of the Republic of Niger. *Plant Foods Hum. Nutr.* 52 (1): 17–30.

Seo, K. I., Y. H. Moon, S. U. Choi, and K. H. Park. 2001. Antibacterial activity of S-methyl methanethiosulfinate and S-methyl 2-propene-1-thiosulfinate from Chinese chive toward *Escherichia coli* 0157:H7. *Biosci. Biotechnol. Biochem.* 65: 966–8.

Shao, H., R. A. Dixon, and X. Wang. 2007. Crystal structure of vestitone reductase from alfalfa (*Medicago sativa*). *J. Mol. Bio.* vol. 149(4) 2007.

Shishoo, C. J., S. A. Shah, I. S. Rathod, and S. G. Patel. 1997. Determination of vitamin C content of *Phyllanthus emblica* and chyavanprash. *Indian J. Pharm. Sci.* 59: 238–70.

Siddaraju, M. N., and S. M. Dharmesh. 2007. Inhibition of gastric H(+), K(+)-ATPase, and *Helicobacter pylori* growth by phenolic antioxidants of *Zingiber officinale*. *Mol. Nutr. Food Res.* 51 (3): 324–32.

Siddhuraju, P., and K. Becker. 2001. Species/variety differences in biochemical composition and nutritional value of Indian tribal legumes of the genus Canavalia. *Nahrung* 45 (4): 224–33.

Siegmund, G. 1958. Cabbage (*Brassica oleracea*) as a medicinal plant. *Hippokrates* 29 (19): 628–9.

Simon, J. E., A. F. Chadwick, and L. E. Craker. 1984. *Herbs: An annotated bibliography, 1971–1980*. Hamden, CN: Shoe-String Press.

Simoons, Frederick J. 1990. Nutritional and medicinal perspectives. In *Food in China: A cultural and historical inquiry*, 559. Boca Raton, FL: CRC Press.

Sinclair, C. J., and J. D. Geiger. 2000. Caffeine use in sports: A pharmacological review. *J. Sports Med. Phys. Fitness* 40: 71–9.

Singh, D. R. 2006. West Indian cherry (*Malpighia glabra*): A lesser known fruit for nutritional security. *Nat. Prod. Radiance* 5: 369–72.

Singh, P. P. 1973. The oxalic acid content of Indian foods. *Plant Foods Hum. Nutr.* 22 (3/4): 335–47.

Siqueira, E. M., S. E. Arruda, R. M. deVargas, and E. M. de Souza. 2006. Beta-carotene from cassava (*Manihot esculenta* Crantz) leaves improves vitamin A status in rats. *Comp. Biochem. Physiol. C Toxicol. Pharmacol.* 2007. Jul–Aug 146(1–2) 235–40.

Small, E. 1980. The relationships of hop cultivars and wild variants of *Humulus lupulus*. *Can. J. Bot.* 58: 676–86.

———. 2006. *Culinary herbs*. 2nd ed. Ottawa: NRC Research Press.

Small, E., and P. M. Catling. 1999. *Canadian medicinal crops*. Ottawa: NRC Research Press.

Smith, T. K., E. K. Lund, R. G. Clarke, R. N. Bennett, and I. T. Johnson. 2005. Effects of brussels sprout juice on the cell and adhesion of human colorectal carcinoma cells (HT29) in vitro. *J. Agric. Food Chem.* 53 (10): 3895–901.

Smith-Warner, S. A. 2001. Intake of fruits and vegetables and risk of breast cancer. *JAMA* 285: 769–76.

Song, K., and J. A. Miner. 2001. Heating garlic can reduce some of its biological activity, study says. *J. Nutr.* 2001 (supp.): 1054–7S.

Soucek, J., J. Skvor, P. Pouckova, J. Matousek, J. Slavik, and J. Matousek. 2006. Mung bean sprout nuclease and its biological and antitumor effect. *Neoplasma* 53 (5): 402–9.

Stuart, G. A. 2004. *Chinese herbal medicine: Materia medica*. 3rd ed. Taipei, Taiwan: Oriental Book Store, Southern Materials Centre.

Suleman, A., and N. H. Siddiqui. 2000. Haemodynamic and cardiovascular effects of caffeine. *Pharmacy On-Line, Int. J. Med.* www.priory.com/pharmol/caffeine.htm.

Summanen, J. O. 1999. *A chemical and ethnopharmacological study on* Phyllanthus emblica L. (Euphorbiaceae). Helsinki: Helsingin yliopiston verkkojulkaisut. http://ethesis.helsinki.fi/julkaisut/mat/farma/vk/summanen/.

Suzuki, R., Y. Okada, and T. Okuyama. 2005. The favorable effect of style of *Zea mays* L. on streptozotocin induced diabetic nephropathy. *Biol. Pharm. Bull.* 28 (5): 919–20.

Tan, B. 1989. Palm carotenoids, tocopherols, and tocotrienols. *J. Am. Oil Chem. Soc.* 66: 770–6.

Tanaka, T., M. Ishihashi, H. Fujimoto, E. Okuyama, T. Koyano, T. Rowithayakorn, M. Hayashi, and K. Komiyama. 2002. New onoceranoid triterpene constituents for *Lansium domesticum*. *J. Nat. Prod.* 65 (11): 1709–11.

Tao, M., F. Zeng, X. Lu, and W. Zhang. 2005. Hypoglycemic activity of *Opuntia dillenii* polysaccharides. *J. Hunan Agric. Univ.* 31 (6): 612–5.

Taussig, S. J., and S. Batkin. 1988. Bromelain, the enzyme complex of pineapple (*Ananas comosus*) and its chemical application. *J. Ethnopharmacol.* 22 (2): 191–203.

Tengammray, P., K. Pengrunagwong, I. Pheansri, and K. Likhitwitayawuid. 2006. *Artocarpus lakoocha* heartwood extract as a novel cosmetic ingredient: Evaluation of the in vitro, anti-tyrosinase, and in vivo skin whitening activities. *Int. J. Cosmet. Sci.* 28 (4): 269–76.

Thomson, L. A. J., and R. R. Thaman. 2006. Species profiles for Pacific Island agroforestry. http://www.traditionaltree.org.

Tippayakul, C., S. Pongsamart, and M. Suksomtip. 2005. Lipid entrapment property of polysaccharide gel extracted from fruit-fulls of duriang. *Songklanakarin J. Sci. Technol.* 27 (2): 291–300.

Tiwari, K. P., and S. D. Srivastava. 1979. Pigments from the stem bark of *Dillenia indica*. *Planta Med.* 35 (2): 118–90.

Tolo, F. M., G. M. Rukunga, M. Charles, J. Muli, L. K. Keter, and K. T. Mawuli. 2006. Antiviral activity of the extracts of Kenyan medicinal plant *Carissa edulis* against herpes simplex virus. *J. Ethnopharmacol.* 104 (1–2): 92–9.

Tomomatsu, H. 1994. Health effects of oligosaccharides. *Food Technol.* 48: 61–5.

Tripathi, M., M. B. Pandey, R. N. Jha, and V. B. Pandey. 2001. Cyclopeptide alkaloids from *Zizyphus jujuba*. *Fitoterapia* 72 (5): 507–10.

Tshikalange, T. E., J. J. Meyer, and A. A. Hussein. 2005. Antimicrobial activity, toxicity, and isolation of a bioactive compound from plants used to treat sexually transmitted diseases. *J. Ethnopharmacol.* 96 (3): 519–29.

Tsuda, T., Y. Makino, H. Kato, H. T. Osawa, and S. Kawakishi. 1993. Screening for antioxidative activity of edible pulses. *Biosci. Biotech. Biochem.* 57: 1606–8.

Turner, N. J. 2006. *Food plants of coastal first peoples.* Victoria, BC: Royal BC Museum Publ.

Tyler, V. E., ed. 1993. *The honest herbal.* 3rd ed. Binghamton, NY: Pharmaceutical Products Press (Haworth Press).

Tyler, V. E. 1994. *Herbs of choice: The therapeutic use of phytomedicinals.* New York: Pharmaceutical Press.

———. 1999. Herbs affecting the central nervous system. In *Perspectives on new crops and new uses*, ed. J. Janick, 442–9. Proceedings of the fourth national symposium on new crops and new uses, Phoenix, AZ, Nov. 8–11, 1998.

Udayasekhara R. P. 1996. Nutrient composition and biological evaluation of roselle (*Hibiscus sabdariffa*) seeds. *Plant Food Hum. Nutr.* 49 (1): 27–34.

Udayasekhara R. P., and B. Belavady. 1978. Oligosaccharides in pulses: Varietal differences and effects of cooking and germination. *J. Agric. Food Chem.* 26 (2): 316–9.

USDA. 2003. Database for the flavonoid content of selected foods. http://www.nal.usda.gov/fnic/foodcomp.

USDA Agricultural Research Service. 1999. ORAC of common vegetables and fruits. http://www.ars.usda.gov/is/np/fnrb/fnrb499.htm.

Vaccari, A., P. G. Pifferi, and G. Zaccherini. 1981. Anthocyanins of sunflower (*Helianthus annuus*). *J. Food Sci.* 47: 40–2.

Van Dam, R. M., W. C. Willett, J. F. Manson, and F. B. Hu. 2006. Coffee, caffeine, and risk of type 2 diabetes: A prospective cohort study in younger and middle-aged U.S. women. *Diabetes Care* 29 (2): 398–403.

Varalakshmi, P., K. M. Lathika, K. G. Raghavan, and B. B. Singh. 1995. Altered physicochemical characteristics of polyethylene glycol linked beet stem oxalate oxidase. *Biotechnol. Bioeng.* 46 (3): 254–7.

Vimala, S. 1999. Anti-tumour promoter activity in Malaysian ginger rhizobia used in traditional medicine. *Br. J. Cancer* 80: 110–6.

Vinson, J. A., Y. Hau, X. Su, and L. Zubik. 1998. Phenol antioxidant quantity and quality in foods: Vegetables. *J. Agric. Food Chem.* 46: 3630–4.

Volpato, G., and D. Godinez. 2004. Ethnobotany of pru, a traditional Cuban refreshment. *Econ. Bot.* 58 (3): 381–95.

Vuotto, M. L., A. Basile, V. Moscatiello, P. Desole, R. Castaldo-Cobianchi, E. Laghi, and M. T. Icelpo. 2000. Antimicrobial and antioxidant activities of *Feijoa sellowiana* fruit. *Int. J. Antimicrob. Agents* 13 (3): 197–201.

Waffo-Teguo, P., M. E. Hawthorne, M. Cuendet, J. M. Merillon, A. Kinghon, J. M. Pexxuto, and R. G. Mehta. 2001. Potential cancer-chemopreventive activities of wine stilbenoids and flavans extracted from grape cell cultures. *Nutr. Cancer* 40 (2): 173–9.

Wagner, J. 2002. Ingredients to watch in 2002. *Nutritional Outlook* 5: 18–20, 22–5.

Wall, M. E., H. Taylor, P. Perera, and M. C. Wani. 1988. Indoles in edible members of the Cruciferae. *J. Nat. Prod.* 51: 129–35.

Warner, K., and T. L. Mounts. 1990. Analysis of tocopherols and phytosterols in vegetable oils by HPLC with evaporative light-scattering detection. *J. Am. Oil Chem. Soc.* 67: 827–31.

Wattenberg, L. W. 1992. Inhibition of carcinogenesis by minor dietary constituents. *Cancer Res.* 52 (supp.): 2085s–91s.

Weaver, C. M., R. P. Heancy, K. P. Nickel, and P. I. Oackard. 1997. Calcium bioavailability from high oxalate vegetables: Chinese vegetables, sweet potatoes, and rhubarb. *J. Food Sci.* 62: 524–5.

Wei, H., R. Bowen, Q. Cal, S. Barnes, and Y. Wang. 1995. Antioxidant and antipromotional effects of the soybean isoflavone genistein. *Proc. Soc. Exp. Biol. Med.* 208: 124–30.

Welton, A. F., J. Hurley, and P. Will. 1988. Flavonoids and arachidonic acid metabolism. In *Plant flavonoids in biology and medicine*, ed. A. R. Liss, 2: 301–2. New York: Alan R. Liss.

Wen, T., D. X. Lin, Y. Xiao, F. F. Kadlubar, and J. S. Chen. 1999. Chemo-prevention of 2-amino-1-methyl-6-phenylimidazo (4,5-b) pyridine induced carcinogen-DNA adducts by *Brassica chinensis* var. *utilis* in rats. *World J. Gastroenterol.* 1999 Apr 5(2), 138–142.

Werner, D. J., E. P. Maness, and W. E. Ballinger. 1989. Fruit anthocyanins in three sections of *Prunus. HortScience* 24 (3): 488–9.

Wettasinghe, M., B. Bolling, L. Plhak, and K. Parkin. 2002. Screening for phase II enzyme-inducing and antioxidant activities of common vegetables. *J. Food Sci.* 67: 2583–88.

Willard, T. 1992. *Edible and medicinal plants of the Rocky Mountains and neighbouring territories.* Calgary, AB: Wild Rose College of Natural Healing.

Wills, R. B. H., A. W. K. Wong, F. M. Scriven, and H. Greenfield. 1984. Nutrient composition of Chinese vegetables. *J. Agric. Food Chem.* 32: 413–6.

Wu, P., W. S. Chen, T. S. Hu, Z. J. Yao, and Y. L. Wu. 2001. Atemoyacin E, a bis-tetrahydro-furan annonareous acetogenin from *Annona atemoya* seeds. *J. Asian Nat. Prod. Res.* 3 (3), 177–182.

Wu, S. J., J. S. Wang, C. C. Lin, and C. H. Chang. 2001. Evaluation of hepatoprotective activity of legumes. *Phytomedicine* 8: 213–9.

Wu, W. H., L. Y. Liu, C. J. Chung, H. J. Jou, and T. A. Wang. 2005. Estrogenic effect of yam ingestion in healthy postmenopausal women. *J. Am. Coll. Nutr.* 24 (4): 235–43.

Wu, Y. C., Y. C. Hung, F. R. Chang, M. Cosentino, H. K. Wang, and K. H. Lee. 1996. Identification of ent-16, 17-dihydroxykauran-19-oic acid as an anti-HIV principle and isolation of the new diterpenoids Annosquamosins A and B from Annona squamosa. *J. Nat. Prod.* 59 (6): 635–7.

Xue, C. X. 2001a. *The encyclopedia of vegetables and fruits in Taiwan.* Vol. 1. [In Chinese.] Taipei: Taiwan Pu-Lu Publ. Co.

———. 2001b. *The encyclopedia of vegetables and fruits in Taiwan.* Vol. 2. [In Chinese.] Taipei: Taiwan Pu-Lu Publ. Co.

————. 2001c. *The encyclopedia of vegetables and fruits in Taiwan*. Vol. 3. [In Chinese.] Taipei: Taiwan Pu-Lu Publ. Co.

Xue, Y., S. H. Song, H. Chen, Y. Xue, S. H. Song, H. Chen, V. E. Rubatzky, C. Hang, and J. Y. Peron. 1998. Possible anti-tumor promoting properties of bitter gourd and some Chinese vegetables. *Acta Horticulturae* 467: 55–64.

Ya, D. Q., K. L. Chin, F. Malekian, M. Berhane, and J. Gager. 2005. Biological characteristic, nutritional and medicinal values of roselle, *Hibiscus sabdariffa*: circular urban forestry. *Nat. Resour. Environ.* 604.

Yamaguchi, M. 1990. Asian vegetables. In *Advances in new crops*, ed. J. Janick and J. E. Simon, 387–90. Portland, OR: Timber Press.

Yamane, A., J. Fujikura, H. Ogawa, and J. Mizutani. 1992. Isothiocyanates as allopathic compounds from *Rorippa indica* roots. *J. Chem. Ecol.* 18 (12): 1941–54.

Yamashito, K., K. Kawai, and M. Itakura. 1984. Effects of fructo-oligosaccharides on blood glucose and serum lipids in diabetic subjects. *Nutr. Res.* 4: 961–6.

Yanagihara, K., I. Akihiro, and T. Toge. 1993. Antiproliferative effects of isoflavones on human cancer cell lines established from the gastrointestinal tract. *Cancer Res.* 53 (23): 5815–21.

Yang, H. L., W. H. Chang, Y. C. Chia, C. J. Huang, F. J. Lu, H. K. Hsu, and Y. C. Hseu. 2006. *Toona sinensis* extracts induce apoptosis via reactive oxygen species in human premyelocytic leukemia cells. *Food Chem. Toxicol.* 44 (12): 1978–88.

Yang, L. L., C. Y. Lee, and K. Y. Yen. 2000. Induction of apoptosis by hydrolyzable tannins from *Eugenia jambos* L. on human leukemia cells. *Cancer Lett.* 157 (1): 65–75.

Yang, R. Y., S. C. S. Twou, T. C. Lee, W. J. Wu, and P. M. Hanson. 2005. Distribution of 127 edible plant species for anti-oxidant activities by two assays. *J. Sci. Food Agric.* 86 (14): 2395–403.

Yang, S. L., and T. W. Walters. 1992. Ethnobotany and the economic role of the Cucurbitaceae of China. *Econ. Bot.* 46: 349–67.

Yin, M., and W. Cheng. 1998. Antioxidant activity of several *Allium* members. *J. Agric. Food Chem.* 46: 4097–101.

Yoshikawa, M., T. Murakami, H. Shimada, and S. Yoshizumi. 1998. Medicinal food stuffs; 14: On the bioactive constituents of moroheiya; 2: New fatty acids, corchorifatty acids A, B, C, D, E, and F, from the leaves of *Corchorus olitorius* L. *Chem. Pharm. Bull.* 46: 1008–14.

Youdim, K. A., B. Shukin-Hale, and S. MacKinon. 2000. Polyphenolics enhance red blood cell resistance to oxidative stress in vitro and in vivo. *Biochim. Biophys. Acta* 1519: 117–22.

Younis, Y. M., S. Ghirmay, and S. S. al-Shihry. 2000. African *Cucurbita pepo* L.: Properties of seed and variability in fatty acid composition of seed oil. *Phytochemistry* 54: 71–5.

Yu, J. G., D. Liu, L. Z. Xu, and S. L. Yang. 1997. Studies on chemical structures of two iso-acetogenins from *Annona reticulata* seeds. [In Chinese.] *Yao Xue Xue Bao* 32 (12): 914–9.

Zhang, X. G., and O. W. Zhao. 2006. Ethanol extract of adzuki bean has the estrogen-like activities through the estrogen response pathway. *Zhongguo Zhong Yao Za Zhi* 31 (15): 1261–5.

Zhu, X. C. 1989. Plantae Medicinals China *Roreali orientalis*. [In Chinese.] Heilongjiang, China. Heilongjiang Sci. Technology Publ. House.

Index